Stop Blaming Aging for Your Slc

How to Heal Your Metabolism

Learn How the Right Foods, Sleep, the Right Amount of Exercise, and Happiness Can Increase Your Metabolic Rate and Help Heal Your Broken Metabolism

Kate Deering
Holistic Lifestyle and Exercise Coach, CNC, PT

A 180-Degree Shift in Understanding What Is Truly Healthy for Us

Copyright 2015 by Kate Deering. All rights reserved, including the right to reproduce this book or portions of this book in any form whatsoever without the prior written permission of the copyright holder.

Limits of Liability and Disclaimer of Warranty

The author and publisher shall not be liable for your misuse of this material. This book is strictly for informational and educational purposes.

Warning—Disclaimer

The purpose of this book is to educate and entertain. The author and/or publisher do not guarantee that anyone following these techniques, suggestions, tips, ideas, or strategies will become successful. The author and/or publisher shall have neither liability nor responsibility to anyone with respect to any loss or damage caused, or alleged to be caused, directly or indirectly by the information contained in this book.

ISBN-13: 978-1511585620
ISBN-10: 1511585625

How to Heal Your Metabolism

Stop Blaming Aging for Your Slowing Metabolism!

Learn how:

- Eating the right foods
- Eating the right amount of food
- Consuming the right food supplements
- Consuming the right amount of water
- Sleeping and resting
- Doing the right amount of exercise
- Happiness

will increase your metabolic rate and help heal your broken metabolism.

Kate Deering
Holistic Lifestyle and Exercise Coach, CNC, PT

Disclaimer

The information provided in this book is intended to be educational and should not be construed as personal medical advice, diagnosis, or treatment of any health issue whatsoever. No action should be taken based solely on the contents of this book.

Readers are advised to consult their own health professionals regarding the programs, advice, and other information contained in this book.

The information in this book should not replace the consultation with appropriate healthcare professionals on any matter relating to the reader's health and well-being.

The information and opinions provided in this book are believed to be accurate and sound, based on the research and best judgment of the author. Readers who fail to consult appropriate health professionals assume the risk of any injuries. The author and publisher are in no way liable for any damage or injury arising from the reader's use of these materials.

Use of the programs, advice, and other information contained in this book is at the sole choice and risk of the reader.

Get your FREE monthly newsletter

Continued knowledge and education are a must when it comes to your health and fitness. Join Kate's list of thousands of current readers and receive a FREE monthly newsletter with the most updated science-based nutritional information.

You will find information on:
- Why "green juicing" may be doing you more harm than good.
- Why a low-carb diet is killing your metabolism.
- Why avoiding sugar is the worst thing you can do for a high metabolic rate.
- How to increase your sleep time and quality.
- Why too much exercise can encourage a low metabolic rate.

To join the community of "out of the box" nutritionally minded people, go to www.KateDeering.com/blog and enter your name and e-mail. In addition, follow Kate on Facebook and Instagram at Kate Deering fitness for daily tips on everything metabolism.

About the Author

Kate Deering is a respected personal trainer and holistic nutritional, exercise, and lifestyle coach. With more than 20 years experience in the health and fitness industry, she prides herself on her out-of-the-box methods that support metabolic health and improve health and body function.

Kate has committed her life to finding the answers to optimal health, a high metabolism, and true happiness. Her own journey to health and happiness became the foundation of her teachings and helped her understand why health is *not* established with dieting and over-exercising but with self-love and an increase in cellular metabolism—usually achieved with eating more and working out less.

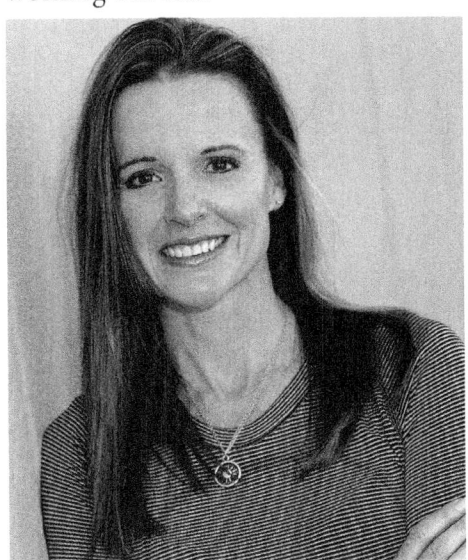

Through continual research and reading, Kate realized a high running metabolism is the foundation to great health, happiness, and longevity. As an author, mentor, consultant, and educator, she coaches people around the world on how to improve their metabolism by using real food, rest, sleep, the right type of exercise and self-love.

Kate holds degrees in psychology and exercise science, is a Certified Nutritional Coach, and is a Holistic Exercise and Lifestyle Coach through the CHEK Institute. Visit www.KateDeering.com for more information.

Acknowledgments

Those who know me know that this book has been a labor of love. Giving up fun weekends, trips, and events to sit home, write, and research was a challenge not only for me but also for the many people in my life that supported me through this process. Thanks to my parents, John and Sue Deering, who have supported me in the constant changes (good and bad) in my life, and who have always been my biggest fans.

Thanks to Dr. Ray Peat for your honesty, time, and knowledge. Without your 40-plus years of research and knowledge, this book would never have been possible.

Thanks to Josh Rubin, who helped guide me on my own healing path. The work you and your wife, Jeanne, put into helping others does not go unnoticed.

Thanks to Heidi Barajas for spending your very valuable time giving me advice on the content, form, and flow of this book.

Thanks to Donna Kozik, my coach and editor, for keeping me on track and helping me make sense of all the knowledge in my head.

And finally, thank you to all my clients who have allowed me to guide them through life changes, exercise programs, and nutritional shifts, especially those who have allowed me to share their stories on the pages in this book.

Contents

Introduction: Why I Wrote This Book 1
Chapter 1: Who Defines Health? 11
Chapter 2: Don't Be Afraid of Saturated Fats 29
Chapter 3: Polyunsaturated Fats: Toxic, *Not* Essential! 40
Chapter 4: The Importance of Carbohydrates—
Especially Sugar 51
Chapter 5: Dump the Grains and Gluten (Your Gut Will
Thank You) 67
Chapter 6: Vegetables: The Good, the Bad, and the Thyroid-
Suppressing 79
Chapter 7: Protein: Why You Need It—Just Not Too Much . 91
Chapter 8: The *Super* Proteins 107
Chapter 9: Dairy and Milk (The Perfect Food) 131
Chapter 10: What About Muscle Meats? 149
Chapter 11: Nuts and Seeds: Too Much of a Good Thing? . . . 157
Chapter 12: Legumes and Soy: Health Foods or Hormone
Disruptors? 167
Chapter 13: Supplementing with Protein Powders 183
Chapter 14: Using *Real* Food Supplements for Nutritional
Support 191
Chapter 15: The Importance of Learning to Balance Your
Blood Sugar 211

Chapter 16: There's More to Healing Than Just Food........ 225

Chapter 17: Be Happy................................. 249

Chapter 18: What a Metabolically Supportive Diet Look Like................................. 255

Chapter 19: Frequently Asked Questions (and Answers) 261

Chapter 20: Recipes................................... 267

Appendix A: Optimal Carbohydrates.................... 287

Appendix B: Best Proteins 289

Appendix C: Best Fats 291

Appendix D: PUFA Oils to Be Avoided 292

References 293

Introduction
Why I Wrote This Book

I want to start off by telling you a story of a childhood friend of mine. Let's call her "Britch Smith." Britch and I have known each other since seventh grade. Britch was beautiful, thin, and smart. We were and are still great friends. Now, I will admit, growing up, I was envious of Britch. Why? Britch was my friend who stayed slender and thin, did little to no activity, and ate whatever she wanted. I, on the other hand, was an athlete. I ran, lifted weights, played tennis, cycled, and played soccer. Yet, past the age of 13, I could never eat anything I wanted and stay thin. I'll admit, I was never overweight and I was pretty fit, but it never came easy. I had to work hard at it each and every day.

I always assumed Britch was one of the lucky ones. I attributed her thin and slender body to good genes. She certainly didn't work out to stay thin, and eating cereal and grilled cheese sandwiches daily didn't really support a thin body (at least that is what I thought). Yet, she was thin, really thin.

Do you have a "Britch" in your life?

And are you wondering: How did Britch stay so thin and not work out? Well, what I now know and understand is that Britch had great cellular respiration. Huh? Cellular respiration? Yes, cellular respiration—or, as most of us know it, metabolism. Now some would say, "Well, of course she had a great metabolism. She was 13 years old. All 13-year-olds have a great metabolism." And I would say, "Look around you. How many 13-year-olds are overweight and obese today?" Fifty years ago, youth was synonymous with being thin. However, in today's world this is no longer true. In today's world the youth are the fastest-growing overweight population around.

So what has happened? Are we just eating more? Are we moving less? Based on the activity level and the diet of my friend Britch, I would say eating more and moving less may play a partial role, but to be honest, she barely moved and ate a ton. And Britch was not obese; she was thin. So what else may be going on here?

Well, I believe, it's the growing epidemic of slowing metabolisms. I believe we are not only being born with slower metabolisms (genetics, cellular mutations, and the effect of our parents' diets), but also that metabolisms are slowing as a result of how people live their lives. This includes the foods we ingest or don't ingest, chemicals, hormones and drugs, the environment, stress level, lack of sleep, exercise level, water consumption, happiness, and purpose. The way we live our lives today is very different from how we lived 50 years ago.

The exercise and fitness explosion has been going on for the last 40 years. Supplements and health food products have become a billion-dollar industry. Low-fat, low-salt, no-sugar, no-carb, low-carb, gluten-free, fat-free, "health" food products have become staples of the average American's diet—yet, we are more overweight, sick, and diseased than ever before. Obviously there must be more to our obesity epidemic than just eating less and working out more. Now, before I start explaining the ins and outs of metabolism and how you can increase or decrease it by the food you eat and the way you live your life, I want to explain a little bit about who I am and how I have come to the realization that staying thin and healthy is not just about eating less and working out more. In fact, I believe staying healthy and thin may be more about *being able* to eat more and work out less.

Let me explain.

I have been an athlete my entire life. I have played competitive tennis and all-star soccer, participated in dozens of running races, including the Las Vegas Marathon, hiked the Grand Canyon rim-to-rim and Mt. Whitney, the highest peak in the continental U.S., and have cycled 100 miles to raise money for cancer—twice.

Yet, in my lifetime, I have followed some of the worst and most damaging diet trends with the belief that I was doing something healthy for myself.

My quest for fitness and health started back in my early teenage years—about the same time I started to develop a complex about my body and weight. Growing up, I was never a heavy child, but I wasn't a size 2 either—so as soon as I could read a *Teen Beat* magazine, I became very aware that "thin" was considered cooler, sexier, richer, more attractive, healthier, etc. And who doesn't want to be all those things—especially, at the ripe old age of 15?

It really sucks that society and the media teach our youth these distorted lessons at such a young age. It has taken me 25 years to unlearn these lessons. Life could have been easier and more fun, had the thought of "thin equals happiness" not been ingrained in my head.

My weird food habits started back in my teenage years when I was told fat was bad and all fat was going to make me fat (which we now know is not true). I think my daily diet went something like this: no breakfast, tuna salad for lunch, raw veggie snack with fat-free dressing when I got home, five Diet Cokes, normal homemade dinner from Mom—with no added fat—and a big bowl of popcorn with fat-free butter spray at night while I was studying. Wow. The mere thought of what I used to put in my body now makes me want to gag. Needless to say, I was thin, but certainly not lean—in fact, I remember having my body fat tested in high school and it was an astonishing 28 percent (on the border of being overweight). Looking back, I would be classified as skinny fat—higher body fat but thin looking.

As I entered college, my obsession to be "the perfect size" continued. After I added a quick "freshman 15" pounds due to beer, late-night pizza, and vending machine food, I was exploring new diet trends to achieve the perfectly thin body. Back in the early '90s food manufacturers were focusing on reducing calories in foods, removing fat and sugar, and adding in artificial sweeteners and other non-food additives. Processed weight-loss foods were advertised as fat-free, sugar-free, low-calorie, and reduced fat, sugar, calories—or all three. Americans were led to believe, by great marketing, that eating less and working out more were the answers to a thin and amazing body—and I was on board. My daily calorie intake dropped to about 1,200 calories/day and included low-calorie cereal with skim milk for breakfast, raw veggies for snack, a low-calorie sandwich with fake cheese and meat for lunch, and a frozen Lean Cuisine for dinner—plus lots of tea and water to fill me up. In addition, I would do at least one to two hours of cardio *every day*.

Guess what happened? I lost weight. I dropped down to a very skinny 105 pounds—the smallest I have ever been in my life—and, looking back, the unhealthiest. My body temperature was a degree above freezing. My roommate hated me because I kept a space heater running 24/7, due to my lack of body heat. I assumed I was cold due to my lack of fat—now I know it was due to my suppressed metabolism because of under-eating and over-exercising. In addition, I had constant food cravings and would find myself binging on salty and sweet food weekly. I lost my period for at least six months, and I became increasingly depressed, anxious, and irritated—but I was thin, so I must be healthy, right? How wrong I was.

After I graduated college, I started my first *real* job, working sales at a big health club chain in Atlanta, Georgia. I stayed there for about a year until I left to pursue a career as the general manager of a small local health club. For the next nine years, my beliefs about health and nutrition became heavily influenced by the fitness and nutritional supplement market. With magazines like *Muscle and Fitness, Shape,* and *Oxygen,* I began to believe protein powders and bars, energy drinks, and tons of nutritional supplements were the answers to optimal health and fitness.

At the same time, the soy industry was advertising the health benefits of increased soy intake. And since I was such a "health nut," I jumped on the soy bandwagon: Soy burgers, soy cheese, soy meats, soy-based cereals, and soy desserts became staples in my diet. Lean turkey, egg whites, and chicken also became big parts of my diet. I continued to work out two hours a day: one hour of weights and one hour of cardio, six to seven days a week—an improvement from my two-hour cardio days, but still far from a metabolically stimulating workout program.

You want to know what happened? My weight bumped up to 140 pounds, which I attributed to muscle gain—yet I still carried around extra fat. I honestly couldn't understand why my soy-based and lean meat, protein powder, energy drink, supplement-filled diet wasn't making me thin. If I only knew then what I know now: Soy is anti-metabolic; fake proteins, too much muscle meat, and energy drinks were stressful to my body; and the supplements were just marketed crap that my hypo-metabolic body was unable to break down.

As I entered my late 20s and early 30s, I finally found something to help my weight loss journey: recreational drugs. Sad, but true. I hate to admit it, but I experienced some very dark years in my life. Even while promoting the health and fitness industry I was knee deep in a pretty heavy drug problem. The uppers, ecstasy and cocaine, were top on my list, but anything that kept me *up* was considered okay. Needless to say, these drugs killed my appetite and increased my energy—well, at least for the night and weekend. The fun was later accompanied by exhaustion and depression—but quite honestly I didn't care: I was finally thinner again. It took about three years of weekly drug use for it to finally take its toll on my health. The highs I experienced early on became harder to achieve, and more drugs were needed—which were followed by deeper lows and more depression.

I can remember the day like it was yesterday—the day I realized my drug usage had to stop. My life felt out of control, fake, and confusing. I had lost myself in late-night partying and drug usage. After 48 hours of straight partying I came home to what I *thought* should make me happy: a perfectly decorated house, new furniture, and a nice car. Yet, all I could feel was extreme sadness and a very empty feeling about who I really was and what I really wanted. All the stuff I had accumulated didn't seem to matter. I looked in the mirror and didn't even recognize myself; I looked aged, tired, and worn out. Although I was thin, I was not a good representation of what health should be like. I made a decision that day that my life needed to change. If I wasn't willing to make a *big* change soon, my drug habit was going to make the change for me—and not in a good way.

Six months later, I quit my job, rented out my house in Atlanta, left all my family and friends, and moved across the country to San Diego, California, to find my health and sanity again.

Leaving everything I knew, including my job, home, friends, and family, may seem extreme to some people—but for me, it was the only answer. Sometimes we have to make *big* shifts to find out who we are and what we want out of life. I knew, for me, if I really wanted to heal and get better I needed to remove myself from all tempting situations, places, and people. Doesn't mean trouble can't find you again, but it's a hell of a lot easier to get healthy without the constant temptations.

Although I had moved, my fascination with the human body, nutrition, and the mind—and how they all worked together—continued. Once I arrived in California, I started a one-year program in holistic clinical nutrition. I took some time off work and tried to figure out, at the age of 31, who I was and what I wanted to do with my life. In the meantime, I dove heavily into researching different nutritional modalities: vegan, vegetarian, organic foods, Metabolic Typing Diet, Atkins diet, Barry Sears 40/30/30 diet, the blood type diet, Dr. Mercola's No Grain Diet, The Omega Diet—the list goes on and on. This was the beginning of my realization that *real* food is a far better option than the low-calorie processed foods.

A few years later I began studies at the CHEK Institute (Corrective-Holistic-Exercise-Kinesiology) owned by exercise and nutritional expert Paul Chek. I learned through the CHEK Institute that health is more than just fitness and nutrition. Stress reduction, sleep, reduced toxic load, happiness, and authenticity all have an effect on one's health. At this time, I took on a real organic food diet consisting of *lots* of grass-fed meats; *no* white foods (sugar, salt, and dairy); tons of water, oatmeal, quinoa, organic protein bars and shakes; tons of raw vegetables; some fruits; and omega-3- filled foods like salmon, nuts, and seeds. From this I got lean and I felt pretty darn good—at least for a while.

In 2010, I hit a wall. I was in the middle of training for a few half-marathons, a possible half-Ironman, and a hike up Mount Whitney. I hit the ripe old age of 38, and all of sudden my body was revolting against me. Injuries would not heal, my skin was getting dry, I gained weight, I felt puffy, my hair lost its shine, my sleep was poor, I had digestive issues, my food cravings increased, and I was feeling "blah." How could this be? I was doing all the right things: eating an organic, real-food diet and exercising—a lot. Yet, I hit a physical, hormonal, and emotional wall. The harder I trained and the more restrictive I became with my diet, the worse things became. Everything I believed, practiced, and espoused was no longer working.

This is when I was introduced to the work of many researchers including Dr. Gilbert Ling, Dr. Albert Szent-Gyorgi, Dr. Ray Peat, Dr. Broda Barnes, Dr. Constance Martin, Dr. Hans Selye, Dr. Uffe Ravnskov, Dr. Lita Lee, Chris Masterjohn, Josh Rubin, Danny Roddy, Rob Turner, Matt Stone, and many others. Each one of these medical doctors, PhDs, health practitioners, and nutritional researchers has had an influence on my writing of this book. From their teachings, I began to realize that the very things I was doing—excessive training and eating a restrictive sugar (carb) diet—were "stressing" my body and mind, which was causing my body to break down and revolt against me.

I'm sure you are wondering why I am telling you all of this. Isn't this a health book? Why are we talking about drugs, excessive exercise, and chronic dieting? Well, I want you to understand the depth of my journey to health. I was a metabolic catastrophe—and I was in the health industry. Ironic, isn't it?

You start to realize things are not always as they seem.

Essentially, I had to unlearn everything I thought was healthy and nutritious, and relearn an entirely different philosophy. This new philosophy was based entirely on science and research in human physiology, endocrinology, digestion, detoxification, the immune system, and my own personal experimentation.

Within one year I went from feeling tired, puffy, bloated, and aged to feeling more energized, leaner, more youthful, and happier. After spending significant time reading and researching, and through personal experimentation, I healed my body and my metabolism—with the *right* sugars, fats, proteins, rest, and *reduced* exercise.

Along the way, my entire belief system about what constituted "true health" shifted. I no longer defined good health as how many hours I could work out, run or bike; how much willpower I could have; or how low I could get my body fat. I now define good health by a lack of injuries and sickness, great sleep, good digestion, healthy skin, a sharp mind, strong bones and lean muscles, overall happiness and purpose in life—all of which, I believe, can be supported by a well-working metabolism.

So, what constitutes a well-working metabolism?

Basically when your metabolism works well, glucose (sugar) enters the cells and converts to usable energy (ATP). Without getting too scientific, it's the most efficient way for cells to harvest energy (carbohydrates/fats/proteins) stored in food and utilize it as energy. Thus, the higher your metabolic rate, the more energy/heat your body will produce.

When your metabolism is running optimally you have great energy all day, your sleep is deep and refreshing, you maintain lean muscle mass and a warm body, your hair shines and your skin radiates, you feel happy, you have a healthy libido, you have great digestion and circulation, you are free of sickness and disease, and you can eat well without working out for hours and hours every day.

On the opposite end of the spectrum, when your metabolism is running poorly, you experience low energy and fatigue, restless sleep that leaves you tired in the morning, constipation, bloating, a reduced libido, constant urination, dry skin and hair, decreased muscle mass and increased fat gain, foggy thinking, depression, and a feeling of being cold all the time.

Does this sound like you or someone you know? I'll bet my last dollar most of you said yes. In this book, I am going to educate you on how you can improve your metabolism by eating the right pro-metabolic foods and removing the anti-metabolic foods. You will begin to understand, on a deeper level, which foods, exercise, and lifestyle choices support a well- running metabolism, and which ones hinder your metabolism. You will learn why *all* diets don't work over the long term. You will understand why over-exercising is never a good solution to long-term health. And finally, you'll learn why happiness, and living with purpose and authenticity are essential for optimal health.

My entire purpose for writing this book is to not only share my healing journey and what I have learned along the way, but to teach you how to utilize the information in this book for your own healing process.

I also want you to understand that no matter how damaged you think you are, you can get better. You just need the right tools, an open mind, a desire to get better, and *patience*. Everything in this book contributed to me getting healthy and may help you in your healing journey.

Please understand this book is not a diet. I don't like diets because most are calorie restrictive, and they deprive your body of the sugars, fats, and nutrients your body so desperately needs. Plus, diets make you feel hungry, grumpy, agitated, irritated, and deprived. Additionally, diets tend to imply an "end" to the diet period, while this journey is a way of life. This book is about learning to nourish your body with the food, movement, and love it so desperately craves.

There are no *quick* weight-loss ideas or gimmicks in this book. Healing the metabolism with proper nutrition, movement, and love takes time, patience, and commitment. You must remember you didn't get to where you are today in a few weeks or months. It has taken the last 20, 30, or 40 years of your life for you to be at your current state of health, so allow the process to happen—without expectation of a miracle in 30 days.

Yet, do expect to start feeling better physically and emotionally. Your body will start warming up, and some of your health issues may start to improve. Weight loss is usually the last thing to happen. But do not despair: It can and will happen—all while you are eating more and exercising less.

My two *big* suggestions while reading this book are to be open and to take things slow. Many of the topics I will cover are going to be a 180-degree shift from what many health professionals are going to tell you. In addition, as you learn this new information, don't try to master everything in one week. Give your body time to adjust and relearn your new lifestyle. All successful coaching programs are slow and steady. Take one step at a time, and before you know it you will regain your health and your life.

So, without further ado, let's begin.

Chapter 1
Who Defines Health?

When I asked a group of people to give me their own definition of what health means to them, I got a mix of interesting answers: free of sickness, youth, running a race pain-free, strong and muscular, mental clarity, happiness, low cholesterol, normal blood pressure, medication-free, warm, soft skin and hair, wrinkle free (I guess that means I am not healthy), and—my favorite—a good pooper.

The World Health Organization (WHO) defines health as "a state of complete physical, mental, and social well-being, not merely the absence of disease or infirmity."

French physician Georges Canguilhem, in his 1943 book, *The Normal and the Pathological*, defined health as the ability to adapt to one's environment. Health is not a fixed entity. Canguilhem believed health was defined differently for each person.

Cardiologist Dr. Broda Barnes believed health was synonymous with a high metabolic rate. In his book *Hypothyroidism: The Unsuspected Illness,* Barnes links a healthy metabolism to a warm body (97.8–98.6 degrees F/36.6–37 degrees C), good digestion and daily bowel movements, healthy skin, shiny hair, strong nails, bones, and teeth, the ability to procreate and desire sex, void of PMS and hormonal issues, a healthy heart, clear mind, infrequent urination, deep restful sleep, good energy all day long, a lean muscular body, lack of disease, and a feeling of content and happiness.

Dr. Barnes's breakthrough research showed how hypothyroid (low thyroid/metabolism; *note that low thyroid is synonymous with low metabolic rate*) people, who were treated with thyroid therapy, showed improvements in many health problems and diseases. Treated patients found decreases in heart disease, migraines, fatigue, behavioral issues, infectious disease, skin problems, menstrual disorders, hypertension, elevated cholesterol, cancer, emphysema, obesity, and aging. Dr. Barnes's research displayed a direct correlation between a higher running thyroid/metabolism and improved health.

Personally, I cannot agree more with Dr. Barnes and his research pointing to a correlation between a high running metabolism and health. My life experience is a perfect example of his explanation. Every time I engaged in metabolically suppressing activities, foods, or drugs, my health and metabolism took a dive for the worse. Once I supported my metabolism through rest, the right foods, sleep, self-love, and the right amount of exercise, my health and happiness improved.

Redefining Health as a *High* Metabolic Rate

Dr. Barnes spent 35 years of his life treating his patients with thyroid therapy versus other standard medical drugs and procedures—with much success. Barnes understood that the thyroid gland is the conductor of every metabolic process in the body. Without the thyroid gland and thyroid hormones, metabolism would slowly stop, disorders and disease would follow, and death would be right behind.

What You Need to Know About the Thyroid Gland

Your thyroid is the butterfly-shaped gland located at the front of your neck. The thyroid, the largest endocrine gland, is referred to as a master gland, since it is the conductor of every metabolic process in your body.

The thyroid synthesizes four thyroid hormones: T1,

T2, T3, and T4. Each thyroid hormone is made up of the protein tyrosine and iodine. The number after the T is the number of iodine molecules attached to tyrosine. T4 and T3 are the most abundant thyroid hormones and what we will focus on in this book.

Thyroxine (T4): T4 is the primary thyroid hormone. T4 is the primary hormone because it is **produced four times more than T3 in the thyroid.** Yet, T4 is 1/10th less active than T3. 80 percent of T4 is converted to the more active T3 in the liver, kidneys, pituitary, and spleen.

Triiodothyronine (T3): T3 is the most active thyroid hormone. Yet, very little is produced in the thyroid: 10–20 percent of T3 is produced in the thyroid; the rest is converted from T4 in the liver, kidneys, spleen, and pituitary. **T3 is the most active hormone because it is 10 times more active than T4.**

Calcitonin: The thyroid also produces the hormone calcitonin, which is in charge of calcium regulation along with parathyroid hormone (PTH). Calcitonin is released when blood calcium levels are too high. PTH is released when blood calcium levels are too low.

In the 1950s, Dr. Barnes reported as many as 40 percent of Americans were affected by low thyroid/low metabolic rate. Today, with an increased ingestion of anti-thyroid foods (processed foods, soy, vegetable oils, grains, legumes, and nuts) and the avoidance of pro-thyroid foods (saturated fats, sugars, salt, and animal proteins), I believe that number could be far higher—*although lab testing may tell us differently.* (See the section titled "Current Thyroid Lab Testing" later in this chapter.)

Add in anti-metabolic activities like endurance-fitness events, increased stress levels, increased pharmaceutical drugs usage, increased exposure to radiation, and decreased sleep, and we are looking at a hypo-metabolic epidemic.

Therefore, since we are defining health as a high running metabolism, the million-dollar question is:

Are you healthy?

Ask yourself the following questions:

- What is your body temperature? Do you feel cold all the time? Cold hands, feet, and nose?

- What is your heart rate/pulse?

- How often do you urinate per day? Do you have chronic thirst?

- How often do you have a bowel movement? Constipated? Bloated? Gas? Diarrhea?

- What does your stool look like? Runny? Pebbles? Smelly? Undigested foods?

- How is your sleep? Restless, interrupted, feel exhausted upon waking?

- How are your skin, hair, and nails? Dry and brittle? Slow growing? Do you heal slowly?

- How are your hormones? Could you care less if you ever have sex again? Do you have PMS? Infertility? Low libido?

- How is your energy? Dragging all day? Energy highs and lows? Mid-day crash? Wired at night?

- How is your mood? Anxious? Depressed? Irritated? Sad?

- Do you get sick often? Or not at all?

- Do you gain weight easily? Do you have edema (water-logged)?

- Do you have a hard time losing weight, even with diet and exercise?

If, you answered yes to many of the above questions and find you are cold (consistently 95–97 degrees)—especially your hands, feet, and nose—have a low pulse (below 75bpm), urinate all day long (ideal is four to five times), your thirst is never quenched, are constipated (good bowel movement is one to three per day), bloated, and gassy, sleep poorly, are tired, depressed, have no sex drive, have dry nails, skin and hair, have slow healing wounds, are sick often, gain weight easily, and have a hard time losing weight, your metabolism may be on the fritz.

Even if you have just a few of the above issues you may be suffering from a depressed metabolic state.

Signs of a High Metabolic Rate:
- Body temperature with a thermometer:
- 97.8 F (36.6 C) upon waking
- 98.6 F (37 C) mid-day
- Pulse 75–90 bpm
- Warm feet, hands, and nose all day.
- 1–3 bowel movements/day
- Urinating 4–5 times/day, *not* 10–12 times/day
- Good hormone function: healthy sex drive, no PMS, fertile
- Shiny hair, smooth and healthy skin, strong nails
- 7–9 hours deep, uninterrupted sleep
- Feel happy and content
- Have good energy all day
- Maintain your weight without dieting and excessive exercise

Many of you may not even know you are suffering from a slow running metabolism; you may attribute your health issues to age or genetics—and you *may* be right (I'm doubtful), but you *may* be wrong. Over the last four years, my research tells me there is a lot more to aging than just years on this planet. In fact, it's quite possible your lifestyle, stress, toxic load, and diet are affecting your thyroid, metabolism, and overall health—far more than the calendar years are.

Luckily, in the upcoming chapters I'll educate you how you can improve your health, metabolism, and longevity with some "out-of-the-box" nutritional and lifestyle changes.

What Is Metabolism?

Metabolism is the sum of *every* metabolic process in your body. When your body is healthy, every metabolic process (including digestion, immunity, detoxification, sex drive, repair) will be working optimally.

Metabolism runs on carbohydrates/fats/proteins, which are stored in food and utilized as energy. Thus, the higher your metabolic rate, the more energy (food) you need to run efficiently. If your metabolic rate drops, metabolic processes (digestion, detoxification, sex drive, immunity) will suffer, and less energy (food) is needed and utilized.

Simple Tests for Metabolic Function

According to Dr. Barnes, the ideal test for thyroid/metabolic function is not even possible. Damn it—not what you wanted to hear, huh? Ideally thyroid levels should be measured in the cell, not the blood, where thyroid controls the rate of fuel (carbs/fats/proteins) burning in the cell. However, since we have trillions of cells, a test like this would be impossible to design—at least in today's world. However, this does not mean there are no usable tests. In fact, there are a few easy-to-do home tests that can give you quite a bit of information concerning your thyroid function and metabolic rate.

Basal Temperature

Before the creation of TSH (thyroid-stimulating hormone) and other thyroid lab tests, Dr. Barnes would have his patients perform a simple home test to measure metabolic rate by measuring basal temperature (body temperature). Barnes would advise his patients to place a well-shaken mercury thermometer by the bedside before bed. Upon waking, before patients did anything else, they were told to take their temperature, under the armpit, without moving, for 10 minutes. (See NOTE below.) According to Dr. Barnes, a healthy body temperature should be 97.8 degrees Fahrenheit (36.6 degrees Celsius) upon rising. Body temperature should steadily rise during the day and peak mid-day to about 98.6 degrees F (37 degrees C). Anything below that could indicate a sign of a sluggish metabolism.

(NOTE: Today most people are not using mercury thermometers and are unwilling to wait 10 minutes to find basal temperature. Although the mercury thermometer is more accurate, a digital thermometer can be used by mouth to find basal temperature. My advice is to take it a few times to get a more accurate reading.)

Heat is a product of a high metabolic rate. When glucose is oxidized in the cell's mitochondria, the waste products—energy (heat), carbon dioxide(CO_2), and water—are produced. Individuals who burn glucose well will produce more waste products (heat, CO_2, and water), producing a higher body temperature.

> *More glucose burned equals more heat equals a high metabolic rate.*

It should be noted that basal temperature is not the perfect test for thyroid function. Many conditions can produce a higher than normal reading: fever, electric blanket, hot weather, high cortisol, high adrenaline, and hot beverages. In addition, many conditions can produce a lower temperature: starvation, a cold, pituitary gland deficiency, adrenal problems, cooler weather, and cold beverages.

Cold hands, Feet, and Nose

Do you have cold hands, feet, and nose? Cold hands, feet, and nose are a sign of increased adrenaline and decreased thyroid. The thyroid hormones and the adrenal hormones, adrenaline and cortisol, are antagonist to each other.

When your thyroid is running well, your adrenaline and cortisol will be kept at bay. When your thyroid is sluggish or at times of stress, adrenaline and cortisol will increase for immediate heat and energy.

Adrenaline mobilizes stored glycogen (stored glucose) and free fatty acids to increase your body's energy needs. Cortisol will stimulate the breakdown of your body's own tissue (thymus, connective tissue, muscle) through gluconeogenesis to provide glucose to your cells. (*Gluconeogenesis is a metabolic process that generates glucose from non-carbohydrate sources including amino acids [your muscle and ingested protein], glycerol [from triglycerides], pyruvate [a ketone], lactate [glycolysis waste], and certain fatty acids.*) The rise in adrenaline is needed to support your brain and internal organs—while decreasing the circulation to your skin and extremities—producing cold hands, feet, and nose. This stress response is important for short-term survival, but *not* for long-term health.

Pulse/Heart Rate

According to Dr. Ray Peat, nutritional researcher and biologist, ideal heart rates for a healthy metabolism should range between 75 and 90 bpm. Despite popular belief, a low heart rate is not a sign of good health. It is a sign of a fit body—but just because you are fit does not mean you are healthy.

Many fit individuals, especially endurance athletes, have a resting pulse rate anywhere from the mid-40s to the mid-50s. They also have lower body temperature, anywhere from 94.5 to 96 degrees F. Due to their high level of cardiovascular activity, their bodies have adapted to their ongoing stressed state. Yes, exercise is a form of stress. Remember stress hormones rise in a time of stress and thyroid hormones lower, which *long* term, decreases heat production, lowering body temperature and pulse.

Essentially, the athlete's body is becoming more efficient, using less energy to perform the same amount of work. While this is helpful to the athlete while he or she is performing, long term the athlete's slower metabolism will start to have some negative effects, including increased aging, decreased sex drive, decreased immune function, decreased digestion, and slower healing.

Once again the pulse/heart rate test is not 100-percent accurate. There can be other reasons your pulse is high or low, including high blood pressure, low blood pressure, heart problems, diabetes, cancer, etc. Use these tests as guides, not as the absolute of all of testing. Yet, these tests, combined with the above questions, will give you usable information about your current metabolic state, which will be helpful in your healing journey. (Don't worry: I will get there.)

Current Thyroid Lab Testing

Most doctors use thyroid-stimulating hormone (TSH) to test for thyroid function. TSH is the hormone secreted from your pituitary gland in response to low thyroid levels of triiodothyronine (T3) and thyroxine (T4). If TSH is elevated above "normal" levels, you may be hypothyroid (sluggish metabolism).

The biggest problem with TSH testing is many people have normal TSH levels while showing signs of a low thyroid. This is referred to as subclinical hypothyroidism. TSH can be suppressed by stress, infection, fever, and caffeine, showing "normal" levels when the person in fact has low thyroid.

Therefore, more tests may be necessary. TSH is a pituitary hormone and not a thyroid hormone, so it actually seems somewhat illogical to test thyroid function with a pituitary hormone, but doctors do.

Here is a list of other thyroid tests that may be necessary to test the health of your thyroid:

Total T4/Total thyroxine = the amount of T4 bound to a carrier protein and the amount of unbound T4 in the blood. T4 is one-fifth to 1/10 as active as T3. T4 is converted into the more active T3 in the liver and kidneys.

Total T3/Total triiodothyronine = the amount of T3 bound to a carrier protein and the amount of unbound T3 in the blood.

FREE T3 = the amount of unbound T3 in blood. Low levels could mean an underactive thyroid.

FREE T4 = the amount of unbound T4 in blood. Low levels could mean an underactive thyroid.

Anti-TPO = anti-thyroid peroxidase (TPO). TPO is an enzyme needed to produce thyroid hormone. High levels of this antibody are an indication of an autoimmune disorder like Hashimoto's or Graves disease.

Hashimotos attacks the thyroid gland, decreasing thyroid production and creating hypothyroidism (low thyroid).

Graves disease produces too much thyroid hormone producing hyperthyroidism (too much thyroid).

Anti TgAB = Antithyroglobulin (Tg) antibodies. Tg is a protein needed to produce T3 and T4. High levels of this antibody may indicate an autoimmune disorder like Hashimoto's or Graves disease.

RT3 = measures the amount of Reverse T3. RT3, like T3, is created from T4 in the liver. RT3 is inactive. When the body is stressed, more T4 is converted into RT3 to conserve energy. This process lowers the conversion of T4 to T3 (the active hormone). Less T3 equals a lower metabolic rate. The ratio of T3/RT3 is a good indicator of how much active thyroid your body is actually using.

Discuss with your health care provider what testing you feel you may need. With the healthcare system constantly changing, doctors will be advised to perform the least amount of testing possible. However, if you want more tests, ask for more tests. This is *your* health.

What Happens When Your Thyroid Becomes Sluggish?

Besides the fact that your body will become cooler, your pulse rate will be low, and your hands, feet, and nose become icebergs, numerous other health issues can result. Remember: The thyroid is the conductor of every metabolic process in your body, and if it is running low, every system in your entire body can be affected. A sluggish thyroid/metabolism can affect not only your weight, but your immune system, digestive system, detoxification, desire for sex, fertility, cholesterol, blood pressure, sleep, and overall mood.

Weight Gain

Thyroid hormone, specifically T3, is needed for cells to create usable energy. When hormone levels are low, metabolic rate slows, producing less energy (heat), water, and carbon dioxide (CO_2). When less energy is used, more is stored as fat and you become overweight.

In a study in *Metabolism Journal*, researchers found that a drop of 1 degree Celsius in body temperature would lower metabolic rate by 10–13 percent. Therefore, if you are consuming 2,000 calories (kcal) to maintain your weight and are running a cool 36 degrees C (97 degrees F) through the day, you have dropped your caloric expenditure by 10–13 percent, or 200–230 kcal/day.

Therefore, if you raised your body temperature to normal, you could lose weight without eating less or working out more! Does this sound good to you? Then you should keep reading.

Elevated Cholesterol

Thyroid hormone, triiodothyronine (T3), along with Vitamin A, is needed to convert cholesterol into all your steroidal hormones.

The hormones pregnenolone, estrogen, progesterone,

androgens like testosterone, DHEA, glucocorticoids like cortisol, and mineralocorticoids like aldosterone are all products from cholesterol synthesis. As you know, some T3 is produced from the thyroid gland while the rest is synthesized from T4 in the liver, kidneys, pituitary, and spleen. If T3 production is low due to a poor running thyroid or a lack of T4 conversion in the converting organs, the creation of steroidal hormones will suffer and cholesterol levels will rise.

Do you have elevated cholesterol? Did the doctor suggest statin drugs? Before you take anything, maybe you should have your thyroid checked.

Low Sex Drive/Infertility/PMS

When thyroid hormones are low, cholesterol conversion becomes inhibited, resulting in *high* cholesterol and *lower* production of sex hormones. Reduced sex hormones in men and women can lead to lower libido, decreased vitality, dry skin and hair, muscle loss, etc. Women can also experience PMS, ovarian cysts, irregular cycles and heavy bleeding. In addition, women need the sex hormones, specifically progesterone (pro-gestation), to get pregnant (pro-create). If these hormones are depleted, infertility will occur.

It's important to note again that when you are stressed, thyroid activity decreases. Due to high stress, the thyroid you are making will be used to convert cholesterol into cortisol. An over-production of your stress hormone cortisol will occur at the expense of your sex hormones testosterone, estrogen, and progesterone.

Have you ever known a woman who was completely stressed about trying to get pregnant? Tried everything and nothing worked? Finally, after doing everything, she decided it was not going to happen, stopped stressing about it, and then got pregnant? Many think this is the miracle child; I think it's basic human physiology: Reduced stress = increased thyroid = increased sex hormones = pregnancy

With the rise in decreased thyroid function and increased

stress, it makes sense the fertility business is now a more-than-4-billion-dollar industry.

What You Need to Know About the Adrenal Glands

There are two adrenal (ad-*renal*) glands that sit on top of each *kidney*. The adrenal gland's main responsibility is to release hormones in response to stress. However, chronic elevation of any of these hormones will increase aging, lower thyroid function, increase fat gain (especially around the belly), increase lactic acid production, muscle wasting, etc.

Remember: The adrenal gland and thyroid are antagonistic to each other.

Main hormones:

Glucocorticoid: (*gluco*-corticoid) Hormones **Cortisol:** released in times of stress to break down tissue (muscle, thymus, connective tissue) to provide *glucose* to the body. Cortisol acts as an anti-inflammatory to the body, like cortisone shots and creams.

Androgens: testosterone, androstenedione, dihydro-testosterone (DHT)

Testosterone: produced in men and women. Men produce more testosterone in their testes.

Androstenedione: precursor to testosterone and estrogen

DHT: produced from testosterone, linked to male pattern baldness. *(For more on this read* Hair Like a Fox *by Danny Roddy.)*

Catecholamines:

Adrenaline: mobilizes glycogen and free fatty acids for energy

Noradrenaline: increases the heart rate Catecholamines are your fight or flight hormones.

They provide immediate physiological responses to the body under stress. Catecholamines are derived from the amino acid tyrosine, also in thyroid hormones.

Mineralocorticoid Hormones:

Aldosterone: helps regulate blood pressure. Increases in aldosterone will increase blood pressure.

Adrenal Fatigue: A Different View

When your adrenals are not functioning optimally many health practitioners refer to this as adrenal fatigue. The adrenals are "burned out" and can no longer support the ongoing stress of your body. Adrenaline and cortisol are depleted, and the body experiences extreme fatigue, illness, and even disease. Yet, in my opinion the root of the problem is not the adrenals; the root of the problem is a suppressed thyroid.

Imagine your thyroid is your main power system and your adrenals are your (in case of emergency) generator.

When your main power system (thyroid) is working correctly, you don't need your generator (adrenals) as much. However, once your power system fails, your generator kicks in so that you can still get energy.

The generator (adrenals) works when your main power system (thyroid) needs support in a time of crisis (stress). This is a good thing.

The problems start when your generator (adrenals) has to work overtime. The generator (adrenals) is not meant to be your primary system to produce energy—and if it (adrenals) works too hard, the system will die out *very* quickly. This is often referred to as adrenal fatigue.

The common practice to alleviate this "diagnosis" is to fix the adrenals, yet this is *not* the root of the problem. What you need to do is fix the main power source, the thyroid, so the adrenals can take a much-needed break, recover, and *regenerate* from all their hard work. The adrenals will regenerate in the right conditions: with nutrient-rich foods (eggs, liver, oysters) and lower stress.

Fixing the adrenals only is not going to solve the problem—at least, not long term. If you don't fix the thyroid, the adrenals will fall back into dysfunction and the cycle will continue.

Sluggish Liver

The liver, your main detox organ, utilizes its own glycogen (stored glucose) to fuel itself in its more than 500 functions. Thyroid hormone is needed to utilize glycogen stores for the liver to function optimally—just like the liver is needed for optimal thyroid function (T4-T3 conversion). When the liver becomes sluggish, a number of metabolic processes can be affected, including decreased cholesterol synthesis, inhibited carbohydrate, protein, and fat metabolism, and a decreased storage of vital vitamins and minerals, including A, D, K, B12, iron, and copper. In addition, since the liver is our main detox organ, when it slows, the breakdown and excretion of insulin, bile, ammonia, estrogen, pharmaceutical drugs, alcohol, and other toxins decreases. An overburdened liver becomes backed up, allowing these toxins to recirculate through the body, creating an immune response and illness.

Digestive Issues

People in a hypo-metabolic state have low levels of hydrochloric acid (HCL) in the stomach. HCL is needed for protein breakdown. Low levels of HCL will inhibit proper protein breakdown and the absorption of vital minerals, including zinc, copper, iron, and calcium, as well as B12 and folate.

The secretion of HCL is used as a barrier against microorganisms to prevent infections. Seventy percent of your immune system is located in your gut. This high-acidic environment is designed to kill bacteria and viruses. Decreased HCL will allow undigested food and pathogens to enter into the small intestine, leading to bloating, gas, constipation, diarrhea, irritable bowel syndrome (IBS), colitis, celiac disease, or possibly cancer.

Low Immune Function

Increasing evidence supports that T3 and T4 are modulators of the immune response, directly and indirectly.

We already know that low thyroid = low HCL = increased gut pH = less protection from bacteria, viruses, and fungus.

And, as I have said previously, the stress hormones adrenaline and cortisol stay elevated when thyroid activity is suppressed. Although this is life-saving in the short term, chronically elevated stress hormones lower the effects of the immune system. Cortisol breaks down the thymus gland to produce needed sugar for the body. The thymus produces T-cells, which protect the body from foreign bacteria and viruses. A damaged thymus leads to lower immunity.

Increased Blood Pressure

Blood pressure is the force against the wall of the arteries while blood flows through them. When the heart beats, pressure increases (systolic pressure), and when the heart relaxes pressure decreases (diastolic). When your body is stressed, the renin-angiotensin-aldosterone-system (RAAS) triggers your blood pressure to rise. Your body has more energy needs when you are stressed, so heart and blood pressure increase to get nutrients and energy into your cells. Once you are out of stress, blood pressure should decrease. However, in our chronically stressed society, this does not happen, and the result is hypertension.

Remember: When stress increases, thyroid activity drops. Chronically high levels of stress can decrease thyroid function in the long term. Therefore, to decrease high blood pressure and increase thyroid function, decrease stress! This may include lifestyle changes, proper nutrition, sleeping more, etc.

Please note this is just one theory regarding high blood pressure.

There are many unknown reasons for high blood pressure.

Mood Disorders

Feeling sad, moody, depressed, or a general feeling of the "blahs" can be linked to thyroid deficiency. If your thyroid is low, and increased demands are placed on your body, your stress hormones increase to compensate for the much-needed energy. (Yes, I am going to say this about 100 times in this book; it is that important!)

The problems start when stress hormones stay high and thyroid/metabolic rate continues to stay low. Over time, reduced thyroid = less cholesterol conversion = reduced cortisol = reduced energy = fatigue, depression, and the "blahs." You can only stress yourself so long until your crazy, out-of-control, no-sleep, crappy-eating life catches up to you. The "cortisol *high*" you were riding on initially is going to eventually come to a screeching halt. Until you fix the underlying problem of a deficient thyroid, your body is going to feel like a truck has run over it—again and again.

Sleep Issues

If you have low thyroid function/low metabolic rate, stress hormones will stay elevated, which can keep you from falling asleep, wake you up in the middle of the night, or give you insomnia. Sleep issues are a common problem in people getting older, which is why sleeping pills are a billion-dollar industry.

It is common practice for many weight-conscious people to not eat three to four hours before bed. Yet, by doing this they are lowering their stored liver glycogen levels. Liver glycogen is needed in times of sleeping (fasting) to provide energy to the body's cells.

When metabolic rate drops, the ability to store liver glycogen decreases (see the "Sluggish Liver" section above). If the liver is unable to store enough sugar for the body to survive the night, a stress response occurs: Adrenaline and cortisol rise, and you wake up or cannot go to sleep.

Wouldn't you like to know how you could prevent this from

happening? Skip to Chapter 16 on sleep for a quick lesson.

As you can see, there is more to good health than looking good and feeling good. Health is synonymous with a high metabolism and reduced stress. Metabolism and good thyroid function are the conductors to every metabolic process in your body. When they are running low, you will be feeling the effects emotionally, physically, and mentally.

In the upcoming chapters, I will educate you about what foods and lifestyle choices are supportive to a high metabolism and what foods inhibit optimal metabolic function. You will learn why "heart-healthy" fats are anything but that, all while learning why saturated fats are the most metabolically stimulating fats. You will learn why sugars are your body's *best* source of energy and why avoiding them will result in a metabolic shutdown. You will learn why nuts, legumes, and leafy greens are *not* the health foods you thought they were. You will learn which proteins are the most nutritious and metabolically stimulating. And finally, you will learn why quality sleep, the right amount of exercise, water, and finding happiness in life are all very important factors in the healing process and supportive of a high metabolic rate.

Let the healing begin!

Chapter 2
Don't Be Afraid of Saturated Fats

More than ever, it seems people today are confused about what to eat and what is truth when it comes to what is healthy for us. With so much conflicting information *and* changing nutrition advice, we are all at a loss as to what is actually healthy for us and what is not healthy for us.

The truth is, overall, we are still in the infantile stages of understanding food, nutrition, hormonal response to foods, and how this all affects our physiology. Nutrition is such a new science that we've barely touched the surface as to the power it has over our health and well-being. As scientific studies reveal more, we realize that we have mislabeled good things as bad and bad things as good. We have learned that just because something produces a certain result in one person, does not mean it will produce the same result in another person. This is one big reason why the study of nutrition is so complex and challenging.

With that said, I want to talk about a very controversial topic, a topic that up until now has received some very bad press: saturated fat—you know, the evil, artery-clogging, heart attack–promoting stuff that most doctors tell you to eliminate from your diet or lower as much as possible.

I want to present another side of the saturated fat story. I want to discuss with you why I believe saturated fat has undeservingly received a bad reputation. I will discuss why saturated fat can actually be very beneficial to you, why we have been brainwashed into thinking it is unhealthful, and why you should start incorporating it back into your daily diet.

What Are Saturated Fats?

Saturated fats are chains of carbon, hydrogen, and oxygen that are held together by single bonds. Single-bonded chains are very stable and strong (since they are saturated with hydrogen). They do not go rancid or break down when exposed to heat or oxygen. In contrast, poly- and monounsaturated fats have one or more double bonds, which make them more susceptible to oxidative stress and free radical damage.

This is one reason why it is best to cook with saturated fats: They are stable and do not chemically break down. Foods that contain saturated fats are coconut oil, eggs, meats, and dairy (such as milk, cream, butter, and cheese).

What Is the Role of Saturated Fats in the Body?

Interestingly enough, when you understand the role of saturated fat in the body, you realize all the positive effects it has on the body, especially when you understand that 60 percent of your brain and 50 percent of your cells' membranes are composed of saturated fat.

Saturated fats:

- Are resilient to oxidation—meaning they're protecting your body from the harmful effects of oxygen and oxidants such as iron. (In this way, saturated fats need less help from antioxidants and lower your risk of developing many types of cancer.)

- When incorporated into cells, decrease body inflammation in comparison to poly- and monounsaturated fats.

- Boost your metabolism (especially coconut oil).

- Help regulate blood sugar by slowing the absorption of carbohydrates.

- Contain high amounts of essential fat-soluble vitamins (A, D, and K2). These fat-soluble vitamins are found primarily in animal fats. Consuming a diet with adequate dairy, eggs, meat and fish would be the best way to meet these nutritional needs.

- Can help detoxify and protect the liver, kidneys, and pancreas.

- Help protect the heart.

- Decrease levels of endotoxins in the gut, thus increasing gut health and digestion. (Endotoxins, also known as lipopolysaccharides (LPS), are toxins kept within the bacterial cell and are released after the destruction of the cell wall.)

- Make food taste better.

Cindy's Story

Cindy was eating a diet high in sunflower oil, sesame oil, grapeseed oil, and canola oil. Cindy's diet was void of eggs, butter, most red meats, dairy, and coconut oil. She avoided these foods due to their saturated fat content, which she believed was unhealthy for her.

Over the last year, Cindy started to gain weight and it seemed that whatever she did, the weight would not go away. Cindy weighed about 140 pounds and was consuming no more than 1,200 calories/day. Cindy exercised almost every day—a long walk or an hour of cardio at the gym. Cindy was constantly cold, tired, and moody, and her sleep was restless—to say the least.

Through weekly coaching, Cindy began to learn the anti-metabolic effects of a low-calorie diet, tons of cardio, and the consumption of the polyunsaturated fats (PUFA).

Cindy's first dietary change was to replace her current PUFA oils with coconut oil and butter. She started with ½ tablespoon and slowly added more each week. Cindy limited her cardiovascular activity to two to three times a week and added in a little yoga. In addition, Cindy added more metabolic-supportive foods to her diet, like eggs, dairy, bone broth, fruits, honey, and gelatin.

Within just two weeks Cindy observed that by just removing the PUFA oils and adding in foods with more saturated fats and eating more, Cindy's body temperature started to heat up. Initially, Cindy was running at a cool 96 degrees with a pulse of 60 bpm. When more body heat (increased pulse and body temperature) is produced, it is a sign of increased metabolic rate. Six months later, Cindy had lost 10 pounds, she was eating more food than she had in years, and she felt far more energized.

So Where Did it All Go Wrong?

Why has saturated fat received such a bad rap? Well, back in the 1950s a biologist/researcher named Ancel Keys "proved" that saturated fats cause heart disease, and then later showed that saturated fats raise cholesterol levels. I say "proved" because when you look at all the research data, including all the omitted data, you will see that Mr. Keys really didn't prove anything at all. Yes, he reviewed seven countries that had high saturated fat intake and high incidences of heart disease. The problem is that he failed to report on the other 16 countries that did not support his hypothesis. In fact, many of these countries proved quite the opposite: they refuted his theory. Some countries, including France and Holland, had a very high saturated fat intake and had extremely low rates of heart disease. And other countries like Chile had a very low saturated fat intake and a high incidence of heart disease. Essentially, Keys developed a *hypothesis*, which made a correlation between high saturated fat and heart disease. Ancel Keys did not *prove* anything. Unfortunately, his correlation was enough to get him on the cover of *Time*, and that ended up becoming the beginning of the "evil saturated fat" theory.

Since then, subsequent controlled studies have tried to prove that saturated fat raises blood cholesterol levels, and thus increases your chances of heart disease. The Framingham study, one of the longest government-funded studies on heart disease, found that cholesterol levels had very little to do with one's chance of heart disease or heart attacks, finding that 50 percent of people who had heart attacks had low cholesterol. In 2010, a meta-analysis on the relationship of heart disease and saturated fat was published in the *American Journal of Clinical Nutrition*. The study followed the lives of almost 350,000 people and concluded the intake of saturated fat was *not* linked to cardiovascular disease.

What About Cholesterol?

Cholesterol has been blamed for heart disease, heart attacks, and strokes for years, but is cholesterol really the problem? Cholesterol is needed to build and maintain cell membranes, intracellular transport, Vitamin D, and the synthesis of all steroidal hormones, including progesterone, estrogen, testosterone, cortisol, and aldosterone. Low cholesterol levels have been linked to increased cancer rates and increased mortality. Without cholesterol you would die.

Current scientific research understands that increased dietary cholesterol contributes very little to blood cholesterol levels. Research also tells us the total blood cholesterol is a poor depicter of heart disease; more important is the ratio of LDL to HDL cholesterol, and the density of LDL is a far better predictor. Small LDL particles are more prone to oxidation versus the large, buoyant LDL particles. Oxidized cholesterol is a far bigger concern than the total cholesterol in your body.

Dr. Broda Barnes, a world-renowned cardiologist and the author of several books, including *Hypothyroidism: The Unsuspected Illness,* found a direct correlation between high cholesterol and hypothyroidism. The thyroid hormone triiodothyronine (T3) is needed to convert cholesterol into the steroidal hormones. If the thyroid, which produces the inactive thyroid hormone thyroxine (T4) and a small amount of T3 and the liver, which converts the inactive T4 to active T3, are both "sluggish," hormonal production will slow and cholesterol levels will rise. Dr. Barnes treated hundreds of his high cholesterol and heart patients with thyroid medication with amazing results.

We now know that increased total blood cholesterol does not correlate to an increase in artery blockage or an increase in heart disease. We know this because just as many people have heart attacks with high cholesterol as have heart attacks with low cholesterol. A cholesterol increase is an immune system response. It is the symptom of a problem, not the problem itself.

In addition, most studies performed on saturated fat intake are performed on unhealthy individuals. Unhealthy individuals usually have a lot of cellular inflammation, and since saturated fat can help with decreasing inflammation, it may actually raise blood cholesterol levels. An increase in cholesterol is the body's response to an increase in inflammation. Therefore, increasing saturated fat can be seen as a way to help the body heal, since a temporary increase in cholesterol is the body's response in trying to help your body heal. Therefore, saturated fat can promote healing in a very unhealthy individual.

Whew! Confused yet?

You see, saturated fat intake in a healthy individual does not increase cholesterol levels or increase heart disease. In many cultures like the Tokelau (with their 50-percent dietary saturated fat intake) or the Masai (with their diet of meat, blood, and milk) or the Inuit (with their ancestral diet of high blubber animals), we find that they all have superior cardiovascular health with very low rates of heart disease and cholesterol issues—yet they eat diets *very* high in saturated fat.

What Does This All Mean?

Simply put, you shouldn't be scared of saturated fat. Personally, I eat anywhere from 20–30 percent of my calories from fat, most of that being saturated fat. For example, for breakfast I eat two eggs cooked in coconut oil, cooked fruit with butter and cinnamon, orange juice, and coffee with cream and sugar. Now, I know this may be a little shocking to many of you, since it's against popular opinion at the moment. However, nutrition science is evolving as we learn more. And think about this: In the last 60 years we have ingested far less saturated fat and tons more polyunsaturated fat, also known as the "heart healthy fats" (vegetable, seed, and nut oils), and have only gotten fatter, have increased the incidences of diabetes and heart disease, and are just plain less healthy.

My personal journey to eating a diet that did not limit saturated fat was an educational, healing, and enlightening one. Remember back in 2010 when I hit a physical, emotional, and hormonal wall? At the time I was attempting to train for three half-marathons and a half Iron Man. I had incurred a groin injury that was not going away. I was also starting to feel "blah." I gained a few pounds and felt increasingly tired. I was at a loss because I thought everything I was doing was supportive to health.

This is when I started to include small amounts of saturated fats, and then gradually increased them more. I started using healthy sugars (fruit, fruit juice, and root vegetables), and eating the super proteins (organic dairy, shellfish, gelatin, white fish, and a small amount of grass-fed beef). I also began removing many other foods that are currently considered "healthy" by many, including *all* polyunsaturated fats, beans, and grains. I also cut out most nuts and some vegetables.

Initially, I saw my weight and cholesterol rise. Weight gain and increased cholesterol levels—that can't be good, right? Well, let's remember, I was in an inflamed state (from chronic overtraining), and the cholesterol was being released to allow me to heal. The additional weight was also in response to trying to heal my metabolism—a metabolism damaged from years of overtraining and under-nourishing (omitting saturated fat and the right sugars, and eating far less than my body really needed). In a matter of three months, while I allowed my body to heal, my cholesterol dropped more than 40 points, my body weight dropped back to normal, and I started to feel that everything was right in the world again (no more "blah" feeling)—all while eating more than 2,000 to 2,500 calories and 50–100g of fat a day (most of that being saturated fat). Interesting, huh?

Yes, I lost body fat while eating 50–100 grams of fat a day, while exercising less than I had in the previous 20 years of my life. I never made all the planned runs or the half Iron Man. Yet, I'm sure it was for the best. Even today, five years later, I am still healing. Well, to be honest, I have stressed my body with a few endurance events, so I have kept a good balance of healing–breaking down–healing again.

Believe it or not, most highly active individuals have a damaged metabolism, yet most don't understand this. They believe it is *age* that is affecting their metabolism. The truth is, all things that are stressful to your body, including exercise, can affect your metabolism negatively. Now, this does not mean you should not exercise. It just means if you want to heal your metabolism, you need to be doing the right type of exercise for you based on your current state of health.

Please understand: I am not telling you to go out and eat tons of butter, cream, and chocolate to try to lose weight and get healthy. You need to have an understanding as to how, when, and what types of saturated fats you should be eating. Plus, there is a lot more to healing your metabolism than just eating saturated fats. Is it okay to eat all these things? Absolutely! Should you start eating 100 grams of saturated fat like I did without understanding what you are doing? Absolutely not! Saturated fat is a very powerful nutrient. If the proper types are used, in the right amounts, with the right combination of protein and carbs, you can have not only a healing nutrient, but also a nutrient that will allow you to enjoy rich, great-tasting food again.

What Types Are Best?

1. Coconut Oil

In my opinion, if you take just a few things away from this book, a big one is to add coconut oil into your diet. One of the biggest benefits of coconut oil is the increased metabolic rate it gives you, which will help with fat loss and overall heat production. Coconut oil consists of medium-chain triglycerides (MCTs), which digest very differently than other fats. MCTs do not need to be digested by bile salts, and can go straight from your gut to your liver and can be metabolized as quick energy. The main MCT is lauric acid, which is a proven anti-fungal, anti-bacterial, and antiviral agent.

Personally, I use refined organic expeller-pressed coconut oil from Healthy Traditions (www.HealthyTraditions.com). Refined coconut oil has the fibers removed, making it is easier to digest and less of an irritant to the gut. You can add coconut oil to soups, broths, and smoothies, cook with it, make a salad dressing, or just eat a spoonful. My recommendation is to start slowly when adding coconut oil. Start with 1 teaspoon/day. Each week add another teaspoon until you are consuming anywhere from 1 to 2 tablespoons/day. There is no "right" amount for everybody; there is only the right amount for you. Therefore, pay attention to how your body responds. Are you feeling "warmer"? Is your digestion better? Are you less sick?

Coconut oil will help clean out your gut and intestines, so pay attention to your stool. If you find it gets too loose, cut back on the amount of coconut oil, until your body gets used to the amount you are using.

2. Grass-Fed Butter

Yes, butter is good—of course, as long as it is real butter and the only ingredients are cream and salt. Grass-fed is always best. We must remember the food we eat is only as good as the source it comes from. Cows are supposed to eat grass, not grains. Butter from a grain-fed cow is a different food than butter that comes from a grass-fed cow. Grass-fed butter contains short- and medium-chain fatty acids, which like coconut oil protect us against infection. Butter also contains the short-chain fatty acid butyric acid, which has been shown to have antifungal and anti-cancer properties. Butter is rich in vitamins A, E, D, and K2, manganese, zinc, chromium, copper, and selenium.

3. Grass-Fed Ghee

If you don't know what ghee is, well you are about to thank me for introducing it to you. Ghee is clarified butter, or butter that has had the milk solids and water evaporated out of it. What is left is buttery oil that tastes like pure yumminess. Ghee can be used in the place of butter in cooking, and its high smoke point makes it a great choice for frying and sautéing. Ghee is very rich in vitamins A and K2. Vitamins A and K2 are fat-soluble vitamins that are very important to bone health.

4. Cacao

Yes! Finally someone is telling you chocolate is good for you! Raw cacao or raw chocolate is filled with health benefits. Cacao is a great source of magnesium and antioxidants. The saturated fat in cacao is stearic acid, which has been touted as one of the healthiest saturated fats since it has been shown to *lower* cholesterol levels. Stearic acid is also found in the fat of whole organic milk (which I will discuss in more detail in Chapter 9). Raw cacao powder is the best source of cacao. If you are choosing a dark chocolate bar to get your cacao from, make sure it has only *real* ingredients: cacao, sugar, vanilla and salt. A healthy dark chocolate bar should be void of soy lecithin, gums, carrageenan, and other additives.

I want to end with one very important message: All saturated fats should still be eaten in moderation. Eating a stick of butter or an entire bar of dark chocolate, in one night, may not be beneficial to your health or your waistline. I think it's safe to say that 20–30 percent of your diet should contain fat. Some people may need a little more and some a little less; it all depends on you, your health, and your goals.

I hope you can look at eating saturated fat a little differently now. I hope you understand saturated fat is not the evil, artery-clogging fat the nutritional and medical industries have led you to believe. The right saturated fats in the right amounts will not only make your food taste better, but they can be very healing and beneficial to your body. Saturated fat is *not* the enemy, and you should not be scared of it—yet, that doesn't mean *all* fat is good. There are fats that are contributing to your sluggish metabolism. More than likely you are eating them in large quantities every day. Any guess as to what they are? You guessed it: the polyunsaturated fats, also known as PUFA.

Chapter 2:
What You Need to Know

1. Saturated fats are single bonded fats that are fully saturated with hydrogen atoms. They are more stable than mono- and polyunsaturated fats. They are less susceptible to oxidative damage.

2. Saturated fats are ideal to cook with. Coconut oil, butter, and ghee are good options.

3. Saturated fats help increase metabolic rate. Saturated fats help detox the liver, kidneys, pancreas, and gut. Saturated fats are protective against the oxidation of PUFAs.

4. Healthy foods containing saturated fats include eggs, grass-fed beef, lamb, bison, milk, cheese, and dark chocolate. (See Appendix C for the best fats to eat.)

5. Saturated fat is *not* the artery-clogging, heart attack–inducing food we are all led to believe. The right saturated fats can actually decrease your cholesterol, heal your body, and decrease your chances of heart disease and cancer.

Chapter 3
Polyunsaturated Fats: Toxic, Not Essential!

Now that you know that saturated fats are not the enemy and can be very healthy for you, it's important to understand the fats that are actually harmful to you. When I say harmful, I mean contributing to slowing your thyroid, decreasing cellular energy, increasing oxidative damage, and encouraging you to gain weight.

What are these harmful fats? The polyunsaturated fatty acids, also known as PUFAs. These are the same fats promoted by the nutrition and medical industry as "heart-healthy" fats. What? Am I telling you polyunsaturated fats, the very fats your doctor and registered dietician have been telling you to eat, are actually harmful to you? *Yes!* That is exactly what I am telling you. The very fats you have been encouraged to eat for the last 50 years are the very fats that are slowing your metabolism, increasing aging, supporting illness and disease, and helping you gain weight!

Americans, and most people around the world, are consuming PUFAs every day—in dangerously large amounts! And most of you may be consuming them thinking you are doing something helpful for yourself when in fact you are doing anything *but* that. Are you consuming chia seeds, nuts, seeds, flax oil, fish oil, etc.? If so, then you may want to keep reading to find out why these very toxic fats are doing you far more harm than good.

What Are Polyunsaturated Fats and Where Are They Found?

Polyunsaturated fats (PUFAs) are fatty acids with many double carbon bonds (double bonds link four electrons, versus the usual two). PUFAs contain double bonds because they lack several hydrogen atoms. This is why they are referred to as "unsaturated." Remember from the last chapter that saturated fatty acids have only single bonds and are fully "saturated" with hydrogen atoms. Double bonds, although stronger, are more reactive to oxygen than single bonds, making them unstable and susceptible to oxidative stress.

Oxidative stress occurs within the body when oxygen reacts with food to create energy (metabolism) and produces by-products called free radicals. (Free radicals are molecules that have an unpaired electron in the outer shell and are looking to "gain or lose" an electron.) Since PUFAs are unstable, once they are exposed to oxygen, free radicals are created. These free radicals "steal" electrons from other molecules, creating more unstable molecules. Over time, this creates a chain reaction of free radical damage that can cause accelerated aging, hormone imbalance, cancer, and immune disorders. Yikes!

PUFAs can be found in large and small amounts in everything you eat. Yes, everything you eat. PUFAs are primarily found in vegetables, nuts, seeds, legumes (like soy and grains), cold-water fish (like salmon), and poultry, beef, and pork that have been poisoned by a diet rich in PUFAs (grain-, soy-, and corn-fed animals). The biggest offenders of PUFAs are the so-called heart-healthy oils, which include vegetable, nut, seed, and fish oils.

The list of oils with the highest concentration of PUFAs and that can be the most harmful are soybean oil, corn oil, safflower oil, grape seed oil, sesame seed, nut oils (peanut, walnut, almond, etc.), flaxseed, fish oil, cod liver oil, evening primrose, borage oils, and, yes, this even includes Omega-3 (EPA and DHA) and Omega-6, also known as the "essential fatty acids."

Polyunsaturated fats can also be produced by the body, from

Chapter 3: Polyunsaturated Fats: Toxic, Not Essential! 43

saturated fat and sugar, in the form of Mead acid, also known as Omega-9 fatty acid. Mead acid has proven to have anti-inflammatory properties. Mead acid increases in the body on a diet "deficient" in the "essential" fats (Omega-3 and Omega-6). Human cells produce these unsaturated fats when their special desaturase enzymes are not suppressed by the presence of exogenous linoleic (Omega-6) or linolenic acids (Omega-3). Basically, we can make our own, *safer* polyunsaturated fats to be used as regulators or signals, and to activate the formation of stem cells.

To call the polyunsaturated fats essential seems quite ridiculous, since we can never completely avoid them and we can make them (Omega-9) using saturated fats and sugar.

Now, I know what you are thinking: "I thought these 'essential fats' were good for me? I thought these oils were 'heart healthy' according to the USDA, my doctor, and my registered dietitian? How could they possibly be bad for me?" Yes, I know it is mind boggling, especially considering the massive marketing push on fish oils, flax, cod liver oils, chia seeds, and the Omega-3 and Omega-6 oils. Trust me: It took me months and months of research to wrap my brain around it, especially since I used to be an avid fish oil user. So let's go back almost 90 years ago so you can understand what has happened.

I'll start with Mildred and George Burr. In 1929, the Burrs published a paper claiming that the polyunsaturated fat linoleic acid (Omega-6) was essential for the prevention of several diseases and essential for health. The Burrs' study concluded that rats that ingested unsaturated fats were far healthier than the rats that were on a fat-free diet—which, in fact, was true. From this the Burrs coined the term "essential fatty acids (EFA)" and a deficiency in EFAs was known as Burr's disease.

However, over 10 years later, the Clayton Foundation Biochemical Institute found that "Burr's disease" was actually a vitamin B6 deficiency. Back in 1929, the B vitamins were not yet discovered. The new research explained that the PUFAs had actually slowed down the metabolism of the PUFA-fed rats, causing a decreased need for nutrients. Thus, this allowed them to not be as nutrient deficient as the fat-free-diet rats. The non-PUFA-fed rats had a higher metabolic rate. A higher metabolic rate comes with an increase in nutrient demand, especially the B vitamins. And since the demand was not met, the rats became sick. Basically, all Burrs showed was that PUFAs slow your metabolic rate down, allowing you to survive on fewer nutrients. Thus the PUFAs prevented a deficiency on a deficient diet. Interesting, huh?

Let me try to break it down a little more. Think of a high metabolism like a Ferrari car engine. A Ferrari has a high-powered engine (high metabolic rate) and requires premium gasoline (sugars) and oils (the right fats and proteins) to run optimally. Because a Ferrari has a high-powered engine (high metabolic rate), it requires a large amount of gas and oil (the right foods) to get you from point A to point B.

On the other end of the spectrum, you have a Ford Fiesta that uses cheaper gas and oils (PUFAs). The Ford Fiesta actually uses less gas and oil to get from point A to point B, because its engine is small and has less power (low metabolic rate).

Now, if you give your Ferrari engine cheap gas and oil (PUFAs) it will slow down, cause damage, and eventually end in early engine death. Obviously, this is not to say the slower, smaller, Ford Fiesta engine (lower metabolic rate) does not survive on the cheaper gas and oils, because it does—but it will *never* run at the speed, strength, or longevity of the Ferrari. Make sense? Basically, do you want to run like a Ferrari or a Ford Fiesta?

This may explain why people who eat a diet primarily of nuts, seeds, and vegetables can live a long life. Their metabolism is actually slower, so they have fewer nutritional requirements, which allows their bodies to live on very little food. The problem is these people usually have less energy, drive, motivation, and vitality. Ever seen a "healthy"-looking vegan? I sure haven't. In fact, most complain of low sex drive, low energy, muscle loss, low motivation, and sleep problems. Before all you vegans start yelling at me, take a good look at your health—and be honest.

Sally's Story

Sally was 46 years old and had adopted a vegan diet (no animal foods) three years earlier for health reasons. Sally was eating a diet high in fast food and processed food prior to this. After removing the processed and fast foods, Sally's health had initially improved. Her belief was that her new vegan diet had "fixed" her. However, over the last year she started to feel a decrease in vitality, energy, sex drive, and muscle mass, and an increase in body fat. Her diet primarily consisted of soy, nuts, grains, beans, vegetables, fruits, and polyunsaturated fats like sesame and canola oils.

Sally learned that although her current eating plan was better than the processed food diet she had been eating, it was counterproductive to a healthy metabolism. The lack of adequate protein, too much soy, the goitrogenic vegetables and legumes, and the PUFAs in her diet were most likely suppressing her metabolic rate, making her feel cold, tired, and sick.

Over the following few months Sally slowly switched her vegetable oils to coconut oil, added some eggs and cheese, and added more fruits and root vegetables to her diet. Sally reduced her soy intake to organic fermented tempeh eaten once or twice a month, versus once or twice per day. Finally, Sally reduced her nut intake and completely removed grains from her diet.

To Sally's amazement, after only a few weeks her energy started to return. In a few months, Sally's mood improved and her body temperature started to heat back up. With her improved mood and increased energy Sally was able to add weight training back into her weekly workout plan, which helped her improve her muscle mass.

Today Sally is thriving on a diet that is almost void of polyunsaturated fats and much higher in saturated fats. Her energy is back, her mood is happier, her weight has dropped, and her sex drive has finally returned. Sally is no longer a vegan, and her husband is thankful for it.

Some Other Things to Think About

In the 1940s, farmers attempted to use coconut oil (a saturated fat) to fatten their animals. But then they found it only made them lean, active, and hungry. Remember that coconut oil is a food that increases the body's metabolism. It actually increases your body's ability to burn fat. Farmers soon found that corn and soy oils, both almost entirely PUFAs, could be used to fatten their livestock. Why? Corn and soy oils, both polyunsaturated fats, slow down your metabolic rate and become fattening agents. This lower metabolic rate allows these animals to gain weight faster, which allows farmers to spend less money to get their animals fat faster. We must remember farmers don't care about having the oldest, healthiest living animals; they care about producing the fattest animals the fastest way possible.

Another interesting fact is this:

Bears and squirrels hibernate in the winter. They do this by eating lots of nuts, seeds, and berries before hibernation. These nuts and seeds, with their high PUFA levels, allow the metabolic rate of these animals to slow, allowing them to sleep through the cold months of the year. Researchers have found that bears and squirrels given coconut oil (saturated fat) and the right carbohydrates were unable to hibernate, since the animals had an increased metabolic rate and energy level.

And another:

By 1950, it was established that PUFAs suppress the metabolic rate and apparently cause hypothyroidism. Researchers found that PUFAs damage the mitochondria of cells, suppressing respiratory enzymes, and promote excessive oxidative damage in the body. The more PUFAs one eats, the higher the suppression of tissue response to thyroid hormone, the lower the metabolic rate, and the more weight gain. This is one reason hospitals feed soy oil emulsions to cancer patients—to prevent weight loss!

And finally:

According to nutritional researcher Dr. Ray Peat, "The enzymes which break down proteins are inhibited by polyunsaturated fats, and these enzymes are needed not only for digestion, but also for production of thyroid hormones, clot removal, immunity, and the general adaptability of cells. Since the polyunsaturated oils block protein digestion in the stomach, we can be malnourished even while 'eating well'." Bottom line: PUFA oils affect protein digestion, thyroid production, the immune system and the health of our cells.

What About the Omega-3 and Omega-6 Oils?

The Omega-3s and Omega-6s, also known as the essential fatty acids, have been touted as cholesterol-lowering and have shown improvement in pain management and inflammation. Yes, these are all true. Yet we must remember just because something reduces a symptom (pain, cholesterol, and inflammation are all symptoms) does not mean it is good for us—at least long term.

Essential fatty acids (EFAs) do have a cholesterol-lowering effect. The question is: How are they doing this, and is this actually good for us long term?

In the book *Generative Energy* by Dr. Ray Peat, he discusses how these "essential fatty acids" (EFAs) actually suppress the immune system by suppressing the cells that cause inflammation as to why they reduce inflammation and pain. Remember, cholesterol is part of our immune system; its levels are elevated, by the liver, when our bodies are in a state of inflammation to help protect our cells. The EFAs are interacting with the liver enzymes that produce cholesterol, decreasing cholesterol production. I might remind you that one of the "side effects" of statin drugs is liver damage. As the severity of liver damage increases, serum cholesterol levels naturally decrease. Just like statin drugs, all the EFAs are doing is suppressing a symptom. The EFAs are not correcting the actual problem.

In fact, long term, there is increased evidence that EFA's do not help with cardiovascular disease, stroke, or heart attacks. In 2012, a study of more than 70,000 patients found that Omega-3 supplementation did not lower risk of all-cause mortality, cardiac death, sudden death, myocardial infarction, or stroke. In another study in 2014, with more than 600,000 participants, researchers found that the consumption of the Omega-3 oils showed no improvements in heart or cardiovascular health. Finally, the Sydney Health study researched the effects of replacing saturated fat for linoleic acid (Omega-6) in men aged 30–59 who had a recent cardiac event. The study concluded that after eight years, those who replaced saturated fats with PUFA oils had higher levels of cardiovascular disease, coronary heart disease, and death.

The truth is this: Most positive research on the Omega-3 and Omega-6 oils is very short term, ranging from four weeks to the "longer-term" research of six months, which is not very long. Little research shows the effects of consuming Omega-3 and Omega-6 oils over several years and decades. Any research that is coming out is far from favorable. Chris Masterjohn gives a great example in his article "Good Fats, Bad Fats." Chris references the Los Angeles Veterans Administration Hospital Study, which lasted more than eight years. The researchers concluded at the end of the study that the high PUFA diet had no effect on total mortality at the end of the study. However, Chris points out that near the end of the research, non-cardiovascular deaths started to increase rapidly at the end of the study in high PUFA diet, which makes you wonder: If the study had gone on longer, what would the researchers have found?

This brings about the question: What would be the effects of a high PUFA diet over 10 years? Fifteen years? An entire lifetime?

I guess the best study is the one being done on all of us—right now. The entire population of America has been consuming far more polyunsaturated fats and far fewer saturated fats over the last 30 years. And look what has happened: We are a nation that is fatter, sicker, and less healthy than ever before. Is it the increased consumption of polyunsaturated fats? I am sure increased PUFA intake is playing a role, but PUFA intake is not the only culprit. Another misconception of the nutritional world is also having a *big* effect on our metabolic rate: the carb-free, sugar-free craze.

Chapter 3:
What You Need to Know

1. Polyunsaturated fats (PUFAs) are unstable fatty acids that have a high level of oxidation.

2. PUFAs can accelerate aging, decrease immune function, slow your metabolism, increase weight gain, and cause hormonal imbalance.

3. A high PUFA diet can encourage cancer, autoimmune diseases, diabetes, and heart disease.

4. PUFAs to avoid include sunflower oil, safflower oil, soybean oil, corn oil, cotton seed oil, vegetable oil, almond oil, walnut oil, peanut oil, grape seed oil, canola oil, fish oil, and Omega-3 and Omega-6 oils. (See Appendix D for a complete list of polyunsaturated fats to avoid.)

5. Check your labels. PUFAs are hidden in "healthy" and "organic" pre-packaged and snack foods: crackers, chips, cookies, popcorn, frozen dinners, soups, ice cream, alternative dairy products, and pre-made meals at your healthy grocery store.

Chapter 4
The Importance of Carbohydrates— Especially Sugar

Besides all the myths surrounding saturated fats, I believe carbohydrates are the most misunderstood macronutrient in the world. Even the most health-conscious people have been hypnotized by the media and food manufacturers that carbohydrates, also known as saccharides or sugars, are unhealthy for us to consume. Pick up any health or fitness magazine asking a celebrity or fitness professional about the "diet" that made him or her lean in 30 days, and every one of them will say, "I avoided carbs." The world, especially Americans, have created a society so obsessed with being thin that these so-called healthy people are willing to give up anything, even our best source of energy and metabolic power, otherwise known as carbohydrates, and sugar, to achieve the "ideal body."

Avoiding carbs is not a sustainable diet or a healthy way to live. The *right* carbs are essential for a high metabolic rate, good energy, and a happy life. Yes, if you reduce or remove carbs from your diet you will lose weight and may get lean quickly, but at what cost?

Personally, I am a recovering low-carb eater. Years ago I would eat as little as 50g carbs/day. This is the equivalent to eating about two cups of fruit, a cup of rice, or a bowl of cooked oatmeal. I was cold, had low energy, slept poorly, had awful sugar cravings, and was easily irritated—*but* I was *very* lean. I looked healthy but felt like crap. However, as many of you know, looks can be very deceiving. Depriving myself of carbohydrates was keeping my body in a stressed state and increasing my stress hormones adrenaline and cortisol.

Short term this strategy worked great; I got lean and felt energized. However, over the long run, my thyroid became sluggish, my adrenals got burned out, my liver became over-burdened, my digestive system got backed up, and my sex hormones became non-existent. Yet, I was following the most common trend in the health and fitness industry, which at the time was (and still is) avoiding carbs and sugars.

As I have pointed out many times before, things are not always factual or clear in the health, fitness, and nutrition industry. The truth is some carbohydrates like breads, pasta, processed cakes, crackers, and cookies can contribute to weight gain, diabetes, autoimmune diseases, cancer, and heart disease. Other carbs—the *right* carbs, like fruit, honey, juice, and milk—are necessary for a speedy metabolism and weight loss. The right carbs are needed for proper cellular function, liver detoxification, thyroid function, muscle recovery, brain function, and overall happiness.

I think the carb-free craziness has gone on long enough. Too many people are confused about which carbs they can eat and which ones they should avoid. Most people clump all carbohydrates into one group and try to avoid all of them, which is one of the *worst* things you could do for proper metabolic health. The truth is we need carbohydrates; we just need the *right* carbohydrates.

Back to Basics

What are carbohydrates? In the simplest of terms carbohydrates are our best and most efficient source of energy. Carbohydrates are organic compounds that consist of only carbon, hydrogen, and oxygen. Carbohydrates are a form of energy for humans and other animals. Carbohydrates contain four calories of energy per gram. Carbohydrates consist of two primary groups: simple and complex.

Simple carbohydrates consist of monosaccharides and

disaccharides. Your primary monosaccharides are glucose, galactose, and fructose. Your primary disaccharides, which are two monosaccharides combined, are sucrose, lactose, and maltose. In layman's terms these are the carbs (sugars) naturally found in white table sugar, honey, most fruits, most root vegetables, and milk.

Complex carbohydrates consist primarily of polysaccharides. Polysaccharides consist of starches and non-starches. These include grains like wheat, corn, and rice; legumes such as beans and lentils; and non-grain starches like potatoes and bananas. Starches are made of a long chain of glucose molecules. The non-starches are glycogen and cellulose (indigestible fiber). Cellulose is considered more of a structural polysaccharide, since humans cannot break it down, whereas starch and glycogen are more storage polysaccharides, since they provide large amounts of energy. Sources of foods with cellulose are most above-ground and leafy green vegetables: spinach, lettuce, grasses, seaweed, kale, celery, etc.

At the end of the day all carbs, with the exception of cellulose, turn into glucose. Think of glucose as gasoline for the body. The optimal energy for cars to fuel their engine is gasoline, just like the optimal energy for the cells of the human body is glucose. Cars need gasoline to be delivered to the engine, where it is converted to energy for power. The same principle is true of our metabolism. We convert glucose in our cells to produce energy. The only difference is as humans we can use other sources like proteins and fats for energy. However, carbohydrates (glucose) will always be the most preferred source of energy for our cells.

Using Fats and Protein as Energy

Fats and proteins are a more efficient form of energy, since you need less of them to produce a similar response as glucose. (Glucose is more wasteful due to its increased heat production.) In a car this may be a good thing, but in the human body this equates to a lower metabolism. In an engine this would be called wasteful since excess heat and carbon dioxide are produced. In the human body this is considered a high metabolic rate, and body temperature will increase and the body will be fueled with plenty of energy. When the cells' mitochondria, where energy production occurs (cell's powerhouse), are oxidizing "wastefully" they don't produce as many free radicals that produce oxidative damage. Cells' "efficiency" makes it easy to get fat, because calories are stored instead of wasted as heat. Because the right carbohydrates speed up the engine (the metabolism) you need more fuel (calories) to maintain body mass and good energy.

Think about this: Most young people have a high metabolic rate. They can eat a lot and produce tons of heat and carbon dioxide (waste products of metabolism) and stay very thin.

And isn't this what you want? Wouldn't you like to be able to eat more and weigh less?

In addition, fats and proteins require your own body's resources to break down the fats and proteins. Fats and proteins produce less ATP (energy) and less carbon dioxide (CO_2). CO_2 acts as an antioxidant in our body, decreasing oxidative damage. Protein metabolism produces ammonia and excess tryptophan, both of which can become inflammatory to our body.

However, at rest the skeletal muscles of the body and cardiac muscles of the heart do prefer to use fat as energy. As to why the best way to burn fat, is at rest—not exercise—more on that later.

Why Are the *Right* Carbohydrates So Important?
Brain Power

As I mentioned previously, glucose is the preferred source of energy for almost every cell in the human body. Glucose is the brain's main source of energy. In fact, your brain can use up to one-half of your consumed/stored glucose. The more you think, the more glucose your brain will need. Without carbohydrates you may feel light-headed, scattered, and forgetful. The red blood cells and cells of the retina can only use glucose as energy since these cells lack a mitochondria.

Muscle Power

Glucose is also needed for quick muscle energy. Muscle glycogen (stored glucose) is needed for quick energy, especially when weight training and sprinting. If your body is depleted of muscle glycogen, your body will utilize your own muscle, tissue, organs, and fat to provide energy to your muscles while under stress (exercising). It is important to note that, at rest, your muscles preferred source of energy is fat. Increasing muscle mass is a good argument for helping reduce fat, since the more muscle you have the more fat you will burn at rest. Burning fat at rest is the safest way to get rid of stored fat, since it produces less oxidative damage.

Thyroid Function

For proper metabolism, glucose is needed by the liver to convert thyroxine (T4) to the active triiodothyronine (T3). T3 is needed by all the cells to produce ATP (energy). Without adequate T3 you will have decreased cellular function (slower metabolism). People on low-carbohydrate diets are notorious for having low body temperature and decreased cellular function. This may be attributed to the low intake of carbs (sugars), which will contribute to lower T3 conversion and lower metabolic function.

Liver Detox

In addition, the liver needs glucose to help with proper detoxification. Low levels of stored glucose (glycogen) will encourage a sluggish liver. This is why fasting and detox programs that restrict *good carbs* (fruits, juices, milk) make no sense. These programs may help clean out your colon, but they hinder the performance of your liver. The liver is your main detox organ. If you hinder the liver's performance, how can it help you detox properly?

Kristen's Story

Kristen was recovering from years of water and vegetable juice cleanses. Every few months she would put herself on a "detox" diet, and drink only water and lots of green (juiced vegetables) drinks. Although Kristen lost weight and felt quite energized on these detox programs, the results were short lived and she slowly gained back the weight plus some over the years. Kristen was led to believe, by not only the health food industry but by many health practitioners, that she was helping her body by only drinking water and vegetable juices. Kristen believed this liquid diet was "cleaning out" and "detoxing" her digestive system.

Kristen learned that these "detox programs" had placed her body in a stressed state by depriving her body of adequate energy (proteins, carbs, and fat) and enough nutrition. The stress of her detox program had increased her stress hormones cortisol and adrenaline. Short term, these elevated hormones helped Kristen feel energized. Elevated cortisol and adrenaline also helped her decrease her body weight, but at the cost of her valuable muscle tissue. Long term, this form of detox program had slowed down her metabolism, slowed her digestive system, and decreased her energy level.

Although detox and fasting programs may have some benefits, they can be followed by many negative side effects if performed for too long or too many times. Kristen had been liquid detoxing for 10 years. I am not going to say these detox programs were the sole contributor to Kristen's reduced metabolic rate, fatigue, digestive issues, and weight gain, but they definitely contributed.

Kristen has been working to increase her metabolism for about a year. She has slowly added in fruit juices with gelatin, cooked fruit, dairy, and bone broth to help her gut and digestion.

As her digestive system improved, Kristen could eat more foods like eggs, fish, grass-fed meats, and potatoes and cooked vegetables. Soon her energy increased and her weight decreased. It has taken some time, but Kristen is well on her way to healing her metabolism—without the influence of liquid detox programs.

Which Carbs Are Best?

As you can see, the right carbs are needed for muscle energy, cellular function, and detoxification. However, not all carbs are created equal. Depending on the size and type of the carbohydrate, carbs can affect your metabolism differently. Some can be more pro-metabolic, while others are more anti-metabolic. Now the question is: Which ones are the best?

Simple carbs *(sugars)* are best.

Yes, you heard me. Simple sugars are better than complex carbs for increased cellular function, increased metabolism, and increased energy. You're thinking, "*What?* Sugar is good? Sugar increases my metabolism? I thought sugar just made me fat and prone to disease?" Yes, I know it is a bold statement, so let me explain.

When I am referring to sugar, I am referring to natural, organic foods that contain fructose, glucose, lactose, and sucrose. To be more specific, I am referring to most organic fruits, organic root vegetables like potatoes and carrots, organic dairy, some pulp-free fruit juices, raw organic honey, and, yes, even refined white sugar. I am not referring to carbohydrates or sugars that have been processed. These include processed high fructose corn syrup(HFCS), agave, soda, cookies, cakes, candy, crackers, sports and energy drinks, and frozen desserts. I am also not referring to complex carbohydrates or most starchy carbs like grains, breads, pasta, rice, and corn.

Now, I know what you are thinking. Most of you understand that the processed carbohydrates are bad for you. But I'm sure many people think complex carbs, like whole-wheat grains, are good for you. Right? At least, better for you than juice or white table sugar. I know this is confusing, especially since most registered dietitians, the USDA, and the Big Food giants are promoting six to nine servings of grains every day. (Refer to Chapter 5 for a deeper explanation.) To really understand this reasoning we must first understand the creation of the "glycemic index."

All the madness started back in the 1970s, when dietitians

began talking about the value of including "complex carbohydrates" in the diet. Many dietitians claimed that starches were more slowly absorbed than sugars. The thought process was that starches like rice and corn contained more fibers so their absorption into the blood would be slower than something like a peach or orange juice, which contained high levels of sucrose (sugar). From this understanding, people were told to eat whole grains and legumes, and to avoid fruit juices. It wasn't until 1981 when David Jenkins's glucose testing led to the publication of the glycemic index, which discovered that most starches had a higher glycemic index (GI) than sugar and juices.

According to the American Diabetes Society, "The glycemic index (GI) is a ranking of carbohydrates, on a scale from 0 to 100 according to the extent to which they raise blood sugar levels after eating. Foods with a high GI are those which are rapidly digested and absorbed and result in marked fluctuations in blood sugar levels. Low-GI foods, by virtue of their slow digestion and absorption, produce gradual rises in blood sugar and insulin levels, and have proven benefits for health." Foods that constantly spike blood sugar can lead to fat gain, insulin resistance, obesity, and diabetes. Foods that balance blood sugar can lead to weight loss, constant flow of energy, and overall good health.

So from this we can gather that foods with a higher GI will be worse for us than those with a lower GI. Do you know what the highest-scoring GI foods were? Pure glucose is the highest, followed by white bread, wheat bread, corn, rice, pasta, and pretty much all complex carbs! Pure glucose has a GI score of 100. Thus, the more glucose a food contains the higher the GI rating. All starchy foods are full of glucose, so they enter the blood system far faster than fruit or even pure sugar. For example a piece of wheat bread has a GI rating of 78, milk is around 35, and a cup of orange juice has a GI rating of 52. Sugar or sucrose is 65.

Simple sugary foods (fruit, honey, most root veggies, fruit juice) have a lower glycemic index than bread, pasta, corn, or rice because they contain a combination of both glucose and fructose.

Fructose has one of the lowest glycemic index numbers, hovering around 11 (depending on which table you look at). Fructose, also known as fruit sugar, enters the blood system very slowly and has very little to no effect on insulin. Having fructose in your food will slow the glucose entering into your blood system. This will produce less blood sugar fluctuation and less fat gain. Starchy carbohydrates do not contain fructose.

The Truth About Fructose

In May 2009, endocrinologist Robert Lustig delivered a speech entitled "Sugar: The Bitter Truth." Later that year his speech hit YouTube, went viral and caused a stir in the nutritional and health world concerning sugar, especially fructose. In his speech, Dr. Lustig associated fructose intake with weight gain, non-alcoholic fatty liver disease (NAFLD), increased appetite, and insulin resistance. From his speech millions of people became convinced that the fruit sugar fructose was a "poison" and that it was just as damaging to the body and liver as alcohol.

The truth is normal fructose consumption (10 percent of calories) in humans has very little to do with weight gain, fatty liver disease, increased appetite, and insulin resistance. For fructose to be attributed to weight gain, it would have to be converted to fat via de novo lipogenesis (DNL) at a high level. DNL is the process by which the liver converts carbohydrates to fat. DNL is very low in humans. In fact, some research studies say the DNL of fructose in humans is only 2 percent.

In addition, Dr. Lustig conducts research on mice, not humans. Mice convert sugar to fat (DNL) quite easily: About 50 percent is converted—far more than the 2 percent in humans. Furthermore, the mice in studies were ingesting diets with upward of 60 percent of their total calories coming from fructose. You and I would need to ingest 5 liters of soda to get the same effect—not very realistic.

Research on fructose actually shows it is far more thermogenic (heat producing) than glucose. Therefore, if people on a high-fructose diet are gaining weight, it may be due to the increase in overall calories and not the ingestion of fructose itself.

Additional research studies on fructose have also shown:
- Fructose helps detox the liver from alcohol 80% faster.
- Fructose increases CO_2 and energy production.
- Fructose has little effect on increasing blood sugar and insulin levels. Increased insulin is needed for increased fat storage. Thus, ingestion of fructose has been shown to increase insulin sensitivity and glucose metabolism.
- Fructose can enter the cell without the assistance of insulin and can be used as energy. This makes food with fructose ideal for diabetics.
- Fructose can improve the retention of magnesium and other vital nutrients.

As you can see fructose is not the "poison" Dr. Lustig has made it out to be. Dr. Lustig's research only proves high consumption of fructose in mice can have negative health effects, which is really not applicable to you and me. For humans, a diet containing fructose has shown to improve metabolic rate, help detox the liver, increase insulin sensitivity, and improve retention of vital nutrients. From this we can conclude fructose is vital to a healthy diet, not toxic.

Anything that spikes your blood sugar can promote obesity. Increased blood sugar will always be followed by an increase in insulin. Insulin is used to shuttle the sugar into the cells to be used as energy. If the cells are already full or are unable to metabolize sugars effectively, like in diabetes, the sugars are stored as triglycerides (stored fat) so that they can be used at a later time—or, as many of us know, the sugars may stay stored and added to our hip, waist, and bust lines!

In addition, most fruits, fruit juices, and milk contain a higher level of vitamins and minerals than the starchy grains. Potassium in particular is utilized to help push sugar into the cells. Eating foods with potassium will decrease the effects of insulin, causing less blood sugar fluctuations and ultimately less fat gain.

Fruits, fruit juices, and milk are void of the anti-nutrients: phytates and trypsin inhibitors, which are found in grains, seeds, and legumes. Phytates will inhibit the absorption of many minerals, including calcium. Trypsin inhibitors can block the enzymes that break down protein and can lead to a protein deficiency. Fruits are also low in polyunsaturated fats. Finally, most fruits (sweet and cooked fruits) and pulp-free fruit juices are easier to digest than starchy grains and cellulose-rich vegetables, producing less bacterial overgrowth and less endotoxin. Yes, if you have gut issues, you should eat more easy-to-digest, less fibrous foods, *not* more fibrous foods. Fiber feeds bacteria and when the gut is inflamed, this will only make things worse. Ideal sugars to help a damaged gut are pulp-free orange juice, honey, cooked and skinless apples, peaches, pears, and nectarines, sweet fruits like watermelon, and tropical fruits like papaya.

Carbohydrates–Fats–Protein Is an Essential Combination

Now, I am not saying you should run out and overdose on fruits, fruit juice, milk, sugar, and honey. Eating too many of these foods alone will promote weight gain. Even though these foods have a lower glycemic index than most grains and breads, they should still be eaten in moderation and should never be eaten alone. All carbohydrates should be eaten with a combination of fat and protein. Neither fat nor protein increases blood sugar levels directly. By combining fat and protein with a carbohydrate, you will slow the absorbency of the sugars even more, creating a meal that will produce a constant flow of energy (glucose) into your system. A few examples would be combining fruit with cheese, milk with fruit, or eggs with orange juice.

It should be noted that a meal too high in protein can be just as bad as a meal too high in carbohydrates. A high-protein meal void of carbohydrates will directly increase insulin levels. Insulin is required for protein to enter the cells of the muscle tissue. If the meal is void of carbohydrates (sugars) and you spike your insulin levels, your body will respond with a drop in blood sugar. Have you ever eaten eggs or a piece of meat by itself and then soon felt light-headed? The reason is the spike in insulin and then the drop in blood sugar. This blood sugar drop will produce a stress reaction, causing increased adrenaline and then increased cortisol.

Adrenaline and cortisol are both catabolic hormones that trigger your body to break down fat and muscle to produce glucose (gluconeogenesis). This is how people lose weight on low-carb eating plans: they teach their body to use itself as energy. I know you are thinking, "Isn't this what we want? Isn't this how we lose fat?" Yes, if you are looking for short-term, quick fat loss. No, if you are looking for long-term *health*. Unfortunately, society is so focused on quick results we tend to forget about the damage we may be doing when we try to lose weight by restricting carbohydrates, calories, or some other vital nutrient. (Jump to Chapter 7 on protein for more information on low-carb diets.)

Losing weight by restricting carbohydrates will eventually come at an expense to your health and metabolism. A diet that focuses on quick fat loss will eventually result in decreased muscle mass, sleep problems, irritability, hormonal issues, infertility, and decreased metabolic function. Ask anyone who has been on a low-carb diet for six to 12 months: They may look good, but they usually feel like crap. Remember: Years ago, I was one of these people. Like many in the fitness industry, I was so wrapped up in my outward appearance that I had no idea the damage I was doing to my metabolism and overall health.

Moderation Is *Not* Always the Key

If your body is already in a hypo-metabolic state, adding in even a moderate amount of *any* carbohydrate, good or bad, may have an adverse effect on you. I have talked with many people who feel they cannot handle any sugary-sweet foods at all, even in moderation—and, well, they may be right. However, this is not because their body does not need the sugar (glucose) or because they are genetically prone to sugar "addiction." This just means they may be eating the wrong carbs, eating the wrong fat-protein-carb combination, and/or their cells are not metabolizing glucose properly.

The common short-term answer is to not eat anything sweet or sugary. However, this solution, long term, only creates more dysfunction.

Avoiding all sugars to decrease sugar (glucose) in the body is essentially impossible. If you do not provide your body with enough of the right sugars, your body will break down its own tissue through gluconeogenesis (the breakdown of non-carbohydrate substances like lactate, glycerol, amino acids, and pyruvate) to provide its cells with the needed glucose. You must remember most cells in your body prefer glucose as their primary energy source. Some cells, like your red blood cells and the cells in your eyes, can only use glucose as energy. Your brain, although it can utilize ketones from fat, functions best on glucose. Therefore, avoiding all sugars, including healthy sugars, is not an effective long-term plan for promoting a healthy body.

For the sugar sensitive person, he or she needs to add the right carbs in slowly, combined with the right amount of fats and proteins.

Since you differ from your neighbor, spouse, or parent, and you are in a different state of health from basically everyone around you, the recommendations on how much and how often you should eat carbs is not going to be the same. You need to take your current metabolic state, stress level, activity level, size, and current health into consideration to find out what is going to work for you. I usually find the healthier the individual and the higher the person's metabolism, the higher the percentage of carbohydrates required in his or her diet. For most people, anywhere from 40 to 70 percent of their dietary needs should come from healthy, metabolically stimulating carbohydrates.

In summary, the *right* carbohydrates are essential for a healthy metabolism. You need them for optimal cell function, liver health, and brain function. Simple carbs (most organic fruits, fruit juices, most root vegetables, honey, and organic milk) are best due to their low GI levels, increased mineral content, lack of anti-nutrients, and digestibility. All carbohydrates, whether they are simple or complex, should be combined with a fat and protein. Your carbohydrate intake will depend on your level of health, metabolic rate, stress, energy consumption, and size.

In a world where optimal health is defined by how fast you can run or how low your body fat is, it is important to remember that those are external markers. The real definition of good health comes down to optimal cellular function (warm body, good sleep, energized, healthy sex drive, healthy skin, hair, and nails, happy, good digestion and detox, and a lean body). I have met plenty of people who "look good" yet have all sorts of metabolic issues: insulin resistance, infertility, diabetes, cancer, heart disease, arthritis, MS—the list goes on and on. Understanding the physiology of your body and how it works optimally will help establish good health. And eating the *right* carbs will contribute to optimal cellular function, an increased metabolism, and an increase in overall health!

Chapter 4:
What You Need to Know

1. Carbohydrates are your primary source of energy. Consuming the right carbohydrates is needed for a high metabolic rate, increased CO2 levels, decreased oxidative damage, good brain function, muscle energy and recovery, and detoxing the liver.

2. Simple sugars like fructose, glucose, sucrose, and lactose are your best sources. These include: fruits, honey, milk, white sugar, fruit juices, and root vegetables.

3. Carbohydrates should never be eaten alone. Always combine carbohydrates with a fat and protein (e.g., fruit and cheese, eggs and OJ, and milk and honey). (See Appendix A for a list of optimal carbohydrates.)

4. Low-carb dieting, although effective for quick loss, long term will lead to fatigue, sugar cravings, sleep issues, hormone issues, muscle wasting, and weight gain.

5. When adding sugars back into your diet, start slowly. Even the right sugars added in too quickly will lead to weight gain, bloating, and hormonal issues.

Chapter 5
Dump the Grains and Gluten—Your Gut Will Thank You

Now that you know that fruit, juice, milk, and honey are your best sources of carbohydrates, what about the other forms of carbohydrates? What about grains? Can grains be a part of metabolically stimulating diet? I'll let you decide.

Most Americans will admit they love their grains. Currently the USDA, the Academy of Nutrition and Dietetics, and most registered dietitians recommend six to eight servings of grains a day, with half of those being whole grains. The ADA says Americans need them for B vitamins, minerals, fiber, and vegetable protein. Plus, wheat, corn, and rice are three of America's best-selling crops. Breads, muffins, and cereals are staples at most Americans' breakfast table. Quinoa, rice, oats, millet, and barley are common "healthy" side dishes. If all of this is true, why would being a "grain addict" be such a bad thing? Don't Americans need them for health benefits?

The truth is grains are not a needed or a necessary food for anyone to achieve optimal health or a high running metabolism. In fact, the increased ingestion of grains is currently linked to increased allergies, digestive distress, arthritis, hypothyroidism, bone loss, colitis, celiac, skin issues, irritable bowel syndrome (IBS), insomnia, hypoglycemia, diabetes, PMS, infertility, epilepsy, malnutrition, dementia, cancer—and the list goes on.

This is why I recommend *all* grains be avoided while trying to heal a damaged metabolism. This includes wheat, rice, corn, barley, millet, quinoa, oats, buckwheat, rye, and sorghum.

This may sound extreme. Yet, I assure you the added benefit of a healthy gut, less bloating, increased digestion, weight loss, clear thinking, increased metabolic rate, and overall better health will far outweigh your piece of morning toast.

Before I talk more about that, let's take a step back and define "grain."

What Is a Grain?

Grains are hard, dry seeds used for human or animal consumption. Although legumes are also considered grains, in this chapter I will be referring only to the cereal grains, which are grains that are the seeds of grass. The cereal grains consist of wheat, corn, barley, rice, oats, quinoa, millet, rye, buckwheat, and sorghum. Cereal grains are starchy carbohydrates consisting of many glucose molecules bonded together (polysaccharide). The cereal grains are used as "staples" in the American diet since they are cheap, easily transported, have a long shelf life, and are packed with energy (calories).

The U.S. government, since the mid-1920s, has subsidized grains. Farm subsidies (taxpayer money paid to farmers) were started to help supplement farmers while helping to influence the supply and demand of the grain industry. Basically, increased production leads to increased government subsidies. More subsidized money leads farmers to increase production of a crop. Increased production of grains leads to a decreased price point and a necessity to find a need for all the additional grains. This has allowed "Big Food" giants to produce thousands of cheap, grain- based food products. Basically, food science has found a place for grains in everything. From gluten-enriched breads to wheat pasta, cookies to crackers, soy sauce to salad dressings, ice cream to candy, Americans are becoming grain addicts—and it's affecting the health of everybody.

How are grains affecting your health? Oh, let me count the ways…

Grain Equal Glucose

If we go back to the last chapter, you will recall that the carbohydrate portion of grain is 100-percent glucose. Glucose has a glycemic index of 100, which means it travels into the blood system faster than any other sugar. White and wheat bread have a glycemic index around 70. Remember that sugar is 58. Even though bread has fiber and protein to slow the bread's absorbency, the bread absorbs into the blood faster than pure sugar due to the increased amount of glucose. The more glucose a food contains, the faster blood sugar will rise. Remember: A quick rise in blood sugar will be followed by a quick spike in insulin. Insulin shuttles the sugar into your cells for energy or into fat cells for storage. Thus, a high level of grains (glucose) in the diet can encourage fat storage and a larger waistline.

High Phosphorus-to-Calcium Ratio

Grains, like meat, contain a high amount of phosphorus with very little calcium. The ratio of phosphorus to calcium in the body is important in maintaining bone and teeth health. Phosphorus, an essential nutrient needed for strong bones and teeth, and energy production, in excess will increase parathyroid hormones and cause calcium to leach from the bones. High phosphorus-to-calcium diets can impair the synthesis of vitamin D (needed for calcium absorption), which will disrupt calcium homeostasis.

Grains contain some of the highest levels of the mineral phosphorus. The worst offenders are rice bran, wheat bran, and wheat germ.

Eating a diet high in calcium can help eliminate the negative effects of a high phosphorus diet.

Grains Are Seeds; Seeds Are Filled with Anti-Nutrients

Whether they come from legumes, soy, sunflowers, or grains, seeds are indigestible by animals and humans. Seeds are to be planted and fertilized. Why? Seeds have built-in defense mechanisms and anti-nutrients used to protect them from bugs and animals. Humans forget that all living things have their own lines of defense. Dogs and cats have teeth and claws, birds have beaks and wings, and plants have internal toxins.

What are these anti-nutrients?
Oxalates

Oxalic acid is a natural occurring chemical found in leafy green plants, nuts, grains, and legumes. Oxalic acid causes problems because it binds to calcium (CA) in the body, forming oxalates. Oxalates inhibit CA absorption or, worse, can lead to kidney stones. According to the Chicago Dietetics Association, individuals with kidney stones are told to decrease oxalate intake to lower than 50–60mg/day, and less than 10mg/serving. A study in *The Journal of Food Composition and Analysis* in 2005 found that oxalate content ranged from 37 to 269mg/100g in certain grain flours. Buckwheat and whole wheat were the worst offenders. White and brown rice contained the least amount of oxalates. The study concluded, "Diets which are heavily based on flour products may increase predisposition to calcium oxalate-containing kidney stones in susceptible individuals."

Phytates (Phytic Acid)

Phytates, also found in our good friends soy, seeds, and nuts, are antioxidant compounds found in whole grains. Phytates work by blocking or inhibiting the absorption of other nutrients. Phytates block the uptake of essential nutrients zinc and copper, and, to a lesser degree, calcium and magnesium. Cooking, soaking, or sprouting the seeds can lessen the degree of phytic acid.

Trypsin Inhibitors

Trypsin inhibitors, also referred to as protease inhibitors, can block trypsin and other enzymes needed for proper protein digestion. These enzymes produced by the pancreas can overburden the pancreas and lead to pancreatic disorders. Trypsin inhibitors can also lead to digestive distress and a diet deficient in proper amino acid uptake.

Lectins

Lectins are carbohydrate-binding proteins found in plants, seeds, legumes, grains, and nuts. Foods high in lectins are associated with gastrointestinal distress leading to diarrhea, nausea, bloating, and vomiting. Just like the lectins in leafy greens, the lectins in grains can interfere with mucous repair in the gut lining. Therefore, lectins become toxic to wound healing in the gut. If someone is celiac or has a grain intolerance, lectins would exacerbate the individual's issue. Besides grains, the worst offenders of lectins are the legumes beans and soy, and many vegetables.

Gluten

People all over the world are going crazy on gluten-free diets. Yet, most people don't even know what gluten is and why they should be avoiding it. Gluten is a storage protein in *all* grains. Yes, you heard me: *All* grains including oats, corn, rice, and quinoa contain a form of gluten. Gluten is not just one type of grain protein. Gluten consists of a family of more than a thousand types of different grain proteins consisting primarily of glutelins and prolamins. Both glutelins and prolamins are storage proteins found in the endosperm of a grain's seed.

Gluten is a hard-to-digest protein and can lead to digestive resistance in many people. Since gluten is hard to digest, gluten can feed bacteria in the stomach and cause a bacterial overgrowth. These by-products can damage the gut and lead to intestinal permeability. Increased permeability will allow toxins, bacteria, and undigested food particles to leak through the intestinal walls into the blood. As the gut increases permeability, the body may produce an immune response and the body will start attacking the proteins.

This can lead to a gluten allergy (creates an immune system response) or celiac disease, an autoimmune (attacks its own tissue) disease.

What is Celiac Disease?

Celiac is an autoimmune disorder that attacks the villi of the small intestine. Celiac is more common in genetically predisposed people.

According to the National Foundation of Celiac Awareness (NFCA),

"About 95% of people with celiac disease have the HLA-DQ2 gene and most of the remaining 5% have the HLA-DQ8 gene."

Celiac is caused by an overexposure to gliadin, a prolamine found primarily in wheat gluten. Gliadin overexposure produces an inflammatory response in the small intestine. The villi of the small intestine atrophy, which leads to poor absorption of vital nutrients. Symptoms can consist of fatigue, diarrhea, foggy thinking, depression, weight loss, weight gain, skin issues, joint pain, back pain, constipation, bloating, gas, and thin bones. About 1 percent of Americans have Celiac Disease.

Laura's Story

Laura was seeking relief from low back pain and achy knees. Laura was also looking to lose some weight and reduce her belly size. Laura was not a large woman, but she almost looked pregnant considering the size of her midsection. Laura, from what she believed, was a healthy eater. Laura ate a diet filled with vegetables, fruits, pastured meats, raw dairy, wild fish, and at least six servings of whole grains a day: toast and eggs in the morning, a sandwich for lunch, crackers and hummus for a snack, and some sort of cooked grain with a protein and veggie for dinner. For months, Laura trained physically without much success in relieving her back pain and reducing her gut size. Laura got stronger and lost a little weight, but her gut distension and back pain continued.

After months of hard work, Laura decided to try an elimination diet for 30 days. Laura gave up wheat, barley, rye, and oats (the

primary grains, known at the time to create gluten sensitivity issues). Laura also gave up all processed grains like bread, pasta, cookies, and crackers, even if they were labeled "gluten free." Laura ate fruit and eggs for breakfast, a soup or salad for lunch, and protein, a veggie, and a potato or fruit for dinner.

What happened was amazing.

Laura lost 10 pounds, her back and knee pain went completely away, and her stomach bulge became flat. By removing all grains and processed foods Laura eliminated the inflammation in the gut, joints, and back. Laura, an avid bread lover, attempted to add the gluten back in her diet after the 30 days, but found her symptoms returned. Six months later Laura was tested for celiac disease and the test came out positive. Little did Laura know she had been slowly poisoning herself for years on a gluten-filled diet.

Although 1 percent of the population has celiac disease, it is understood that only 10 percent of people actually know it. Up until five years ago, Laura was one of those people. Recently Laura gave up corn and rice, too. She says she feels her best eating 100-percent grain free. Laura is not alone. Many people do their best going grain free.

Some people who consume gluten do not elicit an immune response, but find they cannot tolerate gluten. These people are referred to as non-celiac gluten sensitive (NCGS). If you are diagnosed as non-celiac gluten sensitive, you will have many of the same symptoms of celiac without as much intestinal permeability and villi atrophy. Once again, these symptoms include fatigue, diarrhea, foggy thinking, depression, weight loss, weight gain, skin issues, joint pain, back pain, constipation, bloating, gas, and thin bones. Individuals who are non-celiac gluten sensitive will not test positive for celiac, but their symptoms will improve on a gluten-free diet. Research shows that 1 in 25, or approximately 6 percent of, Americans have an intolerance to gluten.

Gluten-free diets are the only known cure for celiac and non-celiac gluten sensitivity individuals.

The Hidden Sources of Gluten

Yet, this is no easy venture since gluten is hidden in other foods as a food additive, as a stabilizing agent, and even a meat substitute. Gluten is found not only in breads, cookies, and cakes, but also in beer, soy sauce, ice cream, ketchup, sauces, lunch meat, bouillon cubes, salad dressings, seasoned rice, seasoned chips, fried foods, and some candy. Gluten can be used as imitation meat called seitan. Gluten can even be found in cosmetics, lotions, and hair products. This is why it is imperative that health-conscious consumers become vigilant about reading all food and personal product labels. When someone has celiac or is gluten sensitive, even a tablespoon of gluten-free ketchup can cause digestive disturbances.

Unfortunately, even purchasing "gluten-free" products may not save you from being poisoned by grain-based products. Cross-contamination of grains is a big problem. A 2010 article published in *The Journal of American Dietetic Association* reported that more than 30 percent of gluten-free products are contaminated with more than the allowed gluten levels to be considered gluten free. A Canadian study tested 640 naturally "gluten-free" flours and found almost 10 percent contaminated with wheat gluten.

Even if your "gluten-free" food is actually void of gluten, this does not mean the gluten-free food is healthy for you. Check out the ingredients of this popular gluten-free muffin:

"INGREDIENTS: SUGAR, ENRICHED GLUTEN-FREE BLEND [RICE FLOUR, CORNSTARCH, MODIFIED CORNSTARCH, AMARANTH FLOUR, BROWN RICE FLOUR, QUINOA FLOUR, POTATO STARCH, TAPIOCA FLOUR, THIAMINE MONONITRATE (VITAMIN B1), RIBOFLAVIN (VITAMIN B2), NIACIN, REDUCED IRON, FOLATE], EGGS, BLUEBERRIES, SOYBEAN AND/OR CANOLA OIL, WATER, EGG WHITES (EGG WHITES, YEAST, CITRIC ACID), LEAVENING (SODIUM BICARBONATE, SODIUM ACID PYROPHOSPHATE, CORNSTARCH, MONOCALCIUM PHOSPHATE, CALCIUM SULFATE),

NATURAL FLAVOR, CELLULOSE GUM, DEXTROSE, SALT, SOY LECITHIN, XANTHAN GUM, SODIUM PROPIONATE(PRESERVATIVE), YEAST NUTRIENTS (CALCIUM CARBONATE, CALCIUM PANTOTHENATE, CALCIUM PHOSPHATE, CALCIUM SULFATE, PYRIDOXINE HYDROCHLORIDE), AMYLASE, ASCORBIC ACID. CONTAINS: EGG AND SOY MAY CONTAIN: ALMONDS, COCONUT, HAZELNUTS, PECANS AND WALNUTS"

Thanks to good ol' food manufacturing and the business of making money with food, people are misled into thinking they are doing something good for themselves (eating gluten-free), when in fact all they are doing is eating a muffin full of synthetic vitamins, soy, fillers, gums, natural flavors, and other additives. Essentially you are trading one evil (gluten) for another (additive and fillers).

In addition, we must remember gluten is not only found in wheat, barley, rye, and oats; similar storage proteins are found in the other grains. The prolamins found in corn, millet, sorghum, rice, and even quinoa can have similar effects on the gut as gluten. In a 2013 study, *Nutrients* journal reported that the peptides from corn prolamins elicited inflammatory symptoms similar to those of wheat gluten.

A study from the Children's Hospital at Westmead, Australia, conducted over a period of 16 years and released in 2009, found that children with Food Protein Induced Enterocolitis Syndrome (FPIES) had more episodes caused by rice than any other food. FPIES is a gastrointestinal and immune response to certain food proteins.

The American Journal of Clinical Nutrition released a study in 2012 reporting that even quinoa, a grain low in prolamins, caused intestinal distress in individuals who have gluten sensitivities.

It is interesting to note that most of the research on grains and gluten is fairly new. Lately, with a huge increase in celiac and non-celiac gluten sensitivity, more money is being spent on more research to investigate these illnesses. I believe once researchers look deeper into the storage proteins of all the grains, they will find that none of the grains are healthy for an individual who is suffering from gluten sensitivity. The grains of today are far different from the grains of our grandparents' day. Hybridization, crossbreeding, genetic modified crops, and the mass production of grains have degraded our crops—and now the American people are feeling the effects.

How Do You Know if You Have Grain Sensitivity?

I believe the best and most accurate way to know if grains are affecting your health is to eliminate grains for at least 30 days. According to most scientific research, allergy and food "intolerance" tests are unproven, costly, and misinterpreted. Eliminating grains, although challenging, is cheap, effective, and accurate. The worst that can happen if you have an intolerance, allergy, or sensitivity is you will lose weight, and have better digestion, less bloating, fewer aches and pains, clearer thinking, and overall better health.

And yes, you have to give up all grains, grain products, gluten-free products, and foods that contain gluten additives for at least 30 days. Just reducing grains, or only removing them for a few days, will not allow your body enough time to heal if you have a grain or gluten issue. After 30 days, if you don't feel any health improvements, more than likely you can tolerate grains. Yet, even absent of grain issues, I would never advise anyone to consume six to nine servings of grains a day.

In fact, the only grains I do advise, for healthy individuals, are organic white or jasmine rice, organic slow-cooked oatmeal, sourdough bread, and organic masa harina (dough from specially treated corn-dried masa). I find each of these grains, when eaten in moderation, can be tolerated by most healthy, non-gluten-sensitive individuals.

To sum things up, there are far better food choices for optimal health than grains or gluten-free foods. Remember: All grains contain powerful anti-nutrients including the dreaded gluten.

Grains also contain high amounts of glucose, which stimulates insulin and promotes fat storage. Giving up grains may not be the easiest decision, but I assure you, your flat belly, weight loss, ache-free joints, clarity, and improved brain power will be more than worth it.

Chapter 5:
What You Need to Know

1. Grains contain the sugar glucose. Grains can enter your blood system faster than pure sugar. This is due to the high level of glucose. Increased glucose will increase insulin and increase fat storage.

2. Grains contain anti-nutrients like phytates, trypsin inhibitors, lectins, PUFA, and gluten.

3. Gluten is a broad definition identifying thousands of grain proteins. Some sort of gluten is in *every* grain.

4. Celiac disease is an autoimmune disease that attacks the villi of the small intestine. Celiac is a genetic disease created by an overexposure to gluten.

5. Non-celiac gluten sensitivity describes the 12 million Americans who cannot tolerate gluten but do not have celiac disease.

Chapter 6
Vegetables: The Good, the Bad, and the Thyroid-Suppressing

So far, I have told you that saturated fat is good, the "heart healthy" fats are bad, the right sugars are necessary for a great working metabolism, and grains and gluten are ruining your gut. But I am not done.

I am about to question one of the most widely promoted health recommendations in the United States. I'm challenging the recommendation to "eat more vegetables." This is an interesting topic since most of us have been told all our lives that we need to eat more vegetables. Right?

For most of my life, I have been a huge advocate of eating tons of vegetables, including kale, spinach, lettuce, cabbage, broccoli, cauliflower, etc. Personally, I would eat at least eight to nine servings of vegetables a day—mostly raw. Health-conscious people have been told vegetables are supportive to a healthy body because they contain loads of nutrients, fiber, and antioxidant properties. And this is true; Vegetables are filled with all these health-promoting properties. However, does this mean that *all* vegetables are good for us? Or is there another side to the "eat more vegetable" philosophy?

As I have been sharing throughout this book, years ago I went through a massive transformation in my beliefs about health and nutrition. Along with adding in more saturated fats, removing most polyunsaturated fatty acids (PUFAs), removing most grains (including whole wheat and gluten-free grains), and eating more of the right carbs, I also greatly reduced my vegetable intake, specifically above-ground, leafy vegetables like spinach, kale, lettuce, broccoli, cauliflower, Brussels sprouts, and cabbage.

With every current diet plan telling you to eat more vegetables and raw salads, the decision to eliminate cruciferous and leafy vegetables seemed about the craziest thing I could ever come up with. Yet, as I began to remove 90 percent of the leafy green vegetables from my diet, my digestion improved, my bloated gut was gone, and my stool was a lot prettier (if that is possible).

Let me explain.

Leafy greens and all above-ground vegetables have their own internal toxins. These plants will have a variety of defensive, naturally produced chemicals, all with specific functions to deter animals from consuming them. Above-ground vegetables have leaves, stems, and seeds that are susceptible to attack by insects, birds, and grazing animals. To protect themselves, the leafy plants contain mild toxins. These plant toxins include oxalates, lectins/agglutinins, lignans, and other digestive disruptors like polyunsaturated fats.

Here's some more specific information about these toxins.

Oxalates

Oxalic acid is a naturally occurring chemical found in leafy green plants, nuts, grains, and soy products. Like I explained in Chapter 5 on grains, oxalic acid causes problems because it binds to calcium (CA) in the body, forming oxalates. Oxalates inhibit CA absorption and, worse, can lead to kidney stones. Vegetables, like spinach and kale, contain high levels of CA, yet they also contain high amounts of oxalic acid. Due to this combination, the bioavailability of CA is greatly decreased. Therefore, if you are trying to get your much-needed CA requirements from leafy greens you may want to think again.

Pyridoxine Glucoside

Yes, I know pyridoxine glucoside (PNG) is a mouthful. PNG is a form of Vitamin B6 found in plants, particularly cruciferous vegetables. According to a study in *The American Journal for Clinical Nutrition,* the presence of PNG in plants can decrease the bioavailability of B6 by 75–85 percent. Essentially, although plants contain Vitamin B6, the fact that it is the PNG form makes the B6 hard to get. PNG is also found in grains. Animal sources of B6 (pyridoxal phosphate, and pyridoxamine phosphate) have almost 100 percent bioavailability.

What Is Vitamin B6?

Vitamin B6 is a water-soluble vitamin. It can be found in three forms: pyridoxine glucoside (PNG), pyridoxal phosphate (PLP), and pyridoxamine phosphate (PMP). PNG is found in plants and grains; PLP and PMP are found in animal sources. PLP is the active form of B6 and is the cofactor in a multitude of metabolic functions. These include: protein, fat and sugar metabolism, neurotransmission, hemoglobin and histamine synthesis, and gene expression. The most bioavailable sources are beef, liver, eggs, milk, potatoes, and bananas.

Lectins

Lectins are carbohydrate-binding proteins found in plants, seeds, legumes, grains, and nuts. Foods high in lectins are associated with gastrointestinal distress leading to diarrhea, nausea, bloating, and vomiting. A 2007 study found that lectins could interfere with mucous repair in the gut lining. Therefore, lectins become toxic to wound healing in the gut. If someone is alreadyexperiencing digestive distress, constipation, diarrhea, etc., eating foods containing lectins would not help the issue; it would only make it worse. The worst offenders of lectins are grains, beans, soy, and most vegetables. Cooking your vegetables can lessen the damage of lectins.

Lignans

Lignans are phytoestrogens found in plants. They have estrogenic-like properties and can cause hormonal disturbances. In the following chapter I will go into more depth as to why estrogenic foods can be harmful to you. The biggest offenders are seeds like flax and sesame seeds, and cruciferous vegetables like broccoli, cauliflower, cabbage, and Brussel sprouts.

Polyunsaturated Fats

Although polyunsaturated fats (PUFAs) are not found in massive quantities in most vegetables, PUFAs are present and they can affect proper digestion of foods. According to nutritional researcher and biologist Dr. Ray Peat, "Unsaturated fats themselves are important defenses, since they inhibit trypsin and other proteolytic enzymes, preventing the assimilation of the proteins that are present in seeds and leaves, and disrupting all biological processes that depend on protein breakdown, such as the formation of thyroid hormone and the removal of blood clots."

Along with all the anti-metabolic effects of the above-ground vegetables, they are also very high in fiber. I am sure, as a health-conscious person, you are wondering, "Isn't fiber good for me? Don't I need it for proper digestion?" Well, yes and no. Once again, let me explain.

Pectin

Pectin is a polysaccharide (a long carbohydrate molecule that the body cannot break down). Pectin is a soluble (dissolves in water), fermentable fiber found in the cell walls of above-ground vegetables and fruits (especially the skin). High pectin levels can disrupt digestion and lead to increased endotoxins and serotonin in the gut. Pectin has been linked to increasing carcinogenic tumor size in the colon. Besides vegetables, unripe fruits are also high in pectin, especially pears and apples. As a fruit becomes more "ripe," its pectin levels are lower. Cooking vegetables and fruits will help break down pectin. Ripe and cooked fruits and vegetables are easier for our body to digest and less taxing on your digestive system.

Lignin

Lignin, similar to pectin, is a polysaccharide. Lignin is also a fermentable fiber found in the cell walls of plant algae. Unlike pectin, lignin is an insoluble fiber (it cannot dissolve in water). In a 1998 study in *Nutrition and Cancer,* ingestion of lignins was associated with increased uterine cancer. Lignin is also associated with reproductive issues, enlarged spleen, liver, and stomach issues, and increased level of bile acids, which have been linked to colon cancer. Lignin can be found in vegetables, fruits, and grains. Lignin's negative effects can be decreased with ripe and cooked foods.

Cellulose

Cellulose is also a polysaccharide and is the structural component of the primary cell wall in green plants. Cellulose is an insoluble fiber, also known as *roughage.* Unlike ruminant animals like cows and horses, humans cannot digest cellulose. If you do not believe me, the next time you eat a *big* salad, wait 24 hours and check out your stool; your salad will reappear—intact.

In a healthy person cellulose is a safe fiber; it helps speed up the transient time of stool and acts like a bulking agent. However, in a person with a compromised digestive tract, cellulose may actually increase toxic load, inflammation, and irritation in an already-damaged gut.

In the book *Fiber Menace,* Konstantin Monastyrsky explains how external factors (poor diet, stress, chemicals, processed foods) compromise bowel movements and irritate the gut lining. When the gut is damaged the normal bacteria inside the colon are the first to suffer. Because bacteria make up the most of the bulk of normal stools (75 percent of stool is water), once they're gone, stools harden because the bacteria are no longer there to retain water, soften the stools, and provide stool bulk. After the bacteria are gone, and we become constipated, we are told to start eating more fiber to replace their function.

For a while, the increased fiber will appear to be working. Insoluble fiber makes stools voluminous and not as hard. However, if the gut is not healed and you are just adding more fiber, you are not restoring the gut's natural bacteria. Regularity is not happening by restoring the body's natural bacteria and bulk, but by replacing it with an outside bulking agent: fiber. For a while, the problems are hidden because you don't feel them—yet.

Like so many things in the health industry, adding fiber to a dysfunctional gut, in the form of cellulose, only acts like a Band-Aid. Added fiber does not help heal the gut; it just disguises the dysfunction of the digestion system for a while. Over time, the increased stool size will start to lead to more irritation and inflammation of the intestinal lining. Since most of our nutrients are absorbed through the walls of the small intestine, the increased inflammation will inhibit proper nutrient absorption. And what is one of the biggest reasons, we eat leafy green vegetables? Nutrients! Please don't try to convince me it's due to the taste; the taste of raw kale or spinach without any seasoning or dressing is just plain awful!

In addition, undigested foods like cellulose can become the breeding ground for bacteria, in the damaged gut.. Due to the damaged intestinal area, stools move slower, leading to increased toxic load. The longer your undigested food stays in your body, the more toxic it can become to your system.

If we continue to eat tons of fiber and avoid actually healing the gut, our digestive problems will begin to turn into hemorrhoids, diverticulitis, irritable bowel syndrome (IBS), ulcerative colitis, Crohn's disease, and even colon cancer.

Now, I want to be clear: Cellulose is not bad fiber. It is a safe fiber in a healthy person. As long as cellulose has not been chemically or enzymatically altered, like in many processed foods and juices, it can be consumed and can *help* with digestion. However, in someone who is in a compromised metabolic state and has slow digestion, eating leafy green vegetables seems to only contribute to the problem versus helping to solve it.

Shelly's Story

Shelly wanted to lose some weight and improve her digestion. Shelly was very active, ate fairly healthy (at least she thought so), and was a salad-a-holic. Shelly ate green leafy salads almost every day; some days Shelly ate salads twice a day. Along with her slight weight gain, Shelly complained of gas, abdominal bloating, and constipation. Her doctor recommended adding in extra fiber in the form of Metamucil or bran, which Shelly tried, but this method did not work. Shelly's diet, as do so many health-conscious people, primarily consisted of leafy green salads, oatmeal, chicken, berries, grains, and tons of water.

Slowly but surely Shelly decreased her grains and her raw salads. She added in bone broth and gelatin to help heal her gut. She also started to cook all her vegetables and fruits in either butter or coconut oil. Coconut oil is antifungal and antibacterial. And the cooking made Shelly's foods easier to digest. In addition, Shelly added in eggs and an organic-pastured source of dairy for added fat, protein, and carbs. In as little as two weeks, Shelly had lost 5 pounds and her bloated stomach had disappeared.

It was obvious her gut and intestines were inflamed, and once she removed the very foods causing the inflammation, the gut began to heal and her digestion greatly improved. Shelly continues to eat salads but now they consist of raw carrots, tomatoes, cucumber, onions, and peppers. After only six months Shelly has firm and regular bowel movements, has a flat tummy, and feels satisfied after meals, since her body is able to break down foods and get the vital nutrients Shelly's body needs.

Goitrogens

Finally, many vegetables like the cruciferous vegetables are goitrogens. Goitrogens are substances that suppress the function of the thyroid by inhibiting the formation of the thyroid hormone. Goitrogens are found in all cruciferous vegetables, including but not limited to soybeans, broccoli, cauliflower, bok choy, cabbage, cress, and Brussel sprouts. Eating a lot of raw cruciferous veggies can suppress your thyroid, leading to a slower metabolism and increased metabolic hormone disturbance. Wow, that sounds inviting!

Now, if you're dead set on eating a vegetable stir-fry or any other cooked vegetables, it is important to know that cooking cruciferous vegetables for about 30 minutes can lower the goitrogenic effects. Yes, I know cooking vegetables too long may significantly reduce the levels of some nutrients. But it also increases the bioavailability of other nutrients. As I have been talking about throughout this chapter, there is more to food than just its nutrition content. We must get past the thought that the more nutrients a food contains, the better the food is for us. Nutrients are very important, but how the food reacts to our hormones and metabolism, how the food is digested, and how it supports the other systems of our body are just as, if not more, important.

Does this mean all vegetables are bad for you? No. There are many safe vegetables for you to eat. Interested in knowing which ones?

Root Vegetables

Since root vegetables (potatoes, sweet potatoes, turnips, beets) grow *below* ground, they contain a lower level of the anti-metabolic substances listed above, yet are still high in nutritional content. This makes them an ideal choice if you are in need of a complex carbohydrate for energy and you don't want all the negative effects that grains and legumes can bring. It is important to note that root vegetables have a high starch content, so they should be cooked thoroughly (except the carrot) and eaten with a saturated fat, such as butter or coconut oil. This will enable easier digestion and a slower release into the blood system. In addition, potatoes should be eaten in moderation, especially for those who are trying to lose weight, as the high starch content can make them fattening.

The Importance of the Raw Carrot

The raw carrot, which grows below ground and is root vegetable, contains many powerful fungicides and bacteriostats. For the carrot to protect itself from bacteria in the soil, it produces its own fungicides and bacteriostats. These fungicides and bacteriostats act as a natural antiseptic and antibiotic in the bowel. The long carrot fibers attach themselves to endotoxins (a toxin kept "within" the bacterial cell and to be released only after destruction of the bacterial cell wall), bacteria, and estrogens that have been detoxed by the liver and remove these toxins through the colon in your stool. The raw carrot is a key player in lowering estrogen levels and bringing back proper hormonal balance. I guess Bugs Bunny had it right this entire time.

For best results, the raw carrot can be eaten alone, with a meal, or as a salad combined with coconut oil, vinegar, and salt. At the end of the day, just eat the carrot!

Fruit-Vegetables

Squash, tomatoes, cucumbers, zucchini, peppers, and pumpkin are actually fruits. By definition these fruit-vegetables are considered fruits, since the meat of the plant surrounds the seeds. The fruit-vegetables contain both fructose and glucose so they absorb into the blood system slower than a vegetable of pure glucose. The fruit-vegetables are low in starch and cellulose, and have a low PUFA content. Once again, these foods should still be well cooked and eaten with a saturated fat.

Remember: None of these foods should ever be consumed alone. You should always eat all vegetables and fruits with protein and fat to slow the blood sugar response. Even root vegetables, fruits, and fruit-vegetables eaten individually can throw your blood sugar out of whack.

To summarize, there is more to eating high-fiber, leafy vegetables than the nutritional content. Pectins, lignins, lectins, oxalates, PUFAs, and even cellulose can have an adverse effect on your health if you are unable to process them effectively. Of course, a diet with no vegetables or fiber, but tons of processed garbage, is not a good argument for the benefits of a lower vegetable/fiber diet. Only a diet with the right metabolic foods will convince you that a lower vegetable/fiber diet is a healthier option.

Does this mean you should never eat a salad or side of raw vegetables? Of course not. I still eat salads. I just eat them two to three times per month versus two to three times per day. I eat far smaller quantities of these types of vegetables, but I do not avoid them altogether. They do have some beneficial properties if eaten in smaller quantities and eaten the correct way.

Before I changed to my current diet, I was desperate to feel better. What I was doing was not working. Now, I feel 10 times better with more energy, more focus, fewer cravings, better digestion, healthier skin, and a happier, healthier life. Should you eliminate or cut back on these vegetables? My answer is maybe. Unfortunately, there is no clear-cut answer to "what should *every* person eat?" If you are experiencing digestive issues, have sugar and salt cravings, are gassy and bloated, have allergies, or just dislike leafy vegetables, then giving up your daily raw green salad and adding in a yummy raw carrot salad may be something for you to consider.

Remember I only wrote this book to give you another side to what mainstream media, the USDA, registered dietitians, and many doctors are telling you. I am not here to tell you what to do. I am just here so that you can question your own health, and to create awareness and help you understand that there are two sides to every story—especially in the health, fitness, and nutritional world.

Chapter 6:
What You Need to Know

1. Leafy green vegetables like kale, spinach, chard, and lettuce contain anti-nutrients. They consist of oxalates, lectins, lignans, and polyunsaturated fats.

2. Too much fiber or the wrong type fiber can disrupt proper digestion, increase toxic load, and damage the cell walls of the intestines and gut.

3. Cruciferous vegetables like broccoli, cauliflower, Brussel sprouts, bok choy, and cabbage are goitrogenic. Cruciferous vegetables inhibit proper thyroid function.

4. Root vegetables like sweet potatoes, white potatoes, yams, beets, and turnips, and the fruit-vegetables like pumpkin, zucchini, squash, and tomatoes are safer vegetables. Since the roots grow below ground they have fewer anti-nutrients. Roots should be cooked well and eaten with a fat.

5. Consume one to two organic raw carrots a day for the carrot's anti-fungal, anti-estrogenic, and anti-bacterial properties.

Chapter 7
Protein: Why You Need It—Just Not Too Much of It

The subject of protein is popular in the health, nutrition, and fitness world. Many so-called "health foods" are labeled "high protein" to entice the fitness, health, and weight-loss enthusiast to purchase them. These foods include protein bars, protein shakes, high-protein breads and cereals, and high-protein snacks, which can include everything from protein-filled pretzels to nuts to soybeans and ice cream.

High-protein diets have become popular due to the lean-looking bodies that follow such a lifestyle. Many attribute a high-protein diet to represent the diet of our ancestors, often referred to as a caveman, hunter-gatherer, or paleolithic diet. Other popular higher-protein diets include the South Beach diet and Atkins diet.

Years ago, when I was following my low-carb eating plan with a focus of getting and staying lean, I was essentially eating a high-protein diet. My diet was filled with egg whites, lean chicken, turkey, and fish, whey protein shakes and bars, and nuts. I also consumed low-carb breads, lots of vegetables, no salt, almond milk, and a few servings of fruit. This low-carb, higher-protein diet worked quite well for me for a few years. Yes, I had sugar and salt cravings. Yes I was cold most of the time. Yes, my energy fluctuated daily. Yes, I had gas and bloating. But I was super lean, and isn't that what really matters? Boy, did I have a lot to learn.

As I discussed in Chapter 4, protein is not the best foodsource for daily energy. It does have its value in that it is a vital macronutrient, and people need it to build muscle and collagen, repair cells, construct metabolic processes, detox the liver, and transport other nutrients. But using protein as a main energy source is wasteful since it produces the waste product ammonia and high levels of the inflammatory amino acids tryptophan, cysteine, histidine, and methionine. In addition, too much protein can lead to a decreased metabolic rate, increased stress hormones, sleep problems, fatigue, and muscle breakdown.

Unfortunately, I had to learn this the hard way. Once my body started to break down, my injuries wouldn't heal and my overall health started to suffer. My sleep was restless, I gained weight, my skin became dry, my hormones were all over the place, and I felt worn out. This is when I knew something was wrong. In hindsight, I realized I was over-consuming protein and under-consuming the right fats and carbohydrates. Although my high-protein, low-carb approach was effective in keeping me lean for well more than a year, long-term this dietary approach did not support a healthy lifestyle or body.

Now, I don't want you to think consuming protein is bad. Like I said, protein is a vital macronutrient for life—you definitely need it—but consuming a very high-protein diet is no better than eating a very low-protein diet. Too much protein is stressful to the body, just like too little protein is stressful to the body.

The question becomes: How much protein is right for you? And what proteins are going to work best in your body? You will be able to gauge that for yourself once you understand the functions of your body and how protein works within it. You will know more about how much protein—and which ones—to eat. There are no precise nutritional guidelines for everyone. But there are some things to know to help you make the right decision for yourself.

So let's get started.

To Begin, What Is Protein?

The human body needs protein for growth, structure, and maintenance. Protein is an essential macronutrient for the human body consisting of chains of amino acids. Amino acids are organic compounds consisting of the elements carbon, oxygen, hydrogen, nitrogen, and sulfur. Amino acids are the structural units that make up protein; essentially they are the building blocks of all proteins. In terms of nutrition, humans require 20 amino acids. Eleven amino acids are synthesized by the human body and are referred to as non-essential; the other nine are referred to as essential amino acids, since they are not synthesized in the human body and are required from the diet.

Amino Acids: The Building Blocks of Proteins

These are the nine essential amino acids: leucine**, isoleucine**, valine**, lysine, threonine, tryptophan, methionine, phenylalanine, and histidine.

These are the 11 non-essential amino acids: alanine, asparagine, aspartic acid, glutamic acid, arginine*, cysteine*, glutamine*, glycine*, proline*, serine*, and tyrosine*.

Amino acids are the building blocks of proteins. The human body breaks down incoming protein sources to produce amino acids (essential). The human body also produces its own amino acids (non-essential). These amino acids are then used to produce new proteins in the body that, well, do about everything.

* These amino acids become essential in times of stress, illness, famine, and certain medical issues.
** These are the branched-chain amino acids (BCAAs). BCAAs can be used by the muscles for energy.

In the diet, proteins are found in animal sources like eggs, fish, meat, and dairy. Protein is also found in vegetarian sources like nuts, soy, legumes, grains, beans, fruit, and vegetables. Most vegetarian proteins, like animal proteins, are considered complete proteins, since they contain all the essential amino acids. However, vegetable proteins are usually considered lower quality since the concentration of certain amino acids is much lower. In addition, as I discussed in earlier chapters, vegetable proteins contain many internal toxins that interfere with the digestion of the proteins by animals. Thus, even though one may be eating an adequate amount of vegetable protein, due to internal toxins of the vegetable, nut, legume, or grain, the proteins may not be broken down or absorbed.

A diet deficient in protein or bioavailable protein can inhibit many body functions. Protein is required for almost every function in the body. Thus, too little dietary protein will encourage muscle catabolism, decreased hormone production, a slower metabolism, a compromised immune system, water retention, and overall poor health and vitality.

Why You Need Protein

Structural. Protein is needed to build the structural components of our body. These include muscle, collagen, hair, nails, skin, bone, and organs. Without optimal levels of dietary protein, the body will become catabolic (break down), feeding on itself to get the necessary protein needs. Examples are collagen, elastin, and keratin.

Motor Proteins. Protein is needed to produce muscle contraction and movement. Examples are actin and myosin.

Hormones. Protein is needed for hormone production. Peptide hormones (also known as protein hormones) are synthesized in cells from amino acids. There are almost 100 peptide hormones.

A few to consider are:

- Insulin—decreases blood sugar levels by using the sugars as energy or storing the sugars as glycogen (stored sugar) or fat.

- Growth hormone—stimulates growth and increases fatty acid metabolism (which is good when building muscle and bad when encouraging cancer growth).

- Glucagon—elevates blood glucose levels through gluconeogenesis (the breakdown of amino acids, lactic acid, pyruvate, and glycerol into glucose) and glycogenolysis (the breakdown of glycogen into glucose).

- Prolactin—needed for lactation, but chronic levels are linked to breast cancer. Prolactin plays a role in increasing parathyroid hormone, which is linked to bone breakdown.

- Parathyroid hormone (PTH)—acts to increase blood calcium levels either by increasing reabsorption by kidneys, increasing absorption by the intestines by activating Vitamin D, or by breaking down bone. Chronically high levels of PTH can lead to osteoporosis.

- Thyroid stimulating hormone (TSH)—secreted from the pituitary gland to increase the thyroid hormones (T1, T2, T3, T4).

- Thyroid hormone—although not considered a peptide hormone, thyroid hormones are a combination of the amino acid tyrosine and the mineral iodine. Thyroid hormone is responsible for regulating metabolism.

Transport Proteins.

These proteins are in charge of moving nutrients, hormones or other molecules from one place to another. Here are few examples: Hemoglobin transports oxygen in the blood. Sex hormone binding globulin (SHBG) binds to the sex hormones testosterone and estrogen. Transcortin binds to the corticosteroids, cortisol, and progesterone. Transthyretin (prealbumin), thyroid binding globulin, and albumin are all associated with transportation of thyroid hormone.

During times of starvation, fasting, or stress this protein transportation system suffers and less thyroid, oxygen, sex hormones, and corticosteroids are delivered.

Enzymes. Most enzymes are made of proteins. Enzymes act as catalysts and are needed for basically every metabolic function in the body.

Antibodies. Antibodies are proteins used by the immune system. Antibodies recognize and neutralize antigens of foreign objects like bacteria and viruses.

Oncotic pressure. Oncotic pressure is the pressure exerted by the blood proteins (primarily albumin) to pull fluids into the circulatory system. Low levels of blood proteins will result in reduced oncotic pressure, increasing fluid buildup in the tissue, leading to edema (waterlogged). Albumin, the main blood protein, is also involved in the transportation of thyroid hormone, fatty acids to the liver, and calcium.

Energy. In times of need protein can be used as a source of energy. Like carbohydrates, protein contains 4 kcal/gram. Unlike carbohydrates, protein is not an ideal source of energy. Using protein as energy produces many waste products, is costly, and creates a stress response by the body.

The Downside of High-Protein Diets

Too much protein can be just as bad as too little protein. As I shared with you in the beginning of this chapter, I used to consume a fairly high-protein diet. At least 40–50 percent of my calories, which at the time was about 2 pounds or 200 grams of protein, coming primarily from lean cuts of chicken, turkey, fish, egg whites, whey protein shakes, and protein bars. Looking back, this was about twice as much protein as I needed. But at the time, my entire goal for eating lots of protein and reducing carbohydrates was to get lean.

Nutrition and weight loss research reports that higher-protein diets were linked to quicker fat loss and a leaner look. And after cutting my carbs and increasing my protein, I was getting lean. The research was correct—well, at least that is what I thought.

Most short-term research reports that, when followed for fewer than 24 months, high-protein/low-carb diets produce more fat loss than a standard, moderate-protein/high-carbohydrate diet.

Yet, the longer-term studies show a different story.

A review in the Nutricion Hospitalaria Journal looked at 418 studies on higher-protein diets. Only eight studies followed people for at least 24 months on higher protein to carbohydrate diets. Although more weight loss was reported in the first six months of the higher-protein groups, over time no significance in weight loss was shown after 24 months.

Essentially, when it comes to long-term weight loss, higher-protein/lower-carb diets do not perform any better than moderate-protein/higher-carbohydrate diets. *But,* because high protein/low carbs induces weight loss by stressing the body, not by supporting cellular metabolism, long-term use will lead to a stressed body, leading to muscle breakdown, fatigue, sleep issues, inflammation, and hormonal havoc.

Let me show you how the effects of a high-protein diet can lead to this type of stress on the body.

Kim's Story

Kim, a 40-year-old financial advisor, complained of fatigue, sleep problems, knee and ankle injuries, sugar cravings, body aches and pains, and weight gain. For the past two years Kim has been following a low-carb/high-protein diet consisting primarily of meats and vegetables. Kim was also following a five- to six-day/week intense workout program. Kim was lean and fit, yet Kim's energy, sleep, and mood were all being affected.

Kim began to learn that her current diet and workout regime were very stressful on her body. Throw in a demanding job and busy life, and her body was unable to deal with all the combined stressors. Physiologically, the body treats all stress the same way, so whether it comes from a carbohydrate-deprived diet, a hard workout, or a demanding job, the body reacts chemically the same way. If the combined load becomes too much, energy level, hormones, the immune system, sleep, and muscle recovery will all be negatively affected.

Through coaching, Kim learned that using protein as the body's main energy source was wasteful and inefficient in producing high levels of energy. Kim's body was stressed and the best way to reduce stress in the body is to consume the right sugars, fats, and proteins in the right amounts for you. Adding in fruits, orange juice, honey, and milk, and the right fats and proteins could help reduce the stress hormones created by her current lifestyle. To help reduce her stress, Kim also stopped all intense exercise (for now), allowing only for yoga, swimming, and walking. Intense exercise is very stressful to the body. If the person is healthy, intense exercise can produce beneficial results; in the hypometabolic person, the same exercise can make things worse.

The addition of good carbohydrates (sugars), reduced meat protein, added gelatin and bone broth, the elimination of intense workouts, and more rest allowed Kim to regain her energy and life again. This process took about six months. When she recovered, she was able to return to her intense workouts. The difference is she does two to three workouts a week versus five to six per week. Kim is no longer obsessed with obtaining 13-percent body fat, although she is still lean. It's become more important to her to sleep well, have good energy, and be happy. Kim is a smart girl.

Increased Levels of Stress Hormones

As I talked about in Chapter 4, consuming protein without enough carbohydrates will increase insulin levels. Insulin is needed for protein absorption into the cell. Once protein is consumed, insulin rises. If a meal does not contain enough carbohydrates, blood sugar levels will drop due to the rise in insulin. If carbohydrates are not soon ingested, the body will increase the hormones adrenaline and glucagon, to release glycogen (glycogenesis) from the liver and cortisol to break down fat and protein to be converted into glucose (gluconeogenesis) so that blood glucose levels can rise.

Although glycogenesis and gluconeogenesis are normal

metabolic functions, protein catabolism and muscle wasting for energy production are not optimal for a healthy body.

Increased Bone Loss

Protein-rich foods can be high in the mineral phosphorus. Phosphorus, an essential nutrient needed for strong bones and teeth, and energy production, in excess will cause calcium to leach from the bones. In *Nutrition and Physical Degeneration,* Dr. Weston Price discusses how diets with a high phosphorus-to-calcium ratio are linked to many degenerative diseases, including osteoporosis, inflammation, and tooth decay.

A 2002 study in the *American Journal of Kidney Disease* followed 10 healthy individuals on a low-carb/high-protein diet for six weeks. After only six weeks researchers concluded a measurable decrease in calcium balance, which could increase bone loss.

A 12-week study in *Biofactors Journal* found the correct balance of calcium to phosphorus was estimated at 2:1. Diets with a 2:1 ratio of calcium to phosphorus were found to increase calcium absorption into the bone. Diets higher in phosphorus to calcium were found to do the opposite. Foods high in phosphorus and low in calcium are muscle meats, seeds, Brazil nuts, grains, soy, and colas.

Dairy products, although high in phosphorus, are a safe food due to their high calcium content.

Protein Used as Energy Produces Waste Products

When proteins break down through gluconeogenesis, the removed amino acid (referred to as deamination) is converted to ammonia in the intestines and kidneys, and is then used by the liver to synthesize the waste product urea. High-protein diets increase ammonia production. Too much ammonia can suppress respiration and stimulate glycolysis, which produces lactic acid. High levels of lactic acid are present in cancer patients, diabetics, arthritis, and people with heart disease.

It is important to note that in a healthy body, the production of ammonia and urea (a chemical waste product consisting of nitrogen, oxygen, and carbon) is a normal process. However, a person in a hypo-metabolic state, who is consuming too much protein or even a moderate level of protein, will produce an excessive amount of ammonia, urea, and lactic acid. In a healthy state our bodies can handle the stress of too much protein for quite a long time. However, the longer we eat a high-protein diet, the more stress the diet places on our bodies, and once our bodies become overloaded the body can no longer handle such a restrictive diet. I say this because many people who are reading this may disagree with me due to the fact they may have seen success on a high-protein/low-carb diet plan. And I say this to them: Give it time.

Protein breakdown also increases the blood levels of the amino acids tryptophan, cysteine, methionine, and histidine. Each of these amino acids is linked to inflammatory markers in the body.

Tryptophan

The essential amino acid tryptophan is required for reproduction and growth in young people. With age the need for tryptophan decreases. Tryptophan is the precursor to the neurotransmitter serotonin, also known as 5HTP. Under stress (protein catabolism) large amounts of tryptophan are released, turning into serotonin, which activates the pituitary hormone adrenocorticotropic hormone (ACTH) and stimulates cortisol production.

This process suppresses thyroid function, releasing more stress hormones, and the vicious cycle continues.

Essentially, excess tryptophan in the blood can induce a stress reaction leading to slower metabolism, inflammation, depression, fatigue, and premature aging. Interestingly enough, research studies on hair pigmentation show the highest levels of tryptophan are found in white and gray hairs of aging men and women.

The foods highest in tryptophan are not turkey. Soy products, egg whites, elk, and seaweed are much higher.

Cysteine

The amino acid cysteine, unlike tryptophan, is not an essential amino acid. The human body can produce it. However, like tryptophan, cysteine released in large quantities during stress is anti-metabolic. Cysteine is shown to inhibit the enzyme thyroid peroxidase, needed in the production of thyroid hormone (T4). Cysteine, like tryptophan, is released in large quantities in muscle catabolism or in consuming a diet high in muscle meat.

Methionine

Methionine is also an essential amino acid needed for growth and development. However, when it comes to longevity in life, research has found that rats eating a methionine-restricted diet lived 43-percent longer than those that consume a diet high in methionine. Methionine is known for its thyroid-suppressing properties like cysteine and tryptophan. Egg whites, seeds, meat, and grains are foods high in methionine.

Histidine

Histidine, another essential amino acid, is necessary for growth in babies. Far smaller amounts are needed for adults. Histidine is the precursor to histamine. Histamine is involved in the inflammatory response by the immune system. Histamine is produced when foods with histidine are combined with bacteria and yeast. This can happen in aged, spoiled, or fermented foods. Bacteria and yeast contain the enzyme histidine decarboxylase (HDC), which converts histidine to histamine.

People with chronic coughing, sneezing, watery eyes, and/or breathing issues may have an intolerance to histamine. Avoiding fermented foods and foods high in the amino acid histidine should help alleviate the issue. Fermented foods including wine (sorry), kefir, yogurt, sauerkraut, fermented fish, sausage, and ground meats all are high in histidine.

As you can see, protein has far more complexity than I am sure you ever wanted to know. Too little protein can suppress thyroid function, decrease the immune system, increase edema, and increase muscle catabolism. In addition, too much protein can also suppress thyroid function, affect the immune system, increase inflammation, and increase waste products.

This brings us back to this: How much protein is needed for health and vitality?

Well, like I said in the beginning of this chapter, the amount of protein an individual needs is based on the needs of that individual. Age, sex, muscular size, activity level, metabolic health, stress, and the person's diet all play a role in determining how much protein someone needs.

The National Academy's Dietary Reference states adult men and women should consume a minimum of .80 grams of protein/Kg of body weight. Active individuals and athletes may need to double or even triple this amount. Stress and exercise increase muscle turnover, increasing the need for more protein.

Nutritional researcher and biologist Dr. Ray Peat believes the minimum requirements, for all metabolic functions, is at least 80 grams of protein/day. However, Dr. Peat believes when the metabolic rate is high and the person is not completely sedentary, protein needs should be closer to 130–150 grams of protein/day.

I eat about 100–120 grams of protein/day for my active, 120-pound frame. That's almost half of what I used to eat, but double what the current Recommended Dietary Allowance (RDA) recommends. Protein intake is about 25 percent of my daily calories.

In addition to activity and stress, the health of the person plays a big role in protein needs. A person in a hypo-metabolic (slow metabolism) state may have lower needs for protein than a healthy person, but he still may need to increase his consumption of protein due to the lower levels of hydrochloric acid (HCL) in the stomach. HCL is needed for protein breakdown so that the amino acids can be absorbed and utilized. Low levels of HCL decrease protein breakdown, leading to decreased amino acid absorption. Along with healing the gut, eating more protein, primarily easy-to-digest proteins, will help increase protein absorption in a person with a sluggish metabolism.

Finally, the type of proteins consumed will play a role in how much protein a person may need. At the beginning of this chapter I talked about vegetarian versus animal proteins. The biggest difference between the two is the digestibility of each type of protein. Vegetable proteins like soy, nuts, beans, and grains contain many internal toxins like trypsin inhibitors and polyunsaturated fats that interfere with protein digestion. Therefore, someone consuming primarily vegetable proteins may need far more protein due to the amount that is actually digested. *Don't worry; I will go into more detail in the next chapter about the* best *proteins to consume for healing and metabolic power.*

Here are some basic guidelines to work with:

General Protein Guidelines for a Healthy Person

Weight	Sedentary	Active
100–125 lbs.	60–90g.	90–125g.
126–150 lbs.	70–100g.	100–150g.
151–175 lbs.	80–110g.	110–175g.
176–200 lbs.	100–120g.	120–200g.
Over 200 lbs.	120g. +	180g. +

There is no exact science to protein intake. If you have good overall health (free of disease, pain, and illness), a warm body (average 98.6 degrees Farenheit), a normal pulse (75–90 BPM), good digestion, and restful sleep; can maintain good muscle tone; have a healthy sex drive, feel happy; maintain normal blood pressure (around 120/80); and have healthy bones, teeth, hair, skin, and nails, then I would say you are eating the right amount of protein for you.

If you are having issues with any of the above, then your protein intake may be something to look at. But, remember there is more to a good diet than just the amount of protein in the diet: The combination of the right carbohydrates and fats is just as important. (Jump to Chapter 15 if you want to understand more about combining your foods and balancing your blood sugar.)

As you can see there is more to protein than just adding muscle and increasing strength. Proteins are needed for almost every metabolic function in the body. Without enough protein our immune system, digestion, detox, and structural systems are affected. However, not all proteins are created equal, and when it comes to supporting a high metabolism, good digestion, and immunity, some are better than others. I don't believe the hype of eating a high-protein diet will go away anytime soon, especially since so many lean bodies are recommending it. My only hope is people will begin to understand that more is not better and that not all proteins are created equal.

So what are the best proteins? Keep reading to find out.

Chapter 7:
What You Need to Know

1. Protein is needed for structure (muscle, collagen, hair, skin, nails, bone, organs), movement and muscular contraction, hormones, transporting proteins, enzymes, antibodies, and energy.

2. Protein can increase insulin levels and should not be used as the main source of energy, due to the stress response it will create if not consumed with enough carbohydrates.

3. High-protein diets may contain too much phosphorus to calcium. Consuming adequate dairy will help balance this effect.

4. Certain proteins can be inflammatory. The amino acids tryptophan, cysteine, methionine, and histidine can all produce signs of inflammation if consumed in excess.

5. The amount of protein needed for each individual is person-specific. The amount will depend on the sex, age, and size of the person; his or her energy expenditure, metabolic rate, digestion and overall health; and the type of protein the person is consuming.

Chapter 8
The *Super* Proteins

When it comes to protein, there are six proteins in particular that I would refer to as the *super* proteins. Super proteins are proteins that support a healthy gut, high metabolic function, good energy, restful sleep, and a warm and lean body. These six super proteins are easy to digest and carry a high nutritional value outside of their protein content.

What are these super proteins? They include milk, eggs, liver, shellfish/white fish, potato-protein, and bone broth/gelatin.

Milk

Got milk? The topic of drinking milk seems to remain in perpetual controversy. It seems one day experts say milk makes you fat, bloated, and gassy, and the next day they say drinking milk makes you lean, healthy, and strong. In Chapter 9, I will discuss the truth about milk in its entirety. However, what you need to know right now is milk is a great source of protein. Milk packs about 8 grams of protein per cup. One quart of milk contains about 33 grams of protein. A daily consumption of 3 quarts of milk can meet most people's protein needs for the day.

For many people (myself included), consuming 3 quarts of milk a day can be very limiting and boring. I usually recommend about four servings a day along with other dairy. Four servings of milk will provide about 1/3 of most people's daily protein needs.

I actually consider milk to be a perfect food. Milk is perfectly balanced with protein, fat, and sugars, and it is filled with calcium and numerous other vitamins and minerals. Milk is more than just great protein: It supplies good fat and carbohydrates, and it is filled with nutrients. These are a few of the reasons why I have dedicated an entire chapter on understanding milk and dairy better. For now, you should understand that milk is a great source of easily digested and easily absorbed protein. (For more information on milk and dairy, jump to Chapter 9.)

Pastured Organic Eggs

Just like milk, the "incredible edible" egg has also been one of the most controversial nutrition topics over the last century. One day eggs are the perfect protein; the next day nutritional research is comparing them to cigarette smoking. One day egg yolks are a nutritional powerhouse; the next day egg yolks are the key to coronary heart disease. Many medical doctors and health practitioners are advising health-conscious people to minimize egg eating to one a day due to eggs' cholesterol content, yet current research is saying eggs have a minimal effect on health and blood lipid levels. With all these conflicting views, it's no wonder the average person doesn't know what to make of eggs!

The Truth About Eggs

Eggs are considered a complete protein, since they contain all the essential amino acids. Sixty percent of the protein is found in the egg white, and 40 percent of the protein is found in the egg yolk. Egg whites are 100-percent protein, while the yolk also contains the fat and cholesterol. Egg yolks also contain carotenoids, vitamins A, E, D, and K, calcium, iron, phosphorus, zinc, thiamin, B6, folate, B12, pantothenic acid, choline, potassium, magnesium, copper, manganese, and selenium. The egg white, although not void of nutrients, only contains potassium, magnesium, sodium, and selenium. Most of the nutrients are located in the egg yolk, so throw out the yolk and you are throwing out most of the nutrients and almost half of the protein.

What Is Choline?

Choline is a water-soluble nutrient usually combined with the B vitamins. Choline is found in cholesterol-rich foods like egg yolks, liver, and beef. Choline is needed for cell function, liver metabolism, and nutrient transportation throughout the body. Some choline is produced in the body, but more is needed for optimal body function, so choline is required in the diet. According to a study in *The American Journal of Clinical Nutrition* in 2008, increased intake of choline lowered inflammatory markers like homocysteine and C-reactive protein. High levels of both are linked to heart disease, arthritis, and inflammation. In addition, a choline deficiency (not fructose ingestion) is known to play a role in fatty liver disease. Thus, eating enough foods with choline is imperative to good health.

Eating egg whites only is a practice held by many fitness and weight-loss participants. The purpose of dumping the yolk is to avoid eating the fat and cholesterol, and to avoid unnecessary calories. For years, I ate only egg whites, throwing out the highly nutritious yolk so I could be "healthy." At my peak, I was probably consuming close to one-half dozen egg whites a day. Little did I know, the egg-white-only diet was anything but healthy.

Egg whites are high in the inflammatory amino acids tryptophan, cysteine, and methionine. Consuming the whites alone can eventually lead to digestive upset, inflammation, and slower metabolic rate. The whole egg offers a better balance of amino acids and far more nutrition.

Aren't Eggs Yolks High in Cholesterol?

Yes, egg yolks are a cholesterol-rich food. One egg contains close to 200 mg of cholesterol, which is 65 percent of the Recommended Daily Allowance (RDA). Years ago, the American people including myself, were led to believe eating eggs, due to their high cholesterol, were a fast track to heart disease.

But new research shows a different story.

A recent study in *Nutrients* Journal followed 73 college students for 14 weeks. Half of the students received a cholesterol-rich breakfast including two eggs (an extra 400mg of cholesterol) while the other half received a cholesterol-free breakfast. At all points of measurement blood lipids were equal in both groups, indicating that an additional 400mg of cholesterol does not impact blood lipids.

The 65-year-long Framingham study has been researching coronary heart disease since 1949. In a review of the 912 subjects, the study concluded that egg consumption had no correlation to cholesterol levels or coronary heart disease incidence.

The *Journal of American College Nutrition* researched 167 cholesterol- feeding studies, following more than 3,500 people. The results showed that increased egg intake increased total serum cholesterol by only 2.2mg/dL. The increase came from an increase in large particles LDL (so-called bad cholesterol) and HDL (good cholesterol).

Current research tells us that total cholesterol is a poor depicter of heart disease. More important are the ratio between low-density lipoproteins (LDL) and high-density lipoproteins (HDL) cholesterol, and the actual size of the LDL particle. LDL cholesterol is not bad; you need it to bring cholesterol to the cells. Remember: Cholesterol is needed to build and maintain cell membranes, intracellular transport, Vitamin D, and hormonal synthesis. However, small density LDL is more prone to oxidation than the larger, more buoyant LDL particles. Whole-egg consumption improves the lipid profile by increasing large LDL particles and HDL particles. Although eggs may increase the overall cholesterol number, this type of increase will actually improve your lipid profiles and decrease your chance of heart disease.

Now, before you go out and start eating a dozen eggs every day, remember that *Americans love to do everything in excess*. Let's talk about the quality of your eggs.

Not All Eggs Are created Equal

As with meat and milk, the quality of the egg is very dependent on the diet of the chicken that laid the egg. A chicken locked up in a cage, never seeing the light of day and fed a diet of genetically modified (GM) corn and soy is going to produce a far different egg than a chicken that is pasture-raised, allowed to roam free in the sunlight, and fed a diet of worms, bugs, weeds, and grass.

Dr. Niva Shapira, in a 2008 study, demonstrated how the diet of egg-laying hens could change the nutritional quality of the eggs. She fed one group of hens a diet high in Omega-6 polyunsaturated fats (corn and soy), while the other group of hens received a diet low in Omega-6 fats and additional antioxidants. Dr. Shapira went on to show how eating two high-corn-soy eggs a day elevated oxidized LDL (bad) cholesterol by 40 percent in normal, healthy individuals. The individuals who ate two low-Omega-6 eggs a day had normal levels of oxidized LDL cholesterol.

The study by Dr. Shapira is a great example of how eggs coming from different diets can affect a person's body differently.

Here is a list of best to worse eggs:

Pastured, organic, no soy, no corn-fed. I know it is a mouthful. From my experience most soy- and corn-free eggs come straight from a local farmer who has a real concern for the health of his animals. These chickens are allowed to roam free in pastures, are fed worms, bugs, and grass, and are free of antibiotics and hormones. The best places to find pastured eggs are your local farmers market or www.TropicalTraditions.com.

Organic, free-roaming, vegetarian-fed. These eggs come from chickens allowed to roam outside of their cages. The chickens are free of hormones and antibiotics. Their diet may consist of some worms and grass but primarily the chickens are fed chicken feed, which consists of organic corn, soy, and/or other vegetable matter. These are usually the most expensive eggs at your health food grocery store.

Free-roaming. "Free-roaming" can mean very little when it comes to eggs. There is no official legal definition, so it is loosely used to describe chickens that are allowed to go outside for at least a part of the day. Eggs from free-roaming chickens, if not listed as organic, may have been treated with antibiotics and hormones and given GM feed.

Cage-free. These chickens may be indoors only but are allowed to roam freely in a big barn. As with free-roaming, eggs may be from chickens treated with antibiotics and hormones, and fed a GM diet.

Natural. The word "natural" means very little in the food industry. Natural can mean anything from the eggs have a natural color to the eggs are free of hormones and antibiotics.

Conventionally farmed. Egg containers marked with just "eggs" are more than likely coming from your battery-caged chickens. These chickens are kept in crowded cages, and fed GM corn, soy, meat parts, and even their own feces. Antibiotics and hormones are used on these chickens to produce larger-than-normal eggs. If conventionally farmed eggs are all that are available to you, I would advise limiting your egg intake to two to three per week, versus two to three per day.

Personally, I find that consuming two pastured eggs every day works well for me. I poach or fry my eggs in coconut oil and make sure I have them with a cup of orange juice and a cup of fruit. Eggs are a powerful insulin-stimulant, so eating enough good sugars (fruit and OJ) with eggs is essential for maintaining balanced blood sugar levels.

In my opinion, conventionally farmed eggs are an entirely different food than pastured-organic eggs. This is one big reason why nutritional information is so confusing. The nutritional information given to us never clarifies the type of egg, milk, meat, etc. All we hear is that something is good or bad for us. Unfortunately, research on the benefits of organic eggs is very expensive and the local farmers just don't make the money to fund it. Only Big Food giants could afford such a study, but with nothing for them to gain, I doubt it will ever happen.

Until then, we have to use what we do know. Pastured whole eggs are a great source of protein and nutrients. The intake of quality eggs may marginally increase your cholesterol levels, but there is no conclusive evidence that this is a ticket to the heart specialist. In fact, new research is showing egg intake has a positive effect on blood lipid levels. This is why the "incredible edible" egg is my number two super protein.

Grass-Fed Liver

I can already hear the words coming out of your mouth: "Liver? Yuck!" I know eating liver is not a favorite, or a top-10 food most people love to eat, but hear me out. Liver is one of the most nutritionally packed foods on the planet. Liver, like eggs, is a cholesterol-rich (cholesterol is produced in the liver) food, but as you now know dietary cholesterol does not significantly affect blood cholesterol levels, nor increase chances of heart disease.

Not only does liver give you 25 grams of protein in a 4-ounce serving, but liver supplies you with vitamins D, E, K, folate, thiamin, B6, riboflavin, niacin, pantothenic acid, choline, and copious amounts of vitamins A and B12. In addition, liver is filled with the minerals calcium, iron, magnesium, selenium, copper, zinc, and phosphorus. To really understand the high nutritional value of liver, it takes 5 pounds of fruits to equal the same amount of nutrition content in only 4 ounces of liver. Ounce for ounce, no other food supplies you with this much nutrition.

What Is Vitamin B12?

Vitamin B12 is a water-soluble vitamin. Vitamin B12 is required for normal brain and nervous system function. Vitamin B12 is also needed for blood formation and can result in B12 anemia (pernicious anemia), if someone becomes deficient. B12 deficiency can result from damage to parietal cells of the stomach. The parietal cells are responsible for releasing intrinsic factor, which is needed for proper B12 absorbency. Lack of intrinsic factor will result in a B12 deficiency. Thus, the only way to fix this B12 deficiency is healing the gut, allowing the parietal cells to function properly. Increasing B12 through diet or oral supplementation may not help this problem.

Is Eating Liver Toxic?

Many people are under the assumption that eating liver must be toxic since it is in charge of detoxing the animal, and thus is filled with toxic substances. Yes, the liver is the main detoxifying organ, but it does not store toxins; the liver neutralizes toxins. Small amounts of heavy metals are found in the liver, but these amounts are far too small to be of significance. Most toxins are stored in fat tissue, not the liver. The liver is a storage organ for vitamins and minerals; that's why it is so nutritious to consume.

How Much Liver Should You Eat?

Despite its high nutritional content, liver should be eaten only about once a week. For example, one 3- to 6-ounce serving is recommended every seven to 10 days. Liver is high in the amino acid tryptophan, so eating too much can inhibit thyroid function and increase inflammation. Liver is served best cooked in coconut oil or ghee, and consumed with a cooked vegetable or fruit.

Shellfish and Low-Fat Fish

Shellfish, including mussels, clams, oysters, crab, lobster, shrimp, and scallops, are all good sources of protein. Shellfish contain vitamins A, C, D, and E, and the B vitamins. Shellfish are an exceptional source of vitamin B12, which is required for every metabolic process in the body. In addition, shellfish are good sources of the minerals zinc, copper, selenium, iron, magnesium, sodium, and manganese.

What Is Selenium?

Selenium is an important mineral in thyroid activation. Selenium supports adequate thyroid hormone production and protects the gland from excess iodine exposure. Selenium is also needed to convert inactive thyroid hormone T4 to the active T3. A deficiency in selenium can lead to sluggish metabolism. The best sources of selenium are organ meats like liver, shellfish, dairy, and eggs.

Are Shellfish Safe to Eat?

Shellfish safety is a concern to many people, especially due to the continued pollution of our ocean waters. According to the Centers for Disease Control, you have a 10-times-greater chance getting sick from chicken than you do from eating fish or shellfish. Yet, the most common food-borne illness is eating *raw* shellfish. Therefore, safety should not be an issue as long as you cook your shellfish.

According to the FDA, shellfish are low in mercury and should be consumed up to 12 ounces per week. I recommend eating shellfish one or two times per week, depending on preference. Cook your shellfish in butter and eat with a well-cooked vegetable or fruit.

As far as fish are concerned, I recommend low-fat fish like tilapia, cod, sole, and white fish. These fish are high in protein, the B vitamins, and the mineral selenium. Low-fat fish are preferred over fatty fish like salmon, mackerel, herring, and albacore tuna because they contain less polyunsaturated fats.

I Thought Salmon Was Good for Me?

Salmon is a cold-water fish that contains high amounts of the Omega-3 fatty acids, which are polyunsaturated fats (PUFAs). The long-chain EPA (eicosapentaenoic acid) and DHA (docosahexaenoic acid) make up the Omega-3s found in salmon. Although most health, nutritional, and medical professionals will tout salmon and the Omega-3 fats as healthy, in reality these fats have a metabolic-lowering effect. Remember from Chapter 3 that, PUFAs, including the Omega-3s (EPA and DHA), can cause immune suppression, increase age pigmentation, kill white blood cells, slow metabolic rate, and inhibit proteolytic enzymes that are needed for proper metabolic function.

Even the FDA Had Concerns About Fish Oils

In 2002 the FDA responded to Dr. Edward Lorio in a letter about fish oil consumption, noting: "The FDA raised concerns about the consumption of high levels of EPA and DHA, which may increase bleeding time, increase levels of low-density lipoprotein cholesterol, and have an effect on glycemic control in non-insulin dependent diabetics (menhaden oil final rule; 62 FR 30751; June 5, 1997). The FDA concluded that a combined intake of EPA and DHA from all added sources does not exceed 3 g/p/d." Three grams a day is equal to about one-half teaspoon, a far cry from the tablespoons of fish oil supplements that are recommended today.

"Although by 1980 many animal diseases were known to be caused by eating oily fish, and the unsaturated oils were known to accelerate the formation of the "age pigment," lipofuscin, many "beneficial effects" of dietary fish oil started appearing in research journals around that time, and the mass media, responding to the industry's public relations campaign, began ignoring studies that showed harmful effects from eating fish oil."

~ Dr. Ray Peat

Interesting how things change when "a fish oil industry" is produced.

Now, this does not mean you can never eat salmon. If you love salmon, you should eat it, just once or twice each month versus the recommended one to two times per week. Frying salmon in butter or coconut oil is the safest way to cook the fish. Poaching and steaming have a longer cooking time, allowing more PUFAs to break down, producing the toxin acrolein (known carcinogen) and other free radicals. Remember: *All* PUFAs are unstable, and heating them produces oxidation and free radicals; the Omega-3s found in salmon are no exception.

Potato Protein

Most people do not realize that potatoes are a good source of quality protein. The very high value of "potato protein" is better than the egg yolk, because there is material besides the actual protein that functions as protein: keto acids. Potato's keto acids are the equivalent of the essential amino acids. In the body, ammonia is added to keto acids, turning them into amino acids.

According to nutrition researcher Ray Peat, PhD, "Two pounds of well-cooked mashed potato has the protein value similar to a liter of milk, about 33 grams of protein. A person would be able to live for a long time on either two or three liters of milk or 4–6 pounds of potatoes per day. The milk drinker would eventually need to supplement iron, the potato eater would need to supplement vitamin A, possibly B12, but both of them are nearly perfect foods." The well-cooked white potato also contains numerous vitamins and minerals, including vitamins C, D, and K, folate, niacin, pantothenic acid, B6, choline, calcium, potassium, magnesium, phosphorus, copper, manganese, iron, and zinc. The potato lacks adequate Vitamin A and B12.

I would never recommend consuming 4–6 pounds of potatoes a day for its protein—and nothing else, especially when other foods like milk, eggs, liver, and gelatin are available. However, for a person who is in a very compromised metabolic state (diabetic, cancer, HIV, celiac, colitis) or is a vegan, a concentrated potato juice would be a beneficial food. A 2008 study in *Food Chemistry Journal* reported potato protein to have antioxidant and blood pressure–lowering effects. Juicing the potato removes all the starch, leaving primarily protein. Potato protein is easy to digest and absorb. Vegetarians, vegans, and anyone with a compromised metabolism would benefit from using potato protein.

If the metabolism is severely damaged, white potatoes like the russet potato or even a "yellow" sweet potato is best. Orange sweet potatoes or yams can be harder to digest due to their high levels of carotene.

How to Make Juiced Potato Protein

Use a quality juicer (centrifugal is best) to juice 2 pounds of white potatoes. Allow the mixture to sit out, so the starch can separate from the juice. Pour the juice (leave the starchy sediment) in a fry pan with a little butter and scramble it like an egg. Drinking the juice raw is an option, but the taste is less than desirable. Cooking the juice with butter and salt and pepper will make it taste like mashed potatoes. Two pounds of potatoes juiced is equal to about 33 grams of proteins.

Gelatin and Bone broth

Did you ever wonder why homemade chicken soup (made from bone broth) was given to you when you were sick? A few cups of homemade soup somehow magically made you feel better. Many would say it's the love that went into making the soup/broth that made you feel better, and that may be true, but bone broths and soups have been used as a medicinal food for centuries. In fact, many traditional cultures, like the Chinese, French, Japanese, African, and Italian, have used broths to treat not only the common cold but gastrointestinal issues, joint pain, depression, constipation, liver support, and anti-aging, as well as improved hair, skin, nails, and bone health.

In today's busy world, making a bone broth seems far too time-consuming and tedious (although it is not). Instead, Americans eat the muscle meat only (the chicken breast, steak, fish filet) and throw out all the bones and other connective tissue (tendons, skin, cartilage). Americans seem to have forgotten, or never learned, there is more to an animal than just the meat. The cooked connective tissue produces a gelatinous, nutrient-filled food containing healing protein (collagen/gelatin) and essential minerals.

What Is Bone Broth?

Bone broth is produced from cooking the connective tissue of an animal in water, vinegar, vegetables, and salt for 3 to 4 hours. The connective tissue includes the bones (knuckle, marrow, oxtail, feet, chicken or fish carcasses), the skin, cartilage, tendons, and ligaments of an animal. The bones and connective tissue from cows, bison, pigs, fish, and chickens can all be used. Personally, I recommend using grass-fed/pastured beef bones (knuckle, feet, oxtail). Grazing animals will produce stronger bones and joints, producing a broth abundant in gelatin and the bone-building minerals, particularly calcium. The bones of grass-fed animals also produce a broth that contains more saturated to polyunsaturated fat. Remember: Saturated fat is safer and less damaging than the polyunsaturated fats. I skim the fat, after refrigeration, to avoid the fat entirely.

Bone broth gets its protein from the collagen (the extracellular framework of the body) in the connective tissue. Collagen is located in the skin, tendons, ligaments, and bones, and allows for more flexibility. Without collagen, bones would be very brittle. Collagen makes up 25–35 percent of the protein in the human body and is the main structural protein of all the connective tissue. When the bones are cooked, the collagen, minerals, glucosamine, and glycosaminoglycans (GAGs) are extracted from the connective tissue into the water. The extracted cooked collagen, referred to as gelatin, makes the bone broth gelatinous (jelly-like).

Why Is Gelatin So Important?

The super protein gelatin has been studied for centuries due to its healing properties. Back in 1937, American researcher Francis Pottenger, MD determined the secret to gelatin's healing properties was its ability to attract and hold liquids (hydrophilic-water loving). Gelatin would attract digestive juices to food, which would help break the food down better. In his book *Gelatin in Nutrition and Medicine*, Nathan Ralph Gotthoffer demonstrated how taking gelatin with wheat, oats, meat, and dairy would improve the digestion of these foods. Better-digested foods means the body will get more of the nutrients it needs to heal and repair.

Gelatin use has been linked to:

- Improved digestion.
- Decreased joint inflammation.
- Improved sleep.
- Increased insulin sensitivity.
- Increased gastric juices in the stomach.
- Muscle sparing.
- Healing the gut lining and protecting the stomach from ulcers.
- Improved allergies.
- Helping to stabilize blood glucose levels.
- Improved memory.
- Improved wound healing.
- Improved liver detoxification.
- Improved the health of your skin, hair, and nails.

- Helping with arthritis.
- Helping with diabetes.

One reason gelatin is such a healing food is its lack of the inflammatory amino acids that are in the other proteins (meat, eggs, dairy, soy). Gelatin is void of the inflammatory amino acid tryptophan. Gelatin also contains very little cysteine, methionine, and histidine. In the last chapter, I explained how all four of these amino acids, in excess, can produce anti-metabolic and inflammatory conditions in the body. Most healthy people, at least for a while, can handle a diet high in the inflammatory amino acids (a high meat diet). However, a high meat diet for a person in a hypo-metabolic state could lead to a list of inflammatory issues, like poor digestion, achy joints, muscle loss, allergies, poor sleep, fatigue, detox issues, headaches, forgetfulness, weight gain, etc. A person with a sluggish metabolism would benefit from a diet low in muscle meat and high in bone broth and gelatin.

Suzie's Story

Suzie was living on a high-protein/meat diet. Her energy was in the toilet and her busy life was starting to wear her down. Suzie was a busy career mom who had no time to be tired. She exercised daily, and to keep her weight "in check" she consumed a low-carb/high-protein (meat) diet. In fact, Suzie ate meat at almost every meal: eggs and bacon for breakfast, chicken salad for lunch, and steak for dinner. Along with her fatigue, Suzie was also experiencing joint pain, back pain, poor digestion, sleep issues, allergies, and forgetfulness.

With some lifestyle shifts that allowed Suzie to slow things down, Suzie started to shift her diet from a very high-protein diet (almost 60-percent protein) to a more balanced diet (around 30-percent protein).

Every week Suzie cut down on her meat intake. Initially, instead of eating meat three times a day, she dropped it to two times a day. She replaced the meat with a few cups of bone broth, coconut oil, Parmesan cheese, and fruit. In addition, for every meal she did consume meat, she drank 1 cup of bone broth. The amino acid profile of the bone broth makes the meat meal far more balanced.

Slowly, over the next four months, Suzie reduced her three times/day meat habit to three times/week. She switched her protein sources to full-fat dairy (easier to digest than low-fat), cheese, potatoes, eggs, broth, and hydrolyzed gelatin (powdered gelatin). In addition, Suzie balanced her meals better with good carbs (fruit, OJ, root vegetables) and good fats (coconut oil, butter).

What happened?

Initially, Suzie's gut improved, as the high-meat diet seemed to be irritating it. Meat is hard to digest, and in a compromised metabolic state it will lead to bloating, gas, and digestive problems. Broth and gelatin can help food digest better due the hydrophilic properties (water-loving). Essentially gelatin attracts the digestive juices to the food. The gelatin also increases gastric juices, all while coating the stomach lining. As her gut healed, Suzie's joint and back pain subsided (no chiropractor necessary), her allergies and sleep improved, and, most importantly, Suzie's energy returned. It's been two years since Suzie shifted her diet, and she continues to consume bone broth daily. Suzie refers to her bone broth as Magic Juice. Magic indeed!

Gelatin Is High in Glycine

Lacking in the inflammatory amino acids, gelatin is rich in anti- inflammatory amino acids alanine, hydroxyproline, proline, and especially glycine. Glycine is the simplest of all the amino acids. Glycine is used for the synthesis of heme, the portion of the blood that carries oxygen. Glycine is used to synthesize creatine, which helps supply energy to the heart and muscle cells. Glycine helps synthesize bile salts and purines and nucleic acids, which are the building blocks of RNA (ribonucleic acid) and DNA (deoxyribonucleic acid), our genetic messengers In addition, glycine is needed in detoxification. Glycine is one of three amino acids that make up glutathione, one of the key detoxifying enzymes.

Due to all its functions, increased intake of glycine has shown improvements in tissue repair by improving energy and oxygen to the cells. Glycine has shown to accelerate liver recovery in an alcohol-induced liver injury. Glycine enhances gastric acid secretion in the stomach, improving digestion and stomach ulcers. Glycine has shown promise in preventing cancerous tumor growth. Glycine is referred to as an "inhibitory" neurotransmitter since it has anti-stress properties. Increased intake of glycine has shown to improve sleep, memory, and learning.

I recommend using 8 ounces bone broth, salt, and ½ cup fruit *or* 6 ounces orange juice, a dash of salt, and 1 tablespoon hydrolyzed gelatin (powdered gelatin) as a natural sleep aid. The added glycine, in a stressed body, calms the system and allows for deeper sleep. I never recommend taking glycine by itself to receive its benefits. I feel amino acids work better in their natural food source. Thus, drinking broth and/or adding powdered gelatin to your food or drink is the best way to add more glycine to your diet.

What About Powdered Gelatin?

Powdered gelatin is gelatin that has been dried and processed into a powder. This type of gelatin is used to make Jell-O, custards, mousses, ice cream, gummy candy, soups, and sauces. Most powdered gelatins are made of only the skins or hides of the animals. Because of this, powdered gelatin lacks the minerals, glucosamine, and glycosaminoglycans (GAGs) found in homemade broths.

However, powdered gelatin still contains the same amino acid profile as the gelatin you get from broth, so it is still a beneficial protein. There are some benefits of using the powdered gelatin: Gelatin can be added to smoothies, soups, sauces, and workout drinks to increase protein intake, it is easy to travel with, and it takes no effort to make.

Types of Powdered Gelatin

1. Bovine (beef) gelatin. Bovine gelatin comes from the hides of grass-fed cows. It can be used to add thickness and creaminess to foods. Use this gelatin to make gummy candies, marshmallows, ice cream, custards, soups, sauces,

and mousses. Bovine gelatin must be melted in warm water to thicken properly. Do not use this gelatin in cold drinks or smoothies, as it will not dissolve.

2. Porcine (pig) gelatin. Porcine gelatin comes from the skin of pigs. It carries the same properties of bovine gelatin. It is best to dissolve in warm water before using.

3. Hydrolyzed gelatin. Hydrolyzed gelatin has been processed more so that it can dissolve in cold water. Hydrolyzed gelatin works best in smoothies, workout drinks, and coffee (unless you want really thick coffee). Hydrolyzed gelatin will not thicken, even when added to warm liquids.

My personal preference for grass-fed gelatin is Great Lakes Gelatin (www.GreatLakesGelatin.com).

Bone Broth: A Good Source of Minerals

Not only does homemade broth provide the healing effects of gelatin and glycine, but it also provides many essential minerals. Bones and connective tissue are filled with calcium, phosphorus, magnesium, potassium, sodium, and sulfur. When bones are cooked for hours in hot water, vinegar, and salt, the bones break down and the very minerals that made up the bones get absorbed into the broth.

What Is Calcium?

Ninety-nine percent of calcium is stored in the skeletal system (the bones are referred to as Calcium banks). The other 1 percent is located in the soft tissue and blood. Every day there is a transfer of calcium among the bones, cells, and blood. Thus, since we do not make our own calcium within the body, a constant intake of dietary calcium is needed. Without proper intake, the body will pull calcium from our calcium banks (bones) and use it for cellular function. This is one big reason why we need to be ingesting an adequate level of calcium every day.

Calcium is needed for bone and teeth structure, blood clotting, nerve and cell function, muscular contraction, regulating the heartbeat, and lowering blood pressure by down-regulating parathyroid hormone (PTH). Bone broth, along with dairy, are your best sources of calcium.

These essential minerals can help with muscle cramping and relaxation. Calcium, magnesium, sodium, and potassium are all electrolytes needed for proper cell function. A nice warm broth could be used as a pre-during-post workout drink on a cold winter day due its mineral content. Adding a little salt, coconut oil, and a cup of OJ can make a great post-workout meal to help relax the muscles and allow the body to recover.

Finally, bone broth contains glycosaminoglycans (GAGs) and glucosamine. Both are used in the structure of joint cartilage and joint lubrication. They provide the joint with a shock absorber.

Glycosaminoglycans (GAGs)

GAGs are a major component of joint cartilage. GAGs are found in bone broth and act like an additional gelling agent. There are three GAGs found in broth: keratin sulfate, hyaluronic acid, and chondroitin sulfate. Chondroitin sulfate is the most studied and most noted of the GAGs. Most of you have heard of chondroitin. Chondroitin along with glucosamine is the most widely sold non-vitamin/mineral supplement.

Chondroitin sulfate is an important structural compound found in cartilage that provides compression in the joint. Some studies have found the addition of chondroitin into the diet can improve arthritis and joint pain.

Glucosamine

Glucosamine is an amino sugar used as a precursor to synthesize glycosaminoglycans. Glucosamine is found in shellfish, animal bones, and bone marrow. Extensive research has been done on both chondroitin sulfate and glucosamine in their effects on joint repair and people with arthritis. According to the largest clinical trial on glucosamine and chondroitin, the Glucosamine/chondroitin Arthritis Intervention Trial (GAIT), 79 percent of people with moderate to severe joint pain showed significant pain relief with a glucosamine-chondroitin supplement.

Yet, although glucosamine with chondroitin is the most widely consumed non-vitamin/mineral supplement, wouldn't it make more sense to just consume bone broth and get the added bonus of gelatin protein, calcium, magnesium, potassium, sodium, and sulfur? I think so.

How Do You Make Bone Broth?

Although making broth seems like a daunting task to some, in truth it is quite easy. Add bones, water, vinegar, and salt to a pot of water and allow it to simmer for 3 to 4 hours. Add additional vegetables during the last hour.

The keys to a great broth are as follows:

- Make sure to use bones with lots of collagen attached like oxtail, chicken feet, knuckle bones, and chicken necks.

- Always roast the bones prior to adding to water. This will allow the bones to break down better.

- Adding vinegar, lemon juice, and/or orange juice will aid in the bone breakdown.

- Only add enough water to top the bones. Too much water will not allow the broth to gel.

- Do not cook your broth for longer than 4 hours or you risk degrading the amino acids. Excess cooking can also oxidize the nutrients, particularly iron, found in bone marrow bones.

- Use a pressure cooker, crock pot, or covered pot to keep the liquid from escaping.

A complete broth recipe can be found in Chapter 20.

Just so you know store-bought bone broth is a far cry from the homemade version. MSG and other additives are used in store-bought broths to give them a meaty taste. Even the organic varieties don't use actual bones to make the broths. Most are made with skins only, therefore the minerals, GAGs, and glucosamine are missing.

How to Use Bone Broth

All people can benefit from drinking bone broth. For a healthy person, 1–2 cups a day can help keep the gut, liver, and joints healthy and happy. For a person in hypo-metabolic state (low body temperature, tired, fat gain, sleep issues, hormonal issues, low pulse, depression, etc.) 3–4 cups or more of bone broth can be consumed daily.

Drink broth as a meal with added fat and carbohydrates. Broth with coconut oil, Parmesan cheese, and mashed potatoes makes a hearty and healthy meal. Broth can be sipped during the day or at night as a sleep aid. Always add broth to a meal that includes muscle meats to balance the inflammatory amino acids.

Remember if you run out of broth or just don't want to make it, using the powdered gelatin can be a good alternative. Powdered gelatin can be added to sauces, gravies, soups, desserts, smoothies, orange juice, coffee, milk, and tea. For people in a hypo-metabolic state, up to 50 percent of their protein needs can come from bone broth and gelatin. Healthy people should consume 25–35 percent of their protein needs from gelatin and broth.

Wow! Who knew there was so much more to Grandma's chicken soup? Years ago, I had no idea homemade bone broth contained so many healing properties. I just thought it was warm, was easy on the stomach, and tasted good—which are all true. Now I know broth is filled with anti-inflammatory proteins, glucosamine,

GAGs and minerals like calcium and magnesium. Drinking broth daily can improve your digestion, decrease inflammation and pain in the joints, and help you sleep, think, and look better. I don't know about you, but broth seems a whole lot cheaper and healthier than tons of painkillers, antacids, face creams, and sleeping pills. Maybe Suzie was right: Broth is miracle juice!

The super proteins should make up the majority of your protein intake, especially when you are trying to heal your metabolism. Due to their digestibility and high nutritional content, they are perfect foods for anyone trying to regain or maintain great health. Like *all* proteins, super proteins should be consumed with the right carbohydrates and fats to help maintain blood sugar and energy levels. The one exception to that rule—solely because it comes already packaged as the perfect combination of protein, carbs, and fat—is milk.

Chapter 8:
What You Need to Know

1. Milk is the perfect balance of fat, carbs, and protein. It contains high calcium content and is filled with other vitamins and minerals.

2. Pastured-organic eggs are filled with protein, fat, carotenoids, vitamins A, E, D, and K, calcium, iron, phosphorus, zinc, thiamin, B6, folate, B12, pantothenic acid, choline, potassium, magnesium, copper, manganese, and selenium.

3. Grass-fed beef liver is one of the most nutritionally packed foods on the planet, with high levels of vitamin A and the B vitamins. Liver also includes vitamins D, E, and K, calcium, iron, magnesium, selenium, copper, zinc, and phosphorus.

4. Shellfish and low-fat fish are filled with easy-to-digest protein and are filled with vitamins A, C, D, and E and the B vitamins. Shellfish also include zinc, copper, selenium, iron, magnesium, sodium, and manganese.

5. Potato protein is a high-quality protein due to its keto acids. Potatoes also contain vitamins C, D, and K, folate, niacin, pantothenic acid, B6, choline, calcium, potassium, magnesium, phosphorus, copper, manganese, iron, and zinc.

6. Gelatin and bone broth have been used to treat not only the common cold but gastrointestinal issues, joint pain, depression, constipation, liver support, anti-aging, and improved hair, skin, nail, and bone health. Bone broth and gelatin lack the inflammatory amino acids and are rich in anti-inflammatory amino acids alanine, hydroxyproline, proline, and especially glycine.

Chapter 9
Dairy and Milk (The Perfect Food)

Consuming milk after the age of seven seems to be one of the most controversial topics in nutrition today. When I ask health-minded people about milk and why they think milk gets a bad name, I get every kind of answer: *Milk makes you fat, milk encourages mucus, milk has hormones and antibiotics, pasteurization is bad, milk causes gut cramping and gas, I'm lactose intolerant, etc.* Yikes. With thoughts like these, no wonder drinking milk has been shunned by so many health-minded people. Who wants to get fat, gassy, and filled with mucus?

Back in my mid-30s I gave up milk and most dairy for about two years. I was convinced that humans were not meant to drink milk past childhood. What other mammals drink the milk of another animal? None. What other animals drink milk into adulthood? None. Of course, no other mammals drive cars, wear clothes (unless you're my dog), cook their food, or surf the Internet. But, that was beside the point. I was convinced: "I am an adult. It is no longer healthy for me to drink milk." So, instead I consumed copious amounts of almond milk, soymilk, rice milk, or whatever "en vogue" milk was being marketed to me.

I emphasize "marketed to me," because when I look back, I see a good part of my nutrition and dairy choices were influenced *heavily* by food manufacturers, magazine ads, and the USDA. I was told these milk products were healthy for me because they contained "0" cholesterol, were low in saturated fat, low in sugar, high in the "good fats" (polyunsaturated/PUFAs), and were fortified with vitamins and minerals. Well, it is now known that cholesterol and saturated fat are not the enemies. It is also understood that polyunsaturated fats are highly oxidative and damaging. We also know that sugar is needed for a high metabolic rate and that anything synthetic or fortified with nutrients is not the best for us. This is when I began to realize that the manufactured milks (almond, rice, and soy) were anything but healthy for me, so I had to shift my thinking once again.

I also realized that what I knew about dairy was only surface information. Once I started to look deeper, I began to realize dairy is not the problem; the degradation (over-processing and reducing the quality) of dairy is the problem. Quality, organic, pastured dairy is an amazing food. In fact it could, quite possibly, be nature's perfect food.

First, What Is Milk?

Milk is a white liquid produced by the mammary glands of mammals. As far as I know, almonds, rice, and soy do not have mammary glands. Milk from cows, sheep, and goats has tremendous nutritional benefits, including high levels of bone- building calcium. Milk also contains magnesium, potassium, selenium, and vitamins A, B, D, and K. Whole cow's milk contains approximately 87 percent water, 4.6 percent lactose (sugar), 3.4 percent protein, and 4.2 percent fat (most of which is saturated [70 percent] and monounsaturated [25 percent]; less than 2.5 percent of milk fat is polyunsaturated). Higher milk consumption has been linked to lower body fat, lower levels of hyperglycemia (high blood sugar), reduced metabolic syndrome, improved bone density, bone mass, and healthier teeth, and increased milk consumption has been inversely correlated to many cancers including colon and breast cancer. To put it bluntly, milk is one of the most amazing and complete foods you can consume.

Today, I am a big proponent of dairy. I consume milk and other dairy products every day and believe it should be a part of any person's diet, of any age, who is looking for a healthy, metabolically stimulating diet.

However, before I dive deeper into the amazingness of milk, I want to first explain why not all milk and dairy are created equal, and why it is important to understand the health of your own body before guzzling a gallon of milk or eating a pound of cheese.

Not all dairy is created equal.

Organic vs. Conventionally Farmed Milk

Is organic (grass-fed) milk actually better than the conventionally farmed grain-fed milk?

Although there is not a lot of research on the differences between organic milk vs. non-organic, the research that is coming out links the quality of milk to the feeding strategies of the cattle. Knowing cows are designed to eat grass, leaves, and foliage, and not corn, soy, grains, and garbage (yes, conventionally farmed cattle have been fed everything from GMO corn and soy to candy and the candy wrapper), it would make perfect sense that pastured cows produce better milk than conventionally farmed cows. Yet, don't let the obvious convince you. Let's look at the research.

The *Journal of the Science of Food and Agriculture* released a study in 2012 showing that organic dairy produces higher levels of protein and conjugated linoleic acid (CLA). Adequate protein is needed for cellular and muscular repair, hormone and enzyme production, and even blood production. CLA is actually a naturally occurring trans-fat (the hydrogenated trans-fats linked to coronary heart disease are artificially made) that is best known for its anticancer and anti-inflammation properties.

The *Journal of Dairy Science* concluded in a 1999 study that cows grazing on pasture and receiving no supplemental feed had three to five times more CLA in their milk fat than cows fed a grain diet. In many animal and human studies, CLA has been shown to not only slow the growth of cancer on the skin, breast, prostate, and colon, but also to help with weight loss and increased metabolism.

In addition to being more nutritious, pastured milk is less

toxic. Conventionally farmed dairy cattle may be treated with recombinant bovine growth hormone (rBGH). Farmers use rBGH because it can increase a cow's production of milk by 11–25 percent. More milk production equals more money. The problem is milk treated with rBGH has substantially higher levels and more bioavailable insulin growth factor (IGF-1). IGF is absorbed through the gastrointestinal tract, where it has shown growth-promoting effects. Increased levels of IGF have been linked to growth of existing cancer cells, increased aging, and diabetes in humans.

The hormone rBGH has been banned in Canada, Japan, New Zealand, Australia, and the entire European Union—yet, here in the good ol' United States, rBGH is still widely used in the conventional farming dairy industry.

Synthetic Vitamins

Most milk products contain some form of synthetic vitamins A and D. Yes, this is even true for some organic brands. Due to their lower fat content, U.S. law requires that organic low-fat and skim milks must be fortified with additional vitamins A and D. All conventionally farmed milk products, including whole, low-fat, and skim milk varieties, are fortified with vitamins A and D.

The only milk products I have found that have no vitamin additives are all raw organic milk products and some pasteurized whole-milk products. Contact your milk provider if you are unsure of what kind of vitamin additives are in your milk.

Carrageenan

In addition, some milk products, including skim, low-fat versions, and chocolate milk, contain carrageenan. Carrageenan is a natural emulsifier (helps liquids stay together without separating), thickener, and food stabilizer (prevents sugars and ice from crystalizing). Carrageenan is extracted from red seaweed with the use of a powerful alkali solvent. In addition to dairy, Carrageenan is used in most milk alternatives like soy, rice, and almond milks (another reason *not* to consume these milk products). Carrageenan is also used in many meat products and personal hygiene products like toothpaste. Carrageenan has been linked to several types of cancer, arthritis, ulcerations of the intestines, and many other issues. Once again, is it the milk you are drinking *or* is it the additives in the milk that are making it unhealthy for you?

Raw vs. Pasteurized Milk

Pasteurization is a process of heating a food, usually a liquid, to a specific temperature for a specific length of time and then cooling it immediately. The purpose is to kill off all harmful bacteria and pathogens. The problem is that pasteurization also kills the good bacteria (probiotics); alters the enzymes, proteins, fats, and sugar in milk; and creates a less-healthy food.

Food Chemistry published a report in 1994 showing that heated milk has reduced levels of iron, manganese, and copper. The CDC confirms that vitamin C and vitamin B6 are also reduced in pasteurized milk. Beta-lactoglobulin, a milk protein, increases the absorption of vitamin A. Beta-lactoglobulin is heat-sensitive, so pasteurization alters the effects of this protein, decreasing the absorption of vitamin A.

Weston A. Price, a dentist who traveled the world in search of the causes of tooth decay and physical degeneration, reported how isolated indigenous people had healthier straight teeth and far less disease than cultures who had been infected with Western diets. Price reported in his book *Nutrition and Physical Degeneration* how diets of these indigenous cultures contained four times the calcium and minerals, and 10 times the fat-soluble vitamins and minerals. Price attributed the health of these cultures to their unprocessed traditional diets of raw dairy, shellfish, organ meats, fish, and eggs. These diets were free of additive, fillers, and pasteurized dairy.

According to the Weston A. Price Foundation, non-pasteurized (raw) milk consumption has been shown to positively influence the immune system's resistance to the development of asthma, hay fever, and skin allergies. In fact, many of these primitive cultures used raw milk as a homeopathic healing food.

Now, this is not to say all pasteurized milk is bad. Pasteurized milk still contains high levels of calcium and other minerals. Pasteurized milk also contains adequate fat, protein, and sugars to make it a complete food. The downside of raw milk is the cost: Raw milk costs about twice as much as most organic pastured milks. Raw milk also spoils much faster due to it being a live food. In many states raw milk is illegal to buy and sell. Many people find raw milk disagrees with their gut's ecosystem due to the increased levels of live bacteria. For these people pasteurized or even ultra-pasteurized works best.

An organic pastured variety may be your best bet if you live in a state that does not sell raw milk. The key is to find the best available milk to you. For raw milk information check out www.RealMilk.com.

Homogenization

Milk homogenization is defined as an intense blending of milk to create a constant consistency (it blends the fat into the liquid portion by forcing the milk fat at high pressure through small holes/mesh). The fat in non-homogenized milk normally separates from the liquid and rises to the top. Homogenization breaks the fat into smaller particles so that the milk does not separate and has a creamier, more consistent look.

Sounds innocent enough, right? Here is the potential problem:

The homogenization process may damage milk fats, proteins, and enzymes (by breaking them apart). Catherine Shanahan, MD, in her book *Deep Nutrition* talks about how casein micelle complexes, which are held by calcium phosphate, are broken up through homogenization. This exposes the tightly held fat molecules to calcium, producing calcium soaps. These soaps can produce gut irritation and decrease the bioavailability of calcium.

Non-homogenized milk does not have this effect on the

digestive system, since the fats are kept intact. The fats, proteins, and enzymes pass normally through the stomach and digestive tract, and are used properly by our bodies just as Mother Nature designed.

Although most current scientific research will state homogenized milk is just as easy to digest as non-homogenized, I'd rather be safe than sorry. Personally, I don't drink homogenized milk. My ultimate belief is the least amount of food degradation the better.

Whole-Fat Milk vs. Lower-Fat Milks

One of the many reasons milk has received such a bad name is due to its saturated fat content. As I discussed above, milk fat is about 70-percent saturated, 25-percent monounsaturated, and 2.3-percent polyunsaturated. Saturated fat has been linked to increased cholesterol, heart disease, and heart attacks. However, as I discussed in earlier chapters, we now know this is not the case. Saturated fat can be very beneficial to our bodies.

Saturated fat is the most stable of all the fats. Saturated fat can help with metabolism, digestion, thyroid function, and liver detoxification. Some studies show increased milk fat intake can decrease heart disease. A study in *The International Journal of Environmental Research and Public Health,* on 1,800 men over 12 years, found that daily intake of fruit and vegetables was associated with a lower risk of coronary heart disease when combined with a high-dairy-fat consumption but not with a low-fat consumption.

One reason for this may have something to do with the fats in milk being needed for vitamin A and D absorption. Remove the fat, and you remove the nutrients, which is why the government has to add the vitamins back in. As I discussed earlier, milk additives are a known allergen to many people. Using whole milk over a reduced-fat version may rid the milk drinker of the allergy.

In addition, most skim and low-fat versions usually contain some form of dried milk to increase the protein content of the milk. Dried milk has to be heated and pressurized to produce a powdered substance. This process produces oxysterols (oxidized cholesterol).

Oxysterols have been shown to increase atherosclerotic plaques. Even though cholesterol in itself is not bad for you, *oxidized* cholesterol can lead to blocked arteries and heart disease.

There are healthy versions of reduced-fat milks. Some reduced-fat versions do not contain additives or dried milk products. My suggestion is to ask your milk producer directly. The benefits of drinking the lower-fat varieties are sports recovery and increased weight loss. Just make sure your reduced-fat milk is free of dried milk and synthetic milk additives.

Lactose Intolerance

The history of milk tells us that thousands of years ago, most adults were unable to digest milk past the age of seven due to their inability to produce the enzyme lactase. Lactase is an enzyme humans produce in the microvilli of the small intestine. Lactase is released when lactose (milk sugar) enters the intestines. Then, some 9,000 years ago, a genetic mutation spread through Europe that gave people the ability to produce lactase past their adolescent years—thus allowing people to drink and digest milk throughout their entire lives.

When someone becomes "lactose intolerant," more than likely the person's body is no longer producing the enzyme lactase. The question is: Why is this happening? Is it due to the person's heritage and genetics? Possibly. Or, it could be due to their lifestyle choices. An inflamed and damaged small intestine can occur with over-consumption of alcohol, drugs, polyunsaturated fats, grains, processed foods, additives, etc. Once the small intestine becomes damaged, lactase production is inhibited, and thus lactose becomes hard to digest. The result is that milk consumption leads to an inflamed gut that produces gas, bloating, intestinal pain, *and* an inability to digest lactose effectively.

Is Lactose Intolerance Reversible?

The Weston A. Price Foundation conducted a survey of more

than 2,200 people who switched from pasteurized milk to raw milk. Of the 155 people who reported being lactose intolerant before switching to raw, 81 percent reported no symptoms of lactose intolerance after switching to raw milk. The survey concluded the intolerance to milk may be due to the milk processing (versus real, unprocessed milk).

For those who cannot obtain raw milk or do not want to spend the money, healing the gut may be the best bet. Try removing grains and hard-to-digest foods like nuts, raw veggies, and legumes. Add in bone broths, coconut oil, a raw carrot, and gelatin to try to heal the gut and intestinal lining. Biologist, nutrition researcher, and milk advocate Dr. Ray Peat believes you can heal the gut and intestines of lactose intolerance in as little as two weeks. Dr. Peat says first you may want to try adding in a small amount of additive-free cheese (cheese has no lactose). If you can tolerate the cheese, Dr. Peat suggests adding in a little whole, organic, grass-fed milk slowly over time. My suggestion is to start by drinking 1–2 ounces of milk once per day, seven days a week. Each week add another ounce each day until you can drink the desired amount.

Michelle's Story

Michelle is a single career woman turning 40. Michelle has been incredibly active her entire life, working out hard and intense almost every day. Michelle eats a low-carb, no-dairy, no-grain, low-fruit, high-raw-vegetable, high-nut, high-meat protein-type diet. Michelle initially felt great on this program—she lost weight and felt strong—but about a year into the low-carb diet, things began to change.

Michelle complained of fatigue, sleep problems, gas, stomach bloating, lactose intolerance, and fat gain. Michelle was tired of feeling tired and puffy, and she wanted her energy back.

Michelle needed to understand that a low-carb diet is stressful on the body. Too much protein without an adequate amount of carbs increases insulin levels, cortisol, and adrenaline levels. As you now know, good carbs are your body's preferred source of energy. Although the body can survive and get lean on a low-carb plan, long-term this type of diet creates problems.

Michelle's goal was to just feel healthy again, which started with healing her gut. This included a diet filled with bone broth, coconut oil, gelatin, squash and potato soups, a raw carrot, white fish, cooked fruit, salt, and some additive-free cheeses (ricotta and Parmesan Reggiano). Due to Michelle's lactose intolerance, she ate only cheese and a little yogurt.

After the first month, Michelle's energy started to return, her sleep improved, and her stomach was less bloated. At this point, Michelle started to add in a little whole organic milk (2 ounces/day) to see how her body would react. To Michelle's surprise, there was no gas, no bloating, no problem. Whole milk is more tolerable than the lower-fat varieties. Each week Michelle added another 2 ounces of milk, until she reached 3–4 cups a day.

Michelle knew the importance of calcium for her bone health, but she had no idea it could help her sleep better, lose fat, and decrease muscle soreness. Today Michelle drinks milk every day, works out less, eats more, sleeps better, and has maintained her goal weight.

As you can see, there is more to milk than meets the eye. Yes, milk can be considered bad for us. But given the right quality of milk, with the right person, in the right amounts, milk can be very beneficial. I drink milk every day. For me, the benefits of milk far outweigh any negatives.

The Benefits of Drinking Milk

Milk Improves Bone Density

Milk and other dairy products have a high calcium-to-phosphorus ratio. The ratio of calcium to phosphorus in food is very important for bone health. Phosphorus, an important mineral for bone development, in excess can lead to displacing calcium, which will lead to an increase in parathyroid hormone (PTH). Parathyroid hormone is released from the parathyroid gland when blood calcium levels are low. Remember: Calcium is needed not only for healthy bones and teeth but nerve function, blood clotting, and muscle and heart contractions. Due to all its functions, calcium in the blood is closely monitored.

If a person has not ingested sufficient amounts of calcium or too much phosphorus, and the calcium blood levels get too low, parathyroid hormone (PTH) increases and tells the body to absorb more calcium, primarily by pulling calcium from the bones. Chronically high levels of PTH, among other things, will lead to bone breakdown, which will eventually lead to osteoporosis and increased aging. Dairy, with its high calcium and mineral content, helps prevent PTH from rising, decreasing bone breakdown.

According to a 2004 study in *Biofactors Journal,* consuming foods that have double the calcium to phosphorus levels increases calcium absorption and decreases PTH. Milk, with its high level of calcium, makes it an ideal food for healthy bones and teeth. Foods high in phosphorus and low in calcium, like grains, muscle meats, processed foods, and sodas, in excess can inhibit calcium absorption and lead to bone breakdown.

If you want strong, healthy bones consume calcium-rich foods like dairy.

A study in *Osteoporosis International* in 2013 reported higher levels of both bone mass and bone density in 4,800 men and women ages 66–95 who consumed milk regularly throughout their lives.

A study in *Nutrition and Research Practice* reported the relationship between adolescent boys' and girls' bone mineral density and milk consumption: of the 664 adolescent ages 15–17, those who consumed more milk had better bone mineral density without increased weight gain.

Milk Improves Body Mass

Milk, often promoted as a fattening food by milk opponents, is continually linked to people who are less fat. One explanation for lower body mass is the effect calcium has on the body's cells. When adequate amounts of calcium are in the diet, parathyroid hormone

(PTH) is kept low. According to Dr. Ray Peat, "When PTH is kept low, cells increase their formation of the uncoupling proteins, that cause mitochondria to use energy at a higher rate."

The mitochondria of every cell are where the energy is produced. Increasing the mitochondria's energy production increases overall metabolism.

Nutrient Journal reported in a 2013 study of 720 men and women that increased dairy consumption is linked to a more favorable body composition. Current research in Korea, Europe, the United States, and Brazil has also shown a strong correlation between milk drinkers and lower body mass and improved health.

Even in the elderly, a study from the *Journal of Academy of Nutrition and Dietetics* reported in 2013 an association of higher dairy intake to better overall body mass and increase physical performance in 1,456 women ages 70–85.

Milk Helps Regulate Blood Pressure and Improve Cardiovascular Health

David McCarron, a hypertension researcher at Oregon Health And Science University, has done quite a bit of research showing how low calcium can increase blood pressure. Low calcium increases PTH, which decreases calcium in the bone and increases soft tissue calcification. If the heart and blood vessels retain calcium they will not be able to relax fully, leading to an increase in blood pressure.

A study in the *Journal of the American College of Nutrition* in 2009 reported that consumption of dairy foods showed improvements in blood pressure in hypertensive men.

A study in *Hypertension Journal* followed 2,512 men over a 23-year period. The men who consumed the highest level of dairy had significantly lower blood pressure than the men who consumed the lowest amount of dairy.

Several studies including the Helena Study in Europe have shown an inverse relationship between milk consumption and cardiovascular disease (CVD). Countries like France, Sweden, Italy, Greece, Switzerland, and Denmark have some of the highest levels of dairy consumption yet have some of the lowest levels of hypertension and CVD.

Milk's Other Health Benefits

Milk consumption has produced improvements with people who have metabolic syndrome, hyperglycemia, diabetes, and breast and colon cancers. Milk consumption also shows improved absorbency of some vitamins and minerals, including calcium, vitamin A, and vitamin B12—all needed for optimal health and a high functioning metabolism.

Milk: A Complete Food

Milk contains a balanced ratio of fats, carbs, and proteins. Whole milk contains 8 grams of each of these macronutrients. Milk also contains calcium, magnesium, potassium, selenium, and iron, and the vitamins A, B2, B12, K, and D. This makes milk a great blood sugar regulator and a healthy snack between meals. Milk provides the right amount of sugars to maintain good energy, proteins for recovery, and fat for increased satiety.

This is one reason why I recommend drinking milk with added sugar, honey, or cacao post-workout. Milk, especially chocolate milk, has been researched extensively as a post-workout recovery drink. Research shows that milk can improve recovery after an event and can increase performance level for a following event.

Following are my personal recommendations.

Milk
Good health:

This is my order of preference.

1. Raw (non-homogenized, non-pasteurized), grass-fed, organic whole milk is best (no additives).

2. Pasteurized, non-homogenized, grass-fed, organic whole milk (no additives).

3. Pasteurized and homogenized organic, grass-fed whole milk (no additives).

4. Pasteurized and homogenized organic, grass-fed 2% or 1% milk.

Remember: The less processing, additives, and degradation your milk has gone through, the more healthful this food will be for you. Quality is king! Check out www.RealMilk.com for more information on raw dairy.

Sports recovery:

1. Pasteurized, non-homogenized organic, grass-fed 1% or 2% milk with added honey, sugar, or raw cacao.

2. Pasteurized and homogenized organic, grass-fed 2% or 1% milk with added honey, sugar, or raw cacao.

It's important to have the sugars get into your system fast for glycogen replenishment. Milk high in fat will slow this process.

Fat loss:

1. Pasteurized, non-homogenized organic, grass-fed 1% or 2% milk.

2. Pasteurized and homogenized organic, grass-fed 1% or 2% milk.

When looking for fat loss, drinking 3–4 cups of full fat milk can hinder fat loss. Reduced-fat milk can still offer the benefits of increased calcium, magnesium, potassium, vitamins, CLA, protein, sugars, and fat without the added fat calories.

What About Other Dairy?

Cheese

I love cheese and, just like milk, cheese can be a very nutritious food—as long as it is the right cheese. The problem with most cheese is not the fat content but the addition of fillers, including GMO cultures, food coloring, GMO rennet and enzymes, cellulose, artificial and "natural" flavoring, gums, carrageenan, and whey protein. The additives in cheese may become allergenic, which makes most people blame the cheese, not the additives.

As with all foods, your best cheeses are the ones that contain the least amount of additives. Here are my top four cheeses and their ingredients:

1. Organic ricotta cheese: Skim milk, salt, vinegar.

2. Parmesan Reggiano: Milk, salt, and animal rennet.

3. Mascarpone: Heavy cream and lemon juice.

4. Cottage cheese: Whole milk, cream, skim milk, salt, and natural cultures. Make sure your cottage cheese is free of carrageenan and gums. Wash the curds if you are sensitive to lactic acid.

Yogurt

Fermented foods like yogurt can be fine for most in small amounts. I do not recommend eating yogurt as a main source of protein or calcium; milk and cheese are better options. According to Dr. Ray Peat, "The lactic acid in yogurt triggers the inflammatory reactions, leading to fibrosis eventually, and the immediate effect is to draw down the liver's glycogen stores for energy to convert it into glucose." For anyone who is hypoglycemic, has an overburdened liver, or is hypo-metabolic, any type of yogurt may not be an ideal food.

Choose plain Greek 2% yogurt. Greek yogurt has less additives, more protein, and less lactic acid; is high in calcium; and tastes great.

Clean sources of milk and dairy offer so many benefits to people's health it is a shame so many health-conscious people have shunned dairy. Many current diet plans claim milk is fattening, leads to CVD, and can cause cancer. The truth is milk consumption improves body composition, bone density, mineral absorption, blood pressure, insulin sensitivity, and muscle recovery, and may decrease a person's chances of certain cancers. I think it is important to remember that not all milk and dairy are created equal. Additives, pasteurization, homogenization, and fat content can all play a role in how well you tolerate dairy. My advice is to not give up on milk and dairy. Do a little research and find a quality, local source near you, or at the very least buy an organic-grass-fed source. For once the ads are *true*: Milk does a body good!

Chapter 9:
What You Need to Know

1. Dairy and milk are your best sources of usable calcium. Milk also contains magnesium, potassium, and selenium, and vitamins A, B, D, and K.

2. Organic milk is best. Research shows cows that eat grass produce milk with higher levels of CLA and protein. Organic milk is also free of hormones and antibiotics.

3. Raw milk is preferred over pasteurized or homogenized milks for its increased nutritional benefits.

4. Lactose intolerance may be a sign of poor gut function versus the inability to produce lactase. Many people can improve their milk digestibility by healing the gut and adding milk back into the diet very slowly.

5. Milk can improve bone density, body mass, cardiovascular health, metabolic syndrome, hyperglycemia, diabetes, and breast and colon cancers.

Chapter 10
What About Muscle Meats?

There is a lot of gray area when it comes to how much muscle meat (chicken, lamb, beef, turkey, bison, venison) is "okay" in a healthy diet.

Many studies report excessive meat intake leads to heart attacks, bone demineralization, and obesity.

Dr. Colin Campbell, professor of nutritional biochemistry at Cornell University and author of *The China Study*, which promotes a plant-based diet, would lead the reader to believe consumption of muscle meats promotes cancer, autoimmune issues, and increased aging. Dr. Campbell believes the best diet contains zero muscle meat.

The average American consumes 270 pounds of meat per year, most of that coming from a non-grass-fed source. Americans are also overweight, and have increasing rates of heart disease and cancer. So should we conclude that eating muscle meat is a death sentence?

Not so fast.

Dr. Loren Cordain, professor in the department of health and exercise science at Colorado State University and author of *The Paleo Diet*, reports that higher animal protein diets can help with diabetes, kidney stones, osteoporosis, and heart disease. Dr. Cordain believes a healthy diet should consist of 19- to 40-percent protein, primarily lean meats, fish, and organ meats. Cultures like the Masai and Aborigines, who eat a diet high in muscle protein and low in plants, have very little heart disease and cancer.

As you can see, when it comes to meat eating, there are two very conflicting views, both supported by facts and history, which can leave you wondering which view is true. Well, there is some truth to both. If you have realized anything by now, nothing is black and white when it comes to nutritional guidelines. Meat eating can add benefits to the diet of a healthy person. Yet, meat eating, in excess or by a person in a hypo-metabolic state, can produce inflammation, a slower metabolism, and increased disease.

The Downsides of Muscle Meats
High in Inflammatory Amino Acids
Muscle meats are high in the inflammatory amino acids tryptophan, cysteine, histidine, and methionine. As I discussed in Chapter 7 about protein, excess inflammatory amino acids can initiate a stress response in the body increasing the hormone cortisol and lowering thyroid function. The typical American diet of 12 ounces of muscle meat per day, in my opinion, is far too high. Increased muscle meat breakdown allows for increased inflammatory amino acids in the blood. Anyone with an autoimmune disorder like arthritis is advised to stay away from a diet high in meat for this very reason. The increased meat intake will exacerbate their condition due to the inflammatory amino acids. Those with other conditions like gout, diabetes, and cancer are also advised to minimize their meat intake.

High Phosphorus-to-Calcium Ratio
Muscle meats, like grains, are high in phosphorus and low in calcium. The ratio of phosphorus to calcium in the body is important in maintaining bone and teeth health. Phosphorus, an essential nutrient needed for strong bones and teeth, and energy production, in excess will increase parathyroid hormones and cause calcium to leach from the bones. High phosphorus-to-calcium diets can impair the synthesis of vitamin D (needed for calcium absorption), which will disrupt calcium homeostasis.

Wayne Campbell, PhD, of Purdue University, in 2010 performed a study on postmenopausal women, weight loss, bone density, and protein intake. Dr. Campbell found that increased muscle protein intake promoted a decrease in bone density after weight loss. The high protein diets consisted of 26-percent muscle protein from chicken and beef. Since we know muscle meat is high in phosphorus and low in calcium, this conclusion makes perfect sense. However, this does not necessarily mean a diet of 26-percent protein is bad; it just means a diet of 26-percent *meat protein* may be bad. A diet rich in dairy, bone broth, and eggs would have a far different effect due to its high calcium-to-phosphorus ratio, added nutrients, and improved amino acid profile.

This confirms why the majority of one's protein sources should come from the super proteins and not just muscle meats.

Conventionally Farmed Meats

Unfortunately, most of the meat Americans are consuming is coming from conventionally farmed animals. Most conventionally farmed cattle are fed genetically modified (GMO) grains, primarily GM corn and GM soy. Since the farmers' goal is to fatten the cattle, not give it a long and healthy life, the anti-metabolic foods, soy, and corn are used to fatten the cattle *fast*. Farmers are also feeding their cattle what's called "by-product feed-stuff"; this consists of waste products from the manufacturing of human and animal food. This can include same species animals, diseased animals, hooves, skin, hair, manure, other wastes, plastic, bubble gum, candy, and garbage. In addition, conventionally farmed cattle are fed cheap-protein supplements, antibiotics, and other drugs, including growth hormones.

The end result is very sick cattle. Typically, these feedlot cattle farmers try to manage the grain-caused ailments with a medicine chest of drugs, including ionophores (to buffer acidity) and antibiotics (to reduce liver abscesses). An estimated 70 percent of the nation's antibiotics are fed to cattle and poultry to prevent illness and increase growth (just another sign that the drug industry has an unhealthy relationship with the food industry). This means a meat product that is far less superior not only in quality but in nutritional value.

Is Poultry Any Better?

Many nutritionally conscious people think eating lean organic poultry is a healthier option than beef, lamb, or bison due to chicken's lower level of saturated fat. Once again, this is misguided thinking. Chicken and turkeys—even the organic varieties—are consuming a diet high in corn and soy. Due to their corn and soy diets, chicken meat contains more of the metabolism-suppressing polyunsaturated fats. Ruminant animals like cows can convert the unsaturated fats to saturated fats; however, chickens and turkeys are not ruminants and their digestive system does not allow this process, so more polyunsaturated fats will be in the meat. Remember from Chapter 3 that polyunsaturated fats are linked to a suppressed immune system, a sluggish thyroid, and decrease protein digestion.

According to Ray Peat, PhD, "If you depend on chicken for your major protein, it will contribute to suppressing your thyroid and progesterone levels. Meats, other than beef, lamb, venison, and bison, usually contain enough polyunsaturated fat to affect estrogen, testosterone, and energy production."

Years ago, I ate chicken almost every day of my life. Today, I may eat chicken once a month. Pasture-raised organic chicken meat is hard to find; most grocery stores only carry organic chicken. Pasture-raised chickens will consume a natural diet of worms, bugs, and grass, while organic chickens are still fed organic corn and soy.

The Upside of *Grass-Fed* Muscle Meat

Yes, there are some positives to eating muscle meat—as long as it's the right quality of meat. As I have mentioned several times, when it comes to eating food, including meat, quality is king. If you are going to eat meat, make sure your meat comes from a pastured, grass-fed source.

Pastured, grass-fed cattle are fed—are you ready?—grass. Well, to be honest they are fed grass, weeds, shrubs, clovers, and anything that is green and within reach. According to the USDA grass-fed animals must eat as follows: "Grass and/or forage shall be the feed source consumed for the lifetime of the ruminant animal, with the exception of milk consumed prior to weaning. The diet shall be derived solely from forage, and animals cannot be fed grain or grain by-products and must have continuous access to pasture during the growing season."

Ruminant animals such as cows, bison, and sheep, unlike humans, can digest grass and cellulose (grass fiber). The ruminant animals have a unique four-chamber stomach that allows for a re-chewing process (referred to as ruminating) that allows these animals to fully digest and acquire nutrients from highly fibrous foods like grass. This is why grass is an ideal energy source for them. During the normal digestive process, bacteria in the rumen of cattle produce a variety of acids. When animals are kept on grass pastures, they produce copious amounts of saliva that neutralize the acidity. This saliva allows the rumen to remain at a neutral pH, which is ideal for the cow's health.

A study in the *Journal of Animal Science* reported in 2009 that grass-fed beef is better for human health in a number of ways.

Grass-fed beef has:

1. Less overall fat content

2. More beta-carotene

3. More vitamin E

4. More B vitamins: thiamin and riboflavin

5. More minerals: calcium, potassium, and magnesium

6. A more even ratio between Omega-3 and Omega-6 (Less Omega-6 is found in grass-fed beef.)

7. More conjugated linoleic acid (CLA), which is also found in milk from pastured cattle

8. More selenium and iron

Grass-fed meats are far more healthful than the conventionally farmed, grain-fed varieties. However, they should still be consumed in moderation. Grass-fed meats are still high in the inflammatory amino acids and phosphorus. Thus, high consumption of grass-fed muscle meats, without the protective factors of the other super proteins like bone broth and dairy, can lead to inflammation, degenerative diseases, illness, and aging.

How Much Muscle Meat Is "Healthy"?

This can be a complex question, since the answer is based on the health of the person. The healthier the person, the more muscle meat he or she can consume without negative effects. Most healthy people do fine eating muscle meat two or three times per week. You should always, despite your health, consume muscle meat with a cup of bone broth or a tablespoon of added gelatin. Remember: Bone broth produces a better amino acid profile and adds additional calcium. This makes the muscle meat less inflammatory.

I eat muscle meat, primarily lean beef and bison, one to two times per week. This looks very different from the diet I ate years ago, which consisted of daily chicken and turkey consumption. I feel better eating less muscle meat and eating more of the other animal proteins like fish, dairy, eggs, and bone broth.

For someone in a hypo-metabolic state (slow running metabolism), or who has diabetes, arthritis, gout, cancer, or any other inflammatory disease, I would suggest eliminating muscle meat altogether or at least until his or her health improves. When your system is compromised, muscle meat consumption can place a burden on your liver, digestive system, bones, and joints. For these people it is best to stick with the super proteins and limit the muscle meats to special occasions. We must always remember the health of the person when figuring out what "works" for the individual.

I think we can conclude that muscle meat is not the devil, as Dr. Colin Campbell would lead us to believe. Yet, it shouldn't be 40 percent of our diet, as Dr. Loren Cordain concludes. Yes, some cultures may thrive on a high–muscle meat diet, but there are probably other factors influencing their good health other than muscle meat consumption. The Maasai diet, although high in muscle meat, was also high in raw dairy and raw animal blood, and contained no processed foods. The Aborigine people ate a diet high in wild animal meat, but also in shellfish, root vegetables, and fruit. Their diet was also free of processed foods. Therefore we can conclude, grass-fed muscle meats can be a part of a healthy diet—in a healthy person, in moderation, and combined with bone broth and other super proteins.

Here are two good sources of grass-fed meats:
Healthy Traditions: www.HealthyTraditions.com
U.S. Wellness Meats: www.GrasslandBeef.com

Chapter 10:
What You Need to Know

1. Muscle meats consist of chicken, pork, beef, bison, venison, turkey, and lamb.

2. The downsides of muscle meats are their high phosphorus-to-calcium ratio, their high levels of the inflammatory amino acids, and the use of GM corn and soy used in their feed.

3. Grass-fed meats are preferred to conventional farmed meats due to their lower fat content, higher vitamin and mineral content, and higher CLA levels.

4. Consume all muscle meat with bone broth or gelatin to offset the amino acid profile.

5. The amount of muscle meat a person can handle safely is based on his or her size, activity, and metabolic health.

Chapter 11
Nuts and Seeds:
Too Much of a Good Thing?

I used to eat nuts and seeds like an overzealous chipmunk about to hibernate for the winter. Nuts, seeds, nut and seed bars, and nut butters were a big part of my diet. I ate almond butter in my oatmeal in the morning, a bag of nuts for a snack, and a few nuts on my salad for lunch, and ended my day with a scoop of peanut butter in my protein shake. I was told nuts and seeds were highly nutritious and a metabolic-stimulating food. With the average American consuming more than 4 pounds of nuts each year, and me consuming at least 25 times that amount (I am an overachiever), how could I lose with such a tasty nutritious snack? Oh, let me count the ways.

The fact that animals, like chipmunks and bears, eat a lot of nuts and seeds before hibernation, should be an indication that nuts and seeds are not as supportive to a high-running metabolism like Americans have been led to believe. Think about this for a second. Hibernation is characterized as a time of low body temperature, low heart rate, low pulse, low breathing rate, and low metabolic rate. It could be described as a metabolic depression.

Animals that hibernate need to store enough fat and energy to keep them alive for the four to eight months they don't eat. Yes, these animals eat nothing for as long as eight months. A slow metabolic rate is ideal for hibernating animals, but for health-conscious humans, a slow metabolic rate is not ideal or desirable.

Humans are not designed to hibernate. Yet, we continue to eat foods like nuts and seeds that are anti-metabolic. Why? Because the nut and health industry has told us to eat them!

Within the last 10–20 years, nuts and seeds have been advertised as a "healthy" option for protein and "heart-healthy" fat. While the nut crop reached an increasing value of almost $8 billion in 2012, for nut farmers and the companies that sell nuts, it seems to make sense that we are seeing more advertised health benefits of nut eating. The industry promotes nuts as a high-protein, antioxidant-rich food, packed full of healthy unsaturated fats that help lower cholesterol. The question remains: Are these statements completely true?

First, What Are Nuts and Seeds?

To make it simple, nuts are seeds. A nut is defined as "the dry, one-seeded fruit of any of various trees or bushes, consisting of a kernel, often edible, in a hard and woody or tough and leathery shell more or less separable from the seed itself: walnuts, pecans, chestnuts, acorns, etc. are all nuts." The inner part of the shelled nut is considered the seed, and the tough nut casing is considered the fruit. A seed is defined as "the part of a flowering plant that contains the embryo and will develop into a new plant if sown; a fertilized and mature ovule." All cereal grains, including wheat, corn, and rice, and legumes like beans and soy are also considered seeds.

Nuts and Seeds: Good Source of Protein?

Nuts and seeds contain very little usable protein. Many people believe nuts and seeds are a great source of protein. In truth they are anywhere from 5- to 30-percent protein. Most nuts are around 15-percent protein; seeds are even less. Considering nuts and seeds are a calorically dense food, eating them as a primary protein source would be quite fattening. It would take close to 600 calories to get 25 grams of protein from nuts, with most of those calories coming from fat. The rest of the nuts' and seeds' calories come from carbohydrates.

Nuts and seeds, like soy and grains, contain trypsin inhibitors. Trypsin inhibitors are anti-nutrients that inhibit protein digestion. Their function is to protect the seeds of plants from insects by blocking enzyme function. This is a protective mechanism Mother Nature has given seeds and nuts. This is good for the seeds, but bad for the person or animal wanting to eat them. These trypsin inhibitors prevent protease enzymes from digesting protein in the human's or animal's digestive tract. Therefore, the little bit of protein you may think you are getting from your nuts and seeds may not even be digested.

More Anti-Nutrients in Nuts and Seeds
Polyunsaturated Fats(PUFAs)

If you have been paying attention at all, and I know you have, you know I am not a fan of the unsaturated fats, especially the polyunsaturated fats (PUFAs), which include the Omega-3 and Omega-6 oils. PUFAs are commonly found in grains, legumes (soy), *and* nuts and seeds. The PUFAs in nuts and seeds are actually used as protection toward hungry animals and from the cold winter weather. However, what is protective to the seed has been shown to be toxic to the human.

According to Dr. Ray Peat, nutritional researcher and biologist,

"Polyunsaturated oils defend the seeds from the animals that would eat them, the oils block the digestive enzymes in the animals' stomachs. In addition, seeds and nuts are designed to germinate in early spring, so their energy stores must be accessible when the temperatures are cool, and they normally don't have to remain viable through the hot summer months. Unsaturated oils are liquid when they are cold, and this is necessary for any organism that lives at low temperatures. These oils easily get rancid (spontaneously oxidizing) when they are warm and exposed to oxygen.

When the oils are stored in our tissues, they are much warmer, and more directly exposed to oxygen, than they would be in the seeds, and so their tendency to oxidize is very great. These oxidative processes can damage enzymes and other parts of cells, and especially their ability to produce energy (cellular respiration)."

Like Dr. Peat says, PUFAs are highly oxidative, especially under heat and in the presence of oxygen. This can cause decreased cellular function, leading to disease, aging, and a slower metabolism. (Refer back to Chapter 3 for more information.)

Here is a list of the worst to best nuts/seeds based on PUFA content. (Yes, walnuts are the worst.)

1. Walnuts
2. Sunflower seeds
3. Flax seeds
4. Chia seeds
5. Sesame seeds
6. Pecans
7. Brazil nuts
8. Pistachios
9. Almonds
10. Hazelnuts
11. Cashews
12. Macadamia nuts

Oxalates

Remember oxalates from the grains and vegetable chapters? Well, here we are again. Do you see the many similarities in the seeds and nuts? Oxalates are the natural-occurring chemical found in leafy green plants, nuts, grains, and legumes. According to a study in the *Journal of Food Composition and Analysis*, nuts carry one of the highest levels of oxalates, ranging from 42 to 469mg/100g. According to the study, roasted almonds were the biggest offenders, followed by cashews, hazelnuts, pine nuts, peanuts, walnuts, pecans, and pistachio nuts; raw macadamia nuts contained the least amount of oxalates.

Like I explained in the previous chapters, oxalic acid causes problems because it binds to calcium (CA) in the body, forming oxalates. Oxalates inhibit calcium absorption or, worse, can lead to kidney stones. According to the Chicago Dietetic Association, "kidney stone patients who form calcium oxalate-containing stones are advised to limit their intake of foods which contain >10 mg oxalate per serving, with total oxalate intake not to exceed 50–60 mg/day." Using these guidelines, none of the nuts assessed could be recommended for kidney stone patients.

Phytates or Phytic Acid

In Chapter 5, I referenced the anti-nutrient phytates found in grains. Well, phytates are also located in seeds and nuts, which makes sense since we know grains are seeds. Phytates are usually located in the hard outer shell of the seed and nut referred to as the hull.

Phytates are considered antioxidants because they can inhibit other molecules in the body, such as iron, from oxidizing. Iron in excess becomes an oxidant in the body, and phytates can bind to it, thus inhibiting the oxidation of iron. However, many people, especially menstruating women, need iron, so inhibiting iron may not be a good thing. In addition, phytates can also block the absorption of other important minerals like calcium, magnesium, and zinc.

Phytates have a strong affinity for minerals, and any mineral it binds to will become insoluble. This is how phytates leach nutrients from the body. As you know, phytates are found in grains and in legumes (soy and beans). I think it is important to understand that phytate-rich foods may not only inhibit the nutrients within the food itself but also in the foods eaten with the phytate-containing food.

In other words, the phytates in the seeds and nuts added to your fruit and milk smoothie will not only block the nutrients contained in the seeds/nuts, but also the nutrients in the fruit and milk. Cooking, sprouting, or soaking the nuts and seeds can reduce the effects of phytates.

Lectins

As you know from reading about vegetables and grains, lectins are carbohydrate-binding proteins found in plants, seeds, legumes, grains, and nuts. Foods high in lectins are associated with gastrointestinal distress leading to diarrhea, nausea, bloating, and vomiting. Just like the lectins in leafy greens and grains, the lectins in nuts and seeds can interfere with plasma repair in the gut lining. Therefore, lectins become toxic to wound healing in the gut. If you already have a gut issue (celiac, IBS, colitis), nuts and seeds with lectins can exacerbate the issue.

Amy's Story

Amy, a 38-year-old busy career woman, was also a Cross-fitter (Crossfit is common high intensity/weight training workout) and a fairly strict Paleo (lower carb) eater. Amy ate tons of meat and veggies, and loved to chow down on nuts and seeds every minute of the day. Amy was very fit and lean, and looked the part—except for a distended belly that drove her nuts (no pun intended). Amy, like most strict Paleo eaters, focused on wild meats, fish, nuts, vegetables, and some fruits—not a bad diet, but not an easy diet to digest and process, either.

Nuts and raw vegetables can be hard for the body to digest once the metabolism gets "stressed." When the stress hormones are high, digestion is compromised. Crossfitters are known for stressing the body with their very intense workouts and carbohydrate-restricted diet—one reason why they are so "lean" looking. (Remember: Lean and fit does necessarily mean healthy.) Tack on the trypsin inhibitors, lectins, and PUFAs in the nuts and seeds, and Amy had a recipe for "bloated belly."

To fix Amy's distended belly she removed all the foods she was having a hard time digesting, starting with nuts and seeds.

Instead of nuts and seeds, Amy ate Parmesan or ricotta cheese with fruit as a snack. She removed the raw vegetables and added cooked fruit or cooked vegetables. Finally, she added in 2 cups of bone broth daily to help heal her gut. Amy also toned down her workouts and her workload to try to decrease her total stress load. A stressed body has a hard time digesting food properly, especially raw and fibrous foods. Within four weeks, Amy's belly flattened and she began to feel less bloated. Needless to say, Amy is no longer a strict Paleo eater and is better because of it.

What About Roasted Nuts?

The good news about cooking your nuts and seeds is that cooking will decrease the effects of phytates and trypsin inhibitors. Cooking the nuts and seeds allows the fibers to break down and allows for easier digestibility. Problem solved!

If only it could be that easy.

The bad news comes in how the nuts and seeds are cooked. Most nuts and seeds are "roasted," also known as fried. This usually means they were fried and cooked in more vegetable oil, adding insult to injury in the amount of PUFAs you are about to ingest. Some nuts and seeds are dry-roasted, which is better but unfortunately still damages the nut or seed. A study published in the *Journal of Agricultural and Food Chemistry* found that nuts and seeds that were roasted had a higher degree of fat oxidation and increased levels of trans-fats. Research also shows that roasting nuts and seeds at high temperatures denatures the protein. The denatured protein loses its structure and can become harder to digest—one more strike for nuts and seeds as a "good source" of protein.

Are Raw Nuts and Seeds Better?

Many health-conscious people think they are winning the battle over nuts and seeds by eating them raw. I used to be one of those people. However, upon further investigation, I now believe eating raw nuts may be worse than eating the dry-roasted ones. Why? Mostly for the reasons I have already explained. Raw nuts are filled with phytates, lectins, and trypsin inhibitors. Raw nuts are almost indigestible by the human body. They can cause irritation in the gut and small intestine by getting "stuck" in the intestinal micro- filli; this can cause inflammation, bacterial overgrowth, bloating, and gas. Don't believe me? Check out your stool after you eat a load of raw nuts and seeds. They may reappear—intact.

Pesticides and Herbicides

The fats in seeds and nuts have a high affinity for attracting toxic pesticides and herbicides. The high fat content allows nuts and seeds to absorb the toxic chemicals into their seed. Even though seeds have their own defense systems, they are still preyed upon by other animals and bugs. Farmers use toxic pesticides and herbicides to deter the animals. Organic nuts and seeds are usually, but not always, free of toxic pesticides.

What About the Cholesterol-Lowering Effect of Nuts?

Nuts and seeds are filled with polyunsaturated fats (PUFAs), and as I talked about in Chapter 3, PUFAs have an immune-suppressing effect on your body. Cholesterol is part of your immune system. Cholesterol is elevated by the liver when your body is in a state of inflammation to help protect your cells. Your body in flames as a protective mechanism. PUFAs, acting as an immune-suppressive drug, will decrease inflammation *and* lower your protective cholesterol. This is one reason arthritics experience relief on the Omega-3 oils (PUFA oils): because they decrease inflammation.

The polyunsaturated fats (Omega-3s and Omega-6s) in the nuts are interacting with the liver enzymes that produce cholesterol, decreasing cholesterol production. We always have to remember: Just because something suppresses a symptom does not mean it is good for us. Liver disease, malnutrition, malabsorption, and chronic infection can all suppress bad cholesterol, *and* toxins like alcohol and estrogen can increase HDL (good cholesterol).

Don't be fooled into thinking you are doing something healthy by eating tons of nuts to help with your lipid profile. It is better to figure out why your body is inflamed and begin healing the system, versus just eliminating the symptom with nuts, supplements, and drugs.

But, I Love Nuts and I Don't Want to Give Them Up!

If after you read *all* this you still want to consume nuts and seeds, you need to take a few things into consideration:

- Eat organic whenever possible. This is going to cost you—up to $25/pound—but it is worth saving the toxic load.

- Sprout and soak your nuts to decrease the effects of trypsin inhibitors, phytates, and lectins.

- Eat in moderation. Even organic, sprouted, and soaked nuts and seeds contain the anti-metabolic polyunsaturated fats. Instead of daily, restrict your nut eating to one to two times a week.

- Try to consume nuts with the least amount of PUFAs. Hazelnuts, macadamia nuts, and cashews are your best options.

As you can see, nuts and seeds, as a protein source, are not your best option. Nuts and seeds are filled with immune-suppressive, anti-metabolic polyunsaturated fats. In addition, nuts and seeds contain trypsin inhibitors, lectins, and phytates, all of which will disrupt proper digestion and absorption. Big dollars are made in the nut and seed industry, so it is imperative that the industry leaders find "healthy" reasons for you to buy more nuts. As far as I am concerned, none of the short-term health claims have long-term health benefits. So unless you are a hibernating bear or squirrel, there are far better options for a protein source than nuts and seeds.

Chapter 11:
What You Need to Know

1. Nuts and seeds are not a good source of protein. Only 15–30 percent of the nut is protein, seeds even less. In addition, seeds and nuts contain trypsin inhibitors, which inhibit protein digestion.

2. Nuts and seeds contain high levels of polyunsaturated fats (PUFAs). These PUFAs decrease thyroid function, decrease digestive enzymes, and decrease the ability of the cell to produce energy. Macadamia, hazelnuts, and cashews are better nut choices due to their lower levels of PUFAs.

3. Nuts and seeds contain other anti-nutrients like oxalates, phytates, and lectins.

4. Lightly roasting, sprouting, and soaking nuts and seeds can increase their digestibility and decrease their levels of anti-nutrients.

5. Organic nuts are preferred over non-organic due to their lower levels of pesticides and herbicides.

Chapter 12
Legumes and Soy: Health Foods or Hormone Disruptors?

In my book (really in *my* book), legumes are a digestive catastrophe. All I can think about when ingesting legumes is the amount of farting that will soon follow (sorry). In fact, I know very few people who do not have some sort of digestive distress after eating a big serving of legumes—primarily good ol' beans.

The funny thing is when I ask most people about legumes, they are not even sure what they are. Are they a seed? Are they a vegetable? Are they a bean? Well, no fear—I am here to clear the air. (Yes, I can rhyme.) I am sure most of you want to become legume-educated consumers, so here we go.

For the purpose of this book, I'm going to give you a somewhat quick overview of legumes, since they have such similarities to other grains and seeds, and then proceed into what I believe is the worst legume offender: soybeans.

What the Heck Is a Legume?

A legume can be referred to as grain, a seed (yes, another seed), or the fruit of the plant. Legumes are known for their high "fixed nitrogen" content. Nitrogen is a part of all proteins. Legumes convert the fixed nitrogen into protein. Bacteria can break down the plant, releasing the nitrogen back into the soils, which makes legumes useful for fertilization. Popular legumes include peas, chickpeas, soybeans, lima beans, kidney beans, peanuts, lentils, and green beans.

On average, legumes contain anywhere from 10 to 25 percent protein. Most legume calories come from carbohydrates and then fat. The Protein-Digestibility Corrected Amino Acid Score (PDCAA) gives many legumes a high protein rating. The PDCAA is the preferred measure for establishing the measurement of protein value for human nutrition. However, current research has shown that the high level of anti-nutrients in legumes is inhibiting protein digestibility and absorption. Thus, the PDCAA may not be as accurate as previously considered.

Legumes are another food, like grains, seeds, and many raw vegetables, for which we must look past the cover (the nutrition) to really see what's inside (absorption and digestibility). Like these other foods, legumes are high in anti-nutrients, lectins, phytates, protease (trypsin) inhibitors, oxalates, and polyunsaturated fats. Refer back to the chapters on grains, nuts, and vegetables, or jump ahead to the soy section of this chapter to learn more about these anti-nutrients.

Remember that anti-nutrients are located in these foods to help deter pests and animals from eating them. They can cause digestive distress, inhibit the absorption of minerals, interfere with protein digestion, and decrease metabolic function.

Legumes, which are praised for their high fiber content, are very hard for the human body to break down. Even in a healthy body with a high-running metabolism and good gut function (good HCL production, non-inflamed small intestine, and proper enzyme production), a moderate amount of legumes can cause digestive upset, so be prepared. Get the air freshener handy.

Are All Legumes Digestive Disasters?

Although I am not a fan of any legumes, there are a few that are less problematic than others. Cooked green beans and peas seem to digest far easier than a pot of kidney, lima, or black beans. One reason for this is green beans and peas are picked fresh and not dried like other legumes. Green beans and peas are also less starchy than their bean and soy brothers. Thus the body has an easier time digesting them.

Still longing for legumes?

If you are going to consume legumes, be sure to soak or sprout (soaking and allow a tail to form) and cook the legumes; this will allow for easier digestibility. Canned beans, although soft, are not soaked or sprouted. This includes organic canned legumes. Canned beans contain all the anti-nutrients discussed above. Cooking helps the digestibility, but only slightly. In fact, kidney beans retain 92 percent of their phytates after cooking. Soaking and sprouting can reduce the phytate content anywhere from 40 to 70 percent. It should be noted that soaking/sprouting and cooking reduce the anti-nutrient properties, but do not eliminate them.

Therefore, if you are longing for a kidney bean chili or chickpea hummus, purchase your beans and peas fresh, and soak them for the night. Essentially, in a large pot, soak 1 cup beans in 5 cups warm water. Allow the beans to sit overnight. In the morning, discard the phytate-filled water and cook the beans—thoroughly. Consume the beans or peas with a saturated fat, like butter, ghee, or coconut oil, to further the digestibility.

When trying to improve metabolic rate or digestion, high legume consumption is not recommended. Legumes, with their high fiber content and anti-nutrient properties, are not the most digestible or absorbable source of protein—or food, for that matter. Therefore, if you want to take steps toward a healthier gut, metabolism, and body, legume consumption should be reduced to one or two times per month, if not completely avoided until your body is burning fuel like a Ferrari going 100mph.

Still not convinced that most legumes are not that bad? Keep reading so you learn about the worst, most degraded, toxic legume of them all: soy!

Soy

Let's talk about soy—the most degraded and toxic of all the legumes. The topic of soy has been an interest of mine ever since I was a soy addict back in my mid-20s. At the time, I was running health clubs in Atlanta. I was working out more than two hours each day, and I was consuming soy burgers, soymilk, soy cheese, soy protein bars and soy-based dinners like they were going out of style. You would think I would be a twig by the amount of "healthy soy" I was eating and the time I was spending in the gym—yet, I was not. I am not saying I was overweight, but I was a good 15 pounds heavier than I am today.

At the time I believed soy was healthy for me. Soy was low in calories, soy was a complete vegetable protein, soy was…a miracle food! At least, that is what I thought. Yet I was *not* getting the results I felt I deserved based on my "clean soy diet" and my exercise level. It wasn't until years later, when I began to understand how soy metabolizes in your body and the negative effects soy has on your metabolism, that I really understood what I had been doing wrong.

Everything I ate contained soy because I was taught, mostly by the Big Food giants, General Mills, Kellogg's, Nestle and Mondelez to name a few, and the soy industry, that soy was healthy for me. The soy industry reports that this legume helps with weight loss, protects against cancer, enhances immune function, lowers cholesterol, and helps in heart disease prevention.

The real question is: Are any of the above statements actually true? My experience and knowledge have taught me differently. Yet, the FDA and the Big Food giants definitely would like you to believe they are. In 2011, soy farming covered 75 million acres, produced three billion bushels of soy and produced 40 billion dollars in farming sales. Although only 6 percent of the soy grown is used for human consumption, the soy industry grew from a $300 million business in 1995, to a $5.2 billion dollar business in 2011. Profits on soy foods increased almost 2,000 percent in 16 years. From 2000 to 2007 U.S. food manufacturers introduced morethan 2,700 new soy-based foods, with soymilk, meal alternatives, and energy bars topping the charts.

According to the 22nd annual survey on consumer attitudes toward soy foods, 75 percent of consumers perceived soy products to be healthy. A third of Americans are eating soy products at least once a month, 77 percent believe soybean oil is good for them, and 84 percent believe soy will cut their risk of heart disease. Thus far, eating soy has the backing of the soy industry, The Big Food giants, and even the American people. Yet, this very important question still needs to be asked: Does the scientific research about soy confirm America's beliefs and the powerful statements of the soy industry that soy is a healthy food?

Well, let's take a look.

A Little About Soy

Soy (or soybeans) is a type of legume that has been used for more than 5,000 years in China as a food and as a foundation for many drugs. Initially, the soybean did not serve as a food, at least until the discovery of fermentation techniques. The Chinese did not eat unfermented soybeans because the soybean, like grains and some above-ground vegetables, contains large quantities of natural toxins or anti-nutrients. Soy's anti-nutrients include goitrogens, isoflavones (phytoestrogens), hemagglutinin, and phytates. These anti-nutrients can interfere with proper thyroid function, increase the effects of estrogen, and decrease the absorption of protein and other nutrients. Although fermentation helps to reduce most of these anti-nutrients, it does not completely eliminate them.

Soybeans are considered a source of protein, and can be processed into soy protein, soy meal, soy oil, and soy flour. Eighty-five percent of today's soy is processed into soy oil and soy meal, most of which is used for animal feed. This is another great reason to eat grass-fed meats: You should assume if the beef, chicken, or pork you are eating is not pasture-fed or grass-fed, the meat you are about to eat was eating soy.

The main producers of soy products are the United States, Brazil, Argentina, China, and India. The United States is the biggest soy producer, with more than one third of the global market. Today, most soy is considered a "biotech food," along with corn and cotton, because it has been genetically modified. In 1997, about 8 percent of all soybeans grown in the United States were genetically modified. In 2012, the figure had jumped to almost 95 percent.

A Word About GMO Foods

Genetically modified (GMO) foods are foods that have had their DNA directly manipulated by biotechnology to produce a stronger, more resilient food. Many advocates consider GMOs safe and are convinced food technology is the only way to feed the modern world.

The FDA puts the responsibility of "proof of safety" in the hands of the companies who are producing and making money off GMO foods. Critics of GMO foods say GMOs are causing increased allergies, weight issues, and illness. Even after 25 years of testing, the long-term safety of GMO foods has yet to be proven in the human population. I believe if we don't know the long-term effects GMO foods are having on our health, then why risk it? My advice is to always choose organic, local, and GMO-free foods.

In the United States, the FDA recommends Americans should consume 25g of soy a day as part of a healthy diet. According to a 2003 report by UN Food and Agriculture, the Chinese eat an average of 3–4g of fermented soy daily, and the Japanese eat 7–8g/day. However, based on the soy products sold in America, the average American would be getting their soy from processed soymilk, soy meals, and soy bars. Most of these "so-called" food products are genetically modified, highly processed, unfermented, and filled with other additives, preservatives, and fillers—a far cry from the fermented soy of the Asian cultures.

Still, the soy industry continues to claim numerous health benefits. To make health claims based on the history of soy is completely unjustified. The soy of 5,000 years ago, in my opinion, is a completely different food from the soy of today. With the increased mass marketing of this cheap food, people are led to believe eating soy is supportive to a healthy life. Yet Americans are not getting healthier; they are getting sicker, fatter, more depressed, and more diseased. Don't just trust me; let's check out what the research says.

Soy Isoflavones: Are They a Health Benefit?

Soy isoflavones are phytoestrogens (plant estrogens) that are reported to help lower cholesterol and prevent heart disease in humans. Numerous research studies have reported a positive correlation between lower cholesterol and consuming isoflavones. Yet just as many studies have reported no improvements with cholesterol and isoflavones in soy. A U.S. government–sponsored review of 200 different studies on soy and isoflavones, published in 2005, found only a small reduction in "bad" LDL cholesterol. Articles in the *Journal of the American Medical Association, Nutrition Journal, The American Journal of Clinical Nutrition,* and *Annals of Nutrition Metabolism* have reported that isoflavones do not improve cholesterol levels, triglycerides, LDL, or HDL (good cholesterol). And finally, the American Heart Association backtracked on its earlier support of soy, now saying that there is little evidence that soy has a cholesterol-lowering effect or helps with heart health.

According to Dr. Ray Peat, nutritional researcher:

> "The isoflavones (many of which are now being promoted as 'antioxidants' and 'cancer preventives') are toxic to many organs, but they have clear estrogenic effects, and are active not only immediately in the mature individual, but when they are present prenatally, they cause feminization of the male genitalia and behavior, and early maturation of the female offspring, with the tissue changes that are known to be associated with increased incidence

of cancer. The phytoestrogens appear to pose a risk to organs besides the breast and uterus, for example the liver, colon, and pancreas, which isn't surprising, since estrogen is known to be carcinogenic for every tissue."

The fact that certain soy food manufacturers are still promoting the cholesterol-lowering claim is absurd to me, especially since most current research continues to tell us that just as many people have heart attacks and heart disease with high cholesterol as those who have low cholesterol. According to Dr. Stephen Sinatra, a board-certified cardiologist, and Jonny Bowden, PhD, in their book, *The Great Cholesterol Myth*: "Cholesterol has little to do with heart disease and people are spending too much time, energy, and money trying to control it." Dr. Dwight Lundell, a cardiologist who has performed more than 5,000 heart surgeries, says cholesterol is not the culprit when it comes to heart disease; inflammation of the arteries is the problem.

Unfortunately when a billion-dollar industry has been developed to support the cholesterol-lowering theory, little is being done to educate people about what they really need to do to improve their heart health: a metabolically supportive diet, moderate exercise, less stress, sleep, happiness, community, and purpose.

Does Soy Help with Weight Loss?

When people replace a high-fat conventional meat protein with a low-fat soy food they *do* lose weight. Initially, this happens because soy foods contain fewer calories than most meat proteins. However, long-term, soy and its phytoestrogens (plant-derived xenoestrogens that mimic estrogen in the body) are powerful endocrine disruptors. These phytoestrogens inhibit thyroid peroxidase, which produces T3 and T4 from iodine and tyrosine. This will ultimately slow down your metabolism.

Cassy's Story

Cassy, a somewhat-healthy 50-year-old, was a career woman and mother. Cassy complained of sudden weight gain, moodiness, fatigue, and edema (water weight). Cassy exercised regularly, ate lots of fruits and vegetables, consumed almost no fast foods, and loved to cook at home. Yet, Cassy had one big issue: She was consuming close to 50 grams of processed soy and soy products a day. Cassy was not vegetarian. Cassy had read, in a popular health magazine that promoted soy products, that soy and phytoestrogens were very healthy for postmenopausal women.

Believing the marketing claims of the article, Cassy began using soy protein and soymilk in her smoothies, and she ate tofu and soy burgers for dinner and lunch, used soy oils to cook with, and ate soy chips and soy nuts as snacks. The amount of soy Cassy was eating was insane.

Slowly, Cassy started to remove some of her soy-based foods. Cassy substituted organic milk for soymilk; gelatin protein for soy protein; and fish, eggs, and organic tempeh for her soy burgers and tofu; and she started using dried or fresh fruit and cheese as a snack versus soy chips or soy beans. In addition, Cassy added in two raw carrots a day to help decrease endotoxins in her gut and the estrogenic load on her body.

Two months later, Cassy's energy improved, Cassy felt happier, and her mood improved dramatically. Six months later, Cassy had lost her water weight and the additional 10 pounds she had put on. Cassy is no longer a soy food lover, nor is she a reader of that popular health magazine.

Soy Is Goitrogenic

Soy, like flax seeds and cruciferous vegetables, is also a goitrogen. Remember that goitrogens are substances that suppress the thyroid gland by blocking iodine uptake, which can cause the formation of goiters, and can lead to thyroid disease and cancer. Goitrogens interfere with optimal metabolic function. This is one reason farmers feed their pigs, cattle, and chickens soy: It makes the animals fat faster. Soy interferes with proper thyroid hormone production. Thyroid hormones, along with vitamin A and glucose, are the main players in a healthy metabolism. Decreasing thyroid production slows the animals' metabolism, making them gain fat faster. And yes, if soy can slow the metabolism of cows, chickens, and pigs, soy can slow your metabolism as well!

Remember: Most farmers don't care about the longevity of their animals. The farmers just care about the profit they will make by getting the animals bigger faster.

Does Soy Help Decrease Cancer Rates?

You may have heard that soy decreases risk of cancer. Again, this claim seems to be based on old information that is no longer known as truth. In 1997, D. Ingram reported in his paper "Phytoestrogens and Their Role in Breast Cancer" "that women who have cancer are failing to eliminate estrogens, including phytoestrogens, at a normal rate, and so are retaining a higher percentage of the chemicals consumed in their diets." These phytoestrogens, like our own estrogens, suppress the detoxifying systems of the body. If our body cannot detoxify properly, we develop disease, cancer, and get closer to death.

The findings of the Women's Health Initiative (WHI) threw the estrogen drug companies into a tizzy in 2002. At the time, estrogen drug companies were making billions selling women estrogen replacement therapy (ERT) and hormone replacement therapy (HRT) to help decrease cancer, and chances of strokes and heart attacks. They were also sold as a way to decrease hot flashes and increase energy. The problem was that when the WHI findings came out it proved none of the above. In fact, women who took estrogen had increased chances of breast cancer, strokes, and heart attacks. The trial was soon abandoned and estrogen sales plummeted. Truth be told, whether estrogen comes from our own body, ERT, birth control, or soy foods, too much estrogen can be toxic to our body.

Jane's Story

Jane had worked in the health and fitness industry for years. Jane was in her mid-30s and was very fit. She had competed in numerous fitness competitions and was now experiencing the aftermath. Recently Jane was experiencing fatigue, irritability, weight gain, extreme thirst, cold body temperature, and the blahs.

Jane's diet was "clean" by all fitness standards (lots of lean meat, whole grains, egg whites, and steamed vegetables, combined with whey protein and supplements), but she felt like crap and nobody, including her doctors, could figure out what was wrong with her. Jane was also taking a birth control pill that contained estrogen. Jane's doctors told her she was overworked and overstressed, and that she needed more sleep, even though Jane was sleeping 10–12 hours a night.

The high-protein, low-carb diet, excessive exercise, and belief of looking perfect for the fitness industry had become too stressful for her body to handle. (I can 100 percent relate.) Coupled with an increased estrogen load from birth control, and what we see is a tired body, water-logged, unhappy, and irritated woman.

Initially, Jane needed to create a new supportive nutritional foundation, one that would increase her energy and her attitude. Jane cut out the grains, and added in fruit and OJ. Jane added in two carrots per day to help decrease estrogen load. She stopped most supplements and whey protein, and added in bone broth and gelatin. Jane also cut her workouts to no more than three times each week for 30 minutes each.

Jane saw some slow changes at first: better mood, reduced sugar cravings, and less lulls through the day. Then, with the approval and help of her doctor, Jane discontinued her birth control pills. Quite dramatically, Jane's mood and energy significantly improved. Jane felt stronger, happier, and more "normal" again.

Within a few months, Jane's body temperature and pulse increased. We adjusted her daily calories from a very low 1,200–1,500 kcal initially, to almost 2,500 kcal over the next three months. Jane's body was starving for nutrients. Now, I am not going to lie: Jane did add on some weight. This sometimes happens in the healing process.

However, six months later, by leveling her calories out to a comfortable 1,800–2,000 kcal, Jane began to lose the added weight. Most importantly, she feels like she has her life back. With thoughts of a possible baby on the way, Jane promises to never do a fitness competition again.

What Is Estrogen Dominance?

"Estrogen dominance" is a term coined by Dr. John Lee. When estrogen has an unbalanced ratio to progesterone, it leads to estrogen dominance. According to Dr. Lee, a healthy ratio would be somewhere between 50 and 100 times more progesterone to estrogen. Estrogen dominance can be caused by high estrogen production in the body, increased estrogen intake by estrogenic foods or xenoestrogens, poor estrogen detoxification, and/or low progesterone production. Estrogen dominance in men and women can have a number of the following symptoms:

- Fat gain
- Hot flashes
- Depression
- Low energy
- Hypoglycemia
- Foggy thinking
- Sleep issues
- Memory loss
- Cancer
- Osteoporosis
- PMS
- Edema

If you think you have estrogen dominance, talk with your healthcare provider. Prior to that, you can take personal measures to decrease the estrogenic load on your body. These include:

1. Removing all estrogenic food (soy, PUFA, alcohol) from your diet.

2. Stopping the use of xenoestrogens (man-made estrogenic substances), plastics, lotions, makeup, and many soaps that contain phytoestrogens.

3. Decreasing exposure to radiation. Minimize x-rays, cellular use, microwave exposure, and wireless devices.

4. Eating a thyroid supportive diet (like the one described in this book).

5. Reducing stress.

6. Getting off your birth control, ERT, or HRT therapies.*

*Please discuss with your doctor or health care provider before getting off of any medication.

Does Soy Help with Immune Function?

One of the many claims of soy is that it has antioxidant properties. Antioxidants are molecules that inhibit the oxidation of other molecules, which is a good thing. Soy contains phytates. Phytates are antioxidant compounds found in whole grains, legumes, nuts, and seeds. Phytates are also anti-nutrients, meaning they can inhibit the absorption of other nutrients. Phytates block the uptake of the essential nutrients zinc and copper, and, to a lesser degree, calcium and magnesium.

Scientists who have studied the diet of Third World countries (which consist mostly of grains and legumes) are in general agreement that phytates are a big contributor to the widespread mineral deficiency. The soybean has one of the highest phytate contents of any of the grains or legumes. Therefore, despite the fact that calcium, magnesium, iron, and zinc are present in these plant-based diets, the high phytate levels prevent their absorption. This can lead to a mineral-deficient diet and eventually disease. Fermenting soy for a long period of time has been shown to decrease, but not eliminate, the actions of phytates in the soy.

Essentially, there are far better foods to consume if you are looking for antioxidant properties. Fruits, OJ, root vegetables, eggs, dark chocolate, coconut oil, liver, shellfish, and coffee are all great choices.

Trypsin Inhibitors

Soy also contains trypsin inhibitors. These anti-nutrients block trypsin and other enzymes needed for proper protein digestion. This can lead to digestive distress, pancreatic disorders, and a diet deficient in proper amino acid uptake. So if you are using soy as a main protein source, think again. The very food you are eating may be inhibiting the digestion of the protein you are trying to get from it. Trypsin inhibitors have been linked to stunted growth in tested animals.

Hemagglutinin

Finally, soy contains hemagglutinin. Hemagglutinin is a blood clotting substance that causes your red blood cells to clump together. Red blood cell clumping can lead to inadequate oxygen usage by your cells. Anything that impedes your cells' oxygen usage produces problems in cellular respiration and proper metabolic function.

There is a reason so many products these days are displaying "soy free" on the label. Not only is soy *not* the miracle health food we were all led to believe, but soy is linked to decreased cellular respiration, digestive issues, increased estrogen levels, cancer, weight gain, mineral deficiencies, and thyroid issues. These days even "healthy" dog foods are labeled as soy free to help with your pet's digestion and his or her health.

Since the mass production of soy products back in the early 1990s, none of the "improved health claims" have shown up in our culture. If anything, America has more obesity, more cancer, more heart disease, and more autoimmune issues than ever before. Is soy intake the main culprit? That is impossible to say. I think it is a contributing factor. Anytime we start mass-producing a food, the quality always suffers. More processing, more degradation, and more cheaply produced food equals more money, more money, and more money. At the end of the day, we must remember the "big food" companies behind food production are far more concerned about the bottom line than the health of their consumers.

The number-one takeaway from this is to avoid or at least minimize your consumption of soy. I realize that total avoidance of soy may not be possible, so I wanted to tell you which soy products you should eliminate and which others you may consume sparingly.

I recommend avoiding the following products:

Soy Milk	Soy nuts	Soy crackers
Soy cheese	Soy oils	Soy chips
Soy burgers	Soy flour	Soy lecithin
Soy sausage	Soy ice cream	Soy proteins
Soy energy bars	Soy creamer	Tofu
Soy pre-made meals	Edamame	All GM soy

Instead try to consume only the non–genetically modified fermented products, such as tempeh, miso, natto, and gluten-free soy sauce in limited quantities.

I try to avoid all soy, even the fermented soy foods. I feel there are far better options for a good protein source. As you now know, my preferences are organic dairy, eggs, bone broth, liver, wild white fish, shellfish, and gelatin. When it comes to choosing your foods, do not pick a food by what the label reads. Pick a food because it is fresh, is unprocessed, is supportive to your metabolism, and more than likely does not come with a label.

Remember: There is *no* joy in soy. You may love your soymilk or your soy burger, but do not be fooled into thinking these are health products; they are money-making, degraded food products that may be negatively affecting your health. It is up to you to understand *everything* you are putting in your body. Do not count on food manufacturers, the USDA, the FDA, or even your doctor. Personal awareness and self-responsibility are keys to healing your body and becoming the lean, happy, warm, energized being you were meant to be.

Chapter 12:
What You Need to Know

1. Soy is anti-metabolic and is used as a fattening agent of cattle, pigs, and chickens.

2. Most soy in America is genetically modified, highly processed, and a cheap food.

3. Soy is goitrogenic and contains phytoestrogens. Both can inhibit proper thyroid function and slow your metabolism.

4. Soy contains many anti-nutrients, including phytates, which inhibit the absorption of zinc, copper, magnesium, and calcium. Soy contains trypsin inhibitors, which block protein digestion. Soy also contains hemagglutinin, which causes red blood cells to clump together.

5. Avoid all GMO soy products, soy milks, soy cheese, soy meals, soy bars, soy snacks, soy oils, soy flours, and soy lecithin.

Chapter 13
Supplementing with Protein Powders

I don't think the information on protein would be complete without addressing the use of protein powders. I am certainly not a stranger to using numerous different types/brands of protein powders in my lifetime. Remember that I ran health clubs for nine years of my adult life; there was not a day that went by that I wasn't sucking down some sort of protein shake. Fruit protein shakes in morning, maybe a chocolate shake for a midday snack, followed by a protein-made mousse for a post-dinner dessert. Eek. Just the thought of consuming all those processed powdered shakes today makes me want to gag.

More than 30 years ago, when protein shakes became popular in the bodybuilding and fitness world, they tasted like chalky, powdery, vitamin-tasting, gag-while drinking muscle-making food supplements. Food manufacturers hadn't quite honed in on good taste or texture. Today's protein shakes taste far better. Due to the fact that protein powders have become part of a billion-dollar "health food" industry, quite a bit of research and work have gone into creating a better-tasting product. However, does a better-tasting product mean a truly healthy product for you and me? You can decide.

Protein powders are a quick and easy meal when time and convenience are of great importance. In today's busy society, anything that is quick and easy seems to be appealing. There is no time to shop, prepare, and cook real meals anymore, so having a spoonful of protein, some milk/water/almond milk, fruit, and a blender seems like a great alternative to a quick meal. What we are failing to remember is that protein powders are highly processed protein substitutes; they are not real food. And if our goal is to achieve optimal health, a high intake of processed protein powders should not be on the list.

Protein Powders Are Processed Food

According to a study in *The Journal of Nutrition*: "During the processing process, protein powders are treated with heat, oxidizing agents (such as hydrogen peroxide), organic solvents, alkalis, and acids for a variety of reasons such as to sterilize/pasteurize, to improve flavor, texture, and other functional properties, to deactivate anti-nutritional factors, and to prepare concentrated protein products. These processing treatments may cause the formation of Maillard compounds, oxidized forms of sulfur amino acids, D-amino acids, and cross-linked peptide chains (such as lysinoalanine and lanthionine), resulting in lower amino acid bioavailability and protein quality."

The study is essentially saying that the amount of processing that goes into making a protein powder can create many negative effects, ending with decreased protein quality.

Food Additives

Most protein powders contain carrageenan, guar gum, xanthan gum, locust bean gum, and/or Arabic gum, used as a thickener or stabilizing agent. All of these additives are mostly indigestible and can increase gut irritation especially for someone with digestive issues or a sluggish metabolic rate. To increase metabolic rate and increase gut health, you want to consume foods that are easy to digest and absorb. Consuming foods with known gut irritants doesn't support this process.

Soy lecithin is another food additive added to many protein powders—and chocolate, butter alternatives, salad dressings, and cooking sprays. Soy lecithin is a combination of soy oil and phospholipids, used as an emulsifier and/or stabilizer in food. Most soy lecithin is genetically modified, unless otherwise stated.

Using the chemical solvent hexane, soy lecithin is made by extracting soybean oil from raw soybeans. Hexane is a known toxin and ingestion is linked to nausea, vertigo, intestinal irritation, and central nervous system (CNS) problems. A study in *The Journal of the American Oil Chemists' Society* in 2000 found that even after trying to eliminate the hexane from soy oil, the final hexane residue was 1,000 ppm (parts per million). The National Institute for Occupational Safety and Health recommended exposure be limited to 50 ppm. Therefore, it is advisable to avoid products that use hexane as an extracting agent.

Synthetic Vitamins

Most protein powders contain very little natural vitamin and mineral value. Therefore, manufacturers have to make their protein powder seem more desirable, so they add in cheap synthetic vitamins. I am not an advocate of using added vitamin supplements. I find, for most people, they just cause additional digestive distress. Add the vitamins into a powdery-protein powder and the result is an unhappy gut.

Artificial/Natural Sweeteners

Most, if not all, protein powders contain added sweeteners. If you are reading this book, you probably already know the dangers of aspartame (Equal), saccharine (NutraSweet), and sucralose (Splenda). If not, please understand that each of these artificial sweeteners has a long list of negative side effects. The side effects include memory problems, skin issues, cancer, headaches, anxiety, birth defects, and digestive distress. The FDA claims each one of these sweeteners is "generally regarded as safe" (GRAS) at their current level of consumption.

Yet, current research is showing a different story. A study in the *Journal of Toxicology and Environmental Health* found in 2008 that, after 12 weeks of ingesting sucralose, rats showed a reduction in beneficial fecal bacteria and increased fecal pH levels. In numerous studies, aspartame has been linked to mental disorders, and decreased learning and emotional function. Saccharine has been linked to bladder cancer in rats, but current human studies show this to be inconclusive. Still, this is not a reason to run out and buy saccharine-filled foods.

Most people who consume artificial sweeteners are doing it to "save" calories and reduce sugar intake. If you have been paying attention, and I know you have, you know that sugar is not the enemy when it comes to weight gain. Sugar is highly metabolic, and an increased intake shows a rise in metabolic rate. Remember that sugar supports triiodothyronine (T3) production via the liver. Increased thyroid production produces an increase in metabolism. Sugar (combined with fat and protein) also helps balance out blood sugar. If your body is craving sugar, there is usually a reason—it needs sugar; stop trying to ignore your body's signals.

Artificial sweeteners do not have a blood-sugar-balancing effect; in fact, since you are not giving your body what it needs, you will make yourself hungrier. Usually, if our body is craving something sweet, it needs sugar. Give it a fake sugar, and soon you will have an increased craving. A study in the *Yale Journal of Biology and Medicine* in 2010 found that people who consumed more foods and drinks with artificial sweeteners had higher BMIs and increased weight gain. I certainly can attest to that: Many years ago when I consumed diet sodas or sugar-free foods, my "sugar cravings" were never satisfied. I usually consumed twice as much food just to satisfy my cravings—which added up to weight gain and increased sugar cravings.

What About Stevia?

Stevia is an herbaceous family of plants. Stevia is about 250–300 times sweeter than sucrose (sugar). Of all the sweeteners, stevia is the most natural and least toxic. For the most part, stevia seems to be safe. Some studies have even shown stevia can increase insulin sensitivity and reduce blood glucose levels. Yet, I am not convinced it is a better alternative to the real deal—good ol' sugar—especially in a protein shake.

We already know that protein, by itself, will elicit an insulin response. Protein is best consumed with a carbohydrate (sugar) to maintain blood sugar levels. Thus, stevia combined with protein only will lead to an increased insulin secretion, followed by a blood sugar drop, followed by an increase in glucagon, cortisol, and adrenaline (stress reaction). To optimize health and muscle growth, consume regular sugar (sucrose or dextrose) with your protein shake.

Heavy Metals

In 2010 *Consumer Reports* tested 15 protein shakes and powders for cadmium, arsenic, lead, and mercury. Each one of the protein shakes and powders had at least one of the heavy metals. For those of us who want to maintain our health, any amount of heavy metals is too much, especially a daily dose. Ongoing ingestion of heavy metals can affect the kidneys, digestive system, nervous system, cardiovascular system, reproductive system, and blood.

In today's world, we are exposed to hundreds of toxins daily, primarily in the air, water, and food. We cannot avoid exposure, but we can limit it by being aware of the contents of certain foods.

What About Whey Protein?

I feel the need to write a quick blurb about whey protein because it is the most widely used protein powder in the health and fitness world. Let's first remember whey protein was created from the cheese industry, which was discarding it as waste. Like so many other "waste products" (pulpy orange juice and fish oil) whey protein, with a lot of marketing help, became a new health food.

Although whey is an offspring of milk, whey lacks some of the protective qualities of milk, including saturated fats, CLA, sugars, casein, calcium levels, and vitamins A, B, D, and K. Whey also contains high levels of the amino acid tryptophan, which can make whey inflammatory to people who consume it often. Whey protein contains cholesterol, and although I am an advocate of cholesterol, I am not an advocate of oxidized cholesterol. Through the heating process, the cholesterol in whey can oxidize, producing oxysterols. Oxysterols have been shown to increase atherosclerotic plaques.

Now, for some of you reading this I know you are unwilling to give up your whey protein shake—especially due to convenience and time.

Therefore, if you are set on drinking your whey protein shake, I suggest a few a things:

1. Purchase a grass-fed/organic source. If your whey protein is not grass-fed/organic, then you can bet your protein is coming from an rBGH-treated cow.

2. Purchase a raw, low-heated whey or cold-pressed protein powder. This should create less damaged and more bioavailable whey protein.

3. Make sure the protein is void of added sweeteners, additives, vitamins, and artificial flavorings.

As for the rest of the protein powders (rice, hemp, soy, and pea proteins), I am not a fan. Animal-based proteins are far more bioavailable (usable for our system) than vegetarian brands. So note: If you are opting for a vegetarian-based protein powder, you may need to consume twice as much to get a serving of protein in. Your best option is to eat real food.

Are Any Protein Powders Okay?

The only protein powders I ever recommend are hydrolyzed collagen and gelatin by Great Lakes Gelatin (GLG). This powdered gelatin is free of additives, synthetic vitamins, and sweeteners. GLG is also free of monosodium glutamate (MSG). MSG is created during the processing of high-protein foods. Since MSG is not actually added to the protein powder, but a result of the manufacturing process, MSG doesn't have to be labeled on protein powders—so although your protein powder does not say it has MSG, if it has been heated and processed, more than likely it does. Consumption of MSG is linked to obesity, headaches, fatigue, depression, and eye damage.

Gelatin contains a positive amino acid profile void of the inflammatory amino acid tryptophan. For purposes of decreasing inflammation, increasing gut health, improving sleep, decreasing allergies, stabilizing blood sugar levels, improving memory, muscle sparing, liver detoxification, and improving hair, skin, and nails, this is a great thing. Remember: Excess tryptophan is linked to many inflammatory problems. I should note that, for purposes of muscle building, gelatin is not ideal. Dairy, eggs, muscle meats, fish, and shellfish are all better options, since they are all complete proteins.

At the end of the day, when it comes to protein, real food is best—always. Protein powders have their place when convenience is an issue, but they should be used sparingly (not 50 percent of your protein intake). Protein powders have become *big* business in the health and fitness industry, contributing to the billions of dollars we spend on "health products" every year. Yet, can a food product that is overly processed, and contains food additives, synthetic vitamins, heavy metals, and artificial sweeteners be considered healthy? I don't think so—and maybe you shouldn't, either. If you want to obtain a high metabolic rate, with great digestion and a lean body, then consuming unprocessed, *real food* proteins are your best option.

Chapter 13:
What You Need to Know

1. Most protein powders are highly processed. They are heated, and treated with solvents, alkalis, and other oxidizing agents. The result is a protein that may be of lower amino acid bioavailability and protein quality.

2. Most protein powders contain fillers and additives to improve taste and texture. Protein powders containing carrageenan, guar gum, xanthan gum, locust bean gum, soy lecithin, synthetic vitamins, and artificial sweeteners (aspartame, saccharine, and sucralose) should be avoided.

3. The FDA does not regulate for the safety of protein powders. Due to this, heavy metals and other toxins have been found in many name-brand protein powders.

4. Milk is a better option than whey protein shakes due to its protective saturated fat levels, CLA, sugars, calcium, and vitamins A, B, D, and K. If you consume whey protein make sure it comes from a grass-fed cow, is raw or cold-pressed, and is free of additives.

5. Hydrolyzed gelatin is my preferred type of protein powder due to its non-inflammatory amino acid profile. Gelatin can help with decreasing inflammation, increasing gut health, improving sleep, decreasing allergies, stabilizing blood sugar levels, improving memory, muscle sparing, liver detoxification, and improving hair, skin, and nails.

Chapter 14
Using *Real* Food Supplements for Nutritional Support

As you know from the last chapter, I am not an advocate of protein supplements or any non-food supplement. I think the supplement industry has turned into a less-regulated drug industry with a motive to sell products and not to heal the population. The primary concerns of the supplement industry are not health and healing, but money and profit. The nutritional supplement business has become a billion-dollar industry over the last 20- plus years. Protein powders, vitamin and mineral supplements, herbs, probiotics, amino acids, essential fatty acids, etc. have all steadily grown in popularity all with promises of quicker weight loss, improved health, and a happier life. The question is: Are they working?

Well, I don't think so.

And quite honestly current research reports there is very little evidence supporting any long-term health benefits from taking nutritional supplements. One study that covered more than 400,000 participants taking high-dose multivitamins showed no beneficial change in mortality, cardiovascular disease, or cancer. Another study followed 6,000 men over 12 years and found no difference in cognitive function, memory, and performance. And finally, some research concludes taking high doses of individual supplements can actually increase mortality.

Without a strong foundation of good nutrition, adequate sleep, the proper exercise, and happiness, even the best, most natural, cleanest, organic supplements will only have a minimal effect—if any. Nutritional supplements are meant as just that: a supplement to your health, not an answer to health. They are not designed to heal your body, nor are they designed to be taken indefinitely. Supplements, like drugs, can give people a false sense of improved health without ever correcting the underlying problems—leading to more damage over the long term.

So for me, I always suggest using *real* food as your supplement. Food Is An Amazing Composition Of Vitamins, minerals, carbohydrates, protein, fats, antioxidants, etc. that works synergistically to support your health and body. You have already read about the importance of dairy for calcium, vitamin D, and magnesium, liver for vitamins A and E, and the B vitamins, fruit, roots, and orange juice for vitamin C, potassium, magnesium, and manganese, shellfish, and fish for iron, zinc, copper, and selenium. Yet, there are three food supplements (I say food supplement because they should be a small part of your daily diet) I believe deserve to be recognized due to their thyroid- supporting effects and high mineral content.

Over the last 20 years, these food supplements have been very controversial in the media, nutritional, and medical world. Many medical and nutritional professionals have touted these food supplements as being unhealthy for us. Yet, the scientific evidence is just not there, and lately more evidence is supporting the importance of these food supplements and why you should be including them in your daily diet.

What are they?

The food supplements you may need to add into your daily diet are salt, coffee, and eggshell calcium carbonate.

Salt

I admit it: I love salt. I put salt on every savory and even sweet (it's delicious on fruit and in chocolate) thing I eat. Salt can make a tasteless, bland food taste exceptional. In your body, salt can lower inflammation, increase womb healing and metabolic rate, help you sleep, improve muscle function, and positively affect your blood pressure. Yet, salt has been blasted by the medical and nutritional field as being the culprit for high blood pressure and a player in heart disease. Thus, the USDA, FDA, and most RDAs recommend limiting your salt intake to 1,500–2,300mg/day or ½–1 teaspoon salt per day to help keep blood pressure at bay. The question is: Does this recommendation make any sense? Is this recommendation helping us live longer and with less disease? If not, *should* we be eating more salt—and if so, how much?

"In 1972 a paper in *The New England Journal of Medicine* reported that the less salt people ate, the higher their levels of a substance secreted by the kidneys, called renin. Renin sets off a physiological cascade of events that end with an increased risk of heart disease. In this scenario, eating less salt secreted more rennin, leading to heart disease and premature death." ~ Gary Taubes

First, let's look at the research.

In 1979, Dr. Douglas Shanklin and Dr. Jay Hodin proved that pre-eclampsia and pregnancy toxemia could have been corrected by both increased dietary protein and increased salt. Increased dietary protein and increased salt improved circulation, lowered blood pressure, and prevented seizures, all while reducing vascular leakiness.

In a 1980 study by Dr. Gary Nicholls, low salt intake was associated with higher levels of noradrenaline in the blood. Noradrenaline is part of the sympathetic nervous system (SNS). The continuous activation of the SNS can cause hypertension, irregular heartbeats, left ventricular hypertrophy, and coronary vasoconstriction. It can also contribute to the progression of renal disease.

In 1982, Dr. Robert Carey found that as salt increases so do our dopamine levels. He also found that dopamine can suppress the secretion of noradrenaline. Thus, when salt is restricted, dopamine levels fall, lifting the inhibition on noradrenaline and increasing blood pressure. Remember: Noradrenaline is part of the SNS, and any activation of the SNS increases blood pressure.

In 1995, Dr. Michael Alderman showed that in a four-year study of 3,000 people, there was a clear increase in mortality in people who ate less salt. An extra few grams of salt per day was associated with a 36-percent reduction in "coronary events."

Again in 1998, Dr. Alderman studied more than 11,000 people over 22 years and found an inverse relationship between salt intake and mortality.

A 2011 study by a group of Belgium researchers of almost 4,000 people over an eight-year period concluded that healthy people who eat less sodium do not have any health advantage over those who eat more sodium. In fact, these folks had slightly higher death rates from heart disease.

And finally, a 2014 study in the *New England Journal of Medicine* followed more than 100,000 people in 17 countries for more than three years. The study found that those who consumed less than 3,000mg of salt per day had a 27-percent-greater chance of death from a major cardiovascular event. The study found those who consumed an estimated 3,000–6,000mg of salt/day had the lowest level of death and cardiovascular events. Currently the USDA recommends salt consumption of less than 2,300mg/day, and the American Heart Association (AHA) recommends salt consumption of less than 1,500mg/day.

Each and every one of these studies reported no improvements in health when people were placed on a salt-restricted diet. In fact, most issues occurred when salt was restricted. This makes sense when you understand the functions of salt in the body and why you need it.

How Salt Works in Your Body

Salt plays a number of roles in the human body. Salt's primary role is to help maintain blood pressure and volume in the blood.

Have you ever wondered how salt does this? No? Well, the good news is I have and, lucky for you, I am about to tell you.

To really understand the role of salt in the body and its effects on blood pressure, you have to first understand the renin-angiotensin-aldosterone-system (RAAS). The RAAS is a hormonal system that controls blood pressure and water balance in your body.

Three different triggers, all of which bring about the same result—raising your blood pressure—turns on the RAAS system. These triggers are:

1. Low blood pressure. This usually means blood pressure below 90/60. Low blood pressure will contribute to a colder body.

2. Activation of your sympathetic nervous system (adrenaline, cortisol, prolactin, serotonin, growth hormone, and melatonin). This is your flight or fight system that is activated by physical, emotional, and mental stress.

3. Low salt. (please take note of this.)

When your blood pressure is low, you have too little salt or you get "stressed out," your body signals renin from your kidneys to be released into circulation. Renin helps convert angiotensinogen, released by the liver, into angiotensin I. Angiotensin I is then converted into angiotensin II by an enzyme found in the lungs called angiotensin-converting enzyme (ACE). Angiotensin II is the active hormone in this process.

Angiotensin II (A2) is a very powerful vasoconstrictor causing four main things to occur in the body that will increase blood pressure. A2 signals:

1. The arteries in the body constrict, increasing blood pressure.

2. The pituitary gland releases antidiuretic-hormone (ADH), which tells the body to increase water absorption. This will increase stroke volume (the volume of blood pumped from

one ventricle of the heart with each beat), which leads to higher blood pressure.

3. The kidneys directly reabsorb sodium. Increased sodium in the blood will drive more water into the blood and, thus, increase blood pressure.

4. The adrenals to release the hormone aldosterone. Aldosterone increases sodium absorption into the blood and cells, and releases potassium into the urine. Water will follow sodium (Na) into the blood and cells; this increases not only blood pressure but also water retention in the cells (i.e., edema).

Now let's take a step back and notice a very important statement I made a few paragraphs ago: Low blood pressure, stress, and **low salt trigger** the RAAS system to turn on. **High salt does not.** Sodium is involved in increasing blood pressure, but in most cases it is not the reason blood pressure increases. It is just part of a system that helps regulate blood pressure.

We keep putting all the blame on salt, but more than likely salt is *not* the cause of increased blood pressure. Salt retention and increased blood pressure are just results that occur from a system that has become overworked and overstressed. The RAAS hormonal system is a self-regulated, negative feedback system. This means once it has done its job—raising your blood pressure—the RAAS will self-correct and auto-regulate back to normal.

Our body holds on to salt to increase blood pressure when needed; this is a survival technique. Think about it: When you are stressed, you can feel your blood pressure rise. Your body has more nutritional needs so your blood has to circulate more vitamins, minerals, sugars, proteins, and fats to all your body parts. Once your stress has gone away, your blood pressure returns to normal. Problems start occurring when we over-stress our bodies and the RAAS system doesn't turn off. This dysfunction, not salt itself, is what leads to constricted arteries, increased water and sodium retention, hypertension, and quite possibly a heart attack.

Basically salt is the victim of being at the wrong place at the wrong time, and thus gets all the blame for increased blood pressure.

Why Is Salt So Important?

- Salt helps reduce inflammation and cramping.
- Salt helps magnesium absorption.
- Salt suppresses the stress hormone aldosterone and supports thyroid function.
- Salt improves insulin sensitivity.
- Salt increases metabolic rate and heat in the body.
- Salt helps relieve constipation.
- Salt improves sleep.
- Salt is needed for a high metabolic rate. Since we know stress hinders thyroid function, anything that decreases stress hormones should support thyroid function—and salt does this.

Does this mean you should eat endless amounts of salt?

I know how people think: You tell them salt supports metabolic function, and all of a sudden they start downing a daily shaker full of salt. The answer to this question is: It depends on the person and his or her state of health. Sorry—it's just not that black and white. If you start shifting your diet with the recommendations I have already made in this book (eating real food, dairy, super proteins, healthy sugars, saturated fats, etc.), then adding in a clean source of salt should continue to benefit your health and metabolic rate.

If you are experiencing daily stress, you are sedentary, and your current diet is predominately processed foods (which are already high in refined salts), then before you start adding in a clean salt source you should remove the processed foods, clean up the diet, and address the current stressors in your life.

Please note: When you start to increase your salt intake, do it slowly. Your body and kidneys need to get used to the additional salt. Adding in too much salt, too quickly will bring about water retention, bloating, and weight gain, which I am sure you don't want. Salt is an amazing supplement, but in the wrong body, it can have an adverse effect, so talk to your health care provider before becoming a salt addict.

How Much Salt?

My personal recommendation with salt is to eat to taste. Salt your food to your own personal taste. Your food should not taste overly salty just because you are trying to increase your salt intake. If you are working out or are experiencing lots of stress in your life, I recommend adding a little salt to your drinks, like Kate's Miracle Hydrating Beverage (see Chapter 20). A constant flow of good sugars, proteins, fats, and salt throughout the day will help keep your stress hormones at bay, and will allow your body to relax and de-stress easier at night.

What Type of Salt?

Any clean, white sea salt should work. Make sure it is white, not pink or gray. (The pink and gray salts have more impurities.) I prefer to use Morton's Canning and Pickling salt. You can buy it online or at your local Walmart or Target. It's not flashy or organic or in a cool container, but it's clean, and that is what is important.

The salt controversy will be an ongoing discussion. Like the cholesterol theory, there are so many misconceptions and so many unknowns. We must understand that neither cholesterol nor salt are bad for you; you need them both. Both help control vital functions in your body and metabolism. Not understanding their functions and importance, and just avoiding them, can lead to more dysfunction. I am certainly not telling anyone to go out and start consuming heaps of salt. Salt can be a very powerful supplement and should be used mindfully. However, adding a clean, unrefined, non-iodized white salt into your diet, slowly, can be very beneficial to your metabolism and health.

Coffee

I love my morning coffee. Nothing makes me happier in the morning (especially at 6:00 a.m.) than a dark roasted cup of coffee with plenty of cream and sugar. It's warm, it's creamy, it's sweet, and it's just plain delicious. As with salt, there is a lot of controversy surrounding coffee drinking. Many health professionals say coffee is unhealthy and is responsible for killing the adrenal glands, making you nervous, contributing to breast cancer, damaging to your liver, and wrecking your thyroid. Some health professionals may recommend coffee, but only if you drink it black, so you can save yourself the extra calories from the sugar and cream. And then there is me, who will tell you to drink your coffee, every day if you like, with plenty of cream and sugar—because all three are healthy for you.

The truth is coffee is healthy for you. Yay! Current research shows that coffee drinkers have a 40-percent-less chance of getting hepatocellular carcinoma (HCC), the most common type of liver cancer. Some data even concludes that drinking upward of three cups a day can reduce liver cancer up to 50 percent. Coffee also protects the liver from liver-damaging substances like alcohol and acetaminophen. We may attribute this phenomenon to the unexpected effects that caffeine has on liver enzymes. Liver enzymes seem to be the target for the caffeine in coffee, reducing them in the body. High liver enzymes are associated with a damaged liver.

In addition to supporting the liver, coffee drinking is linked to lower levels of thyroid disease, diabetes, Parkinson's disease, and cancer, improvement in Alzheimer's patients, and lower levels of suicide.

Most of the positive research on coffee/caffeine suggests improvements are seen in a daily consumption of three to five cups of coffee. So don't be shy when asking for that second cup of coffee; your health is counting on it.

Essentially, coffee drinkers are just happier people, which makes sense if you have ever seen a person trying to "cleanse" and give up his or her coffee. These are not happy people!

In addition to the benefits of the caffeine in coffee, coffee also contains numerous important minerals, including magnesium, potassium, and B1 and B3 vitamins. Coffee also contains the antioxidant compounds, which include caffeic acid, caffeine, the chlorogenic acids, eugenol, gamma-tocopherol, isoeugenol, p-coumaric acid, scopoletin, and tannic acid. As an antioxidant coffee protects your body from free radical damage, which will ultimately decrease cell damage and death.

Coffee is helpful in relieving constipation (due to its thyroid-supporting effects). Coffee is also an inhibitor of non-heme iron absorption. Anyone with iron overload or who absorbs too much iron should consider adding coffee into the diet. On the other hand, those who are known to have iron anemia should be cautious consuming coffee with foods that contain iron. Drinking coffee one hour before or after an iron-rich meal shows no influence on iron absorption.

And finally, drinking coffee supports thyroid function and increases metabolic rate. Yes, coffee/caffeine increases metabolic rate. Caffeine increases the cellular consumption of glucose, which is caused when metabolism increases. You use glucose faster— which, if you don't know by now, is what you want. You want to be able to use glucose at a very high rate so you can produce more energy, more carbon dioxide, and more heat.

This is why it is so important to consume coffee/caffeine with calories. If you are increasing your metabolic needs and not providing your body with additional energy, you are going to experience a drop in blood sugar, which as you know by now, will elicit a stress response.

Lowering blood sugar will increase adrenaline (due to increased glucose uptake) to bring blood sugar back to normal. This is why many people get jittery, nervous, anxious, or even nauseous while drinking black coffee, especially on an empty stomach. Their increased metabolic rate lowers blood sugar, producing a stress response, thus increasing adrenaline, which leads to all the above symptoms.

What Is the Best Way to Drink Coffee?

The best way to drink your coffee is slowly. Eating and drinking *anything* quickly is stressful to the body, especially if it is hot. Sipping your coffee while reading the paper or talking to a friend is a great way to enjoy a dark-roasted cup of coffee, not speeding down the highway trying to be on time for work.

You should also consume your coffee with plenty of calories. If you like it black, then make sure you consume your coffee with a meal. This will offset the adrenaline response of drinking it alone. You may also add cream, milk, sugar, honey, and even gelatin for a little protein to your coffee. My favorite coffee combination is a 10 oz. of organic dark roast coffee with 2–3 tablespoons cream, 2 tablespoons white sugar, and 1 tablespoon hydrolyzed gelatin. Sometimes I even add a little salt. I sip on this yummy concoction all morning. It warms me up without making me feel jittery or hyped up. I make sure I eat before and after my morning coffee, since the coffee increases my metabolic rate, making my body crave more calories.

To sum it up, coffee is healthy for you. Coffee supports thyroid and liver function. Coffee protects against cancer, diabetes, Parkinson's disease, and Alzheimer's disease. Coffee can be used as a digestive aid and helps with constipation. Coffee is filled with minerals and antioxidants. And finally coffee is best consumed with added calories, either with food or added cream, milk, and sugar. If coffee makes you happy, like it does me, then drink it and know you are supporting your metabolism!

Eggshell Calcium

Calcium is one of, if not the most important minerals when it comes to bone, teeth, and tissue health. Calcium is also involved in blood pressure regulation, nerve and cell function, muscular contraction, weight management, blood clotting, and helping to regulate heartbeat. Without adequate calcium one may experience bone breakdown, high blood pressure, cramping, decreased nerve function, and heart problems. So for optimal health and increased metabolic function, consuming adequate calcium is imperative.

As you already know from Chapter 9, milk and other dairy products are your best sources of calcium. Dairy is the best source of calcium, primarily because calcium is being delivered with all the other supportive nutrients. For optimal calcium absorption adequate levels of vitamins A, D, E, and K, magnesium, fat, protein, and sugars are required. This is why dairy is so important in the diet and should not be avoided—despite what the local juice bar is telling you.

Yet many people, for some reason or another, are not consuming adequate levels of dairy. They may *believe* they are allergic or lactose intolerant (this is usually a gut issue, not a dairy issue), they do not like the taste or texture, they cannot afford quality milk, or they have been tainted by unjustified health claims that dairy is bad for them. For whatever the reason, many people are not consuming enough dairy products, which may produce a calcium-deficient diet. For these people, consuming calcium supplements in the form of eggshell calcium would be beneficial.

What Is Eggshell Calcium?

Eggshell calcium is exactly what it says: calcium that comes from the shell of an egg. Eggshells from your common chicken egg are almost 90-percent calcium carbonate. The other 10 percent of eggshells is a combination of the minerals magnesium, boron, copper, iron, selenium, zinc, and sulfur, and protein and progesterone. Calcium carbonate is about 40-percent calcium. One eggshell is about 6 grams. Thus each eggshell will produce about 2,400mg of usable calcium.

I am not suggesting you should munch on a few raw eggshells to get additional calcium. But if you boil, bake, and grind your leftover eggshells, you can produce a very usable and absorbable form of calcium. (See Chapter 20 for more information.)

Calcium carbonate from eggshells has been shown, in numerous studies, to have positive effects on bone and cartilage health. Research on post-menopausal women has shown that supplementing with eggshell calcium reduced pain, increased mobility, and increased bone density. In addition eggshell calcium has shown to contain lower levels of heavy metals than other natural calcium supplements like oyster shells. This produces a cleaner and safer product for human consumption.

Calcium Carbonate vs. Calcium Citrate

When it comes to usable and absorbable calcium, many doctors and health practitioners like to recommend a calcium citrate supplement, arguing that it absorbs far better than calcium carbonate (eggshells). The belief is that calcium citrate is more absorbable due to its higher acidity. The truth is there is little difference in the amount of absorbable calcium between the two calcium forms. A 2000 study at Osteoporosis Research Center in Omaha, Nebraska, studied 24 post-menopausal women and their absorption of calcium carbonate and calcium citrate. Blood levels of calcium were measured over 24 hours. The researchers concluded that calcium citrate and calcium carbonate were both equally absorbed and bioavailable.

In another study, researchers evaluated the importance of gastric acid secretion in the absorption of dietary calcium. After measuring absorption of calcium with different stomach pH levels (different acidity levels) they found that the level of stomach acid did not play a role in the amount of calcium absorbed. The study concluded that calcium in the form of calcium carbonate, in the form of calcium citrate, or calcium from a food source can be absorbed equally despite stomach acidity.

How Much Should You Take?

As you know dosage depends on the person, what he or she is already eating, her health needs, gut health, size, age, and activity level. For measurement purposes 1 gram of calcium carbonate contains 400mg of calcium. This equals about 1/2 teaspoon eggshell calcium. The RDA recommends adult consumption of calcium to be around 1,300mg. Other researchers, like Dr. Ray Peat, believe calcium consumption should be much higher, closer to 2,400mg. Generally speaking, if you are consuming a low-dairy diet, one to three doses of ½ teaspoon of eggshell calcium (consumed with food) could be added to your diet safely. For specific dosage amounts please consult your healthcare provider.

Bottom line: When it comes to supplementing calcium, calcium carbonate in the form of eggshell calcium proves to be a reliable source. Not only has eggshell calcium proven to be effective in treating osteoporosis, but it also shows improvements in blood pressure, weight management, mobility, and joint health. Eggshell calcium is free of additives, fillers, and binders that other calcium supplements may contain, and is also lower in heavy metals. One-quarter teaspoon eggshell calcium can be taken one to three times per day as a calcium supplement. And finally, calcium supplements purchased at the health food store can be costly; discarded eggshells are far more affordable.

In summary, salt, coffee, and eggshell calcium can be useful food supplements supporting a high metabolic rate and increased health. All three, although controversial in the health and nutritional communities, have substantial scientific research backing their health benefits and metabolism-raising effects. Always remember: The foundation of good health should be established first, before using supplementation—even *real* food supplementation. Food will always be the best supplement for your health. The list below will show you how to use the metabolically supporting foods talked about in this book to obtain all your vitamin and mineral requirements.

Using Food for Your Vitamin and Mineral Supplements

The Vitamins

Vitamin A
Functions:
Needed for:
- Growth and development
- Immune function
- Healthy skin
- Vision
- Cholesterol conversion into the mother hormone pregnenolone

Sources: beef liver, eggs, cheese, milk

Vitamin B
Consists of eight water-soluble vitamins (cannot be stored in the body)

B1: Thiamin
Functions:
- Helps break down sugar and amino acids
- Needed to form the neurotransmitters acetylcholine and GABA

Sources: potato, liver, eggs, pork, coffee

B2: Riboflavin
Functions:
- Needed for fat, ketone, protein, and carbohydrate metabolism

Sources: liver, cheese, eggs, kidneys

B3: Niacinamide
Functions:
- Helps with skin conditions
- Inhibits oxidation of fat in the tissue

Sources: beef and fish

B5: Pantothenic acid
Functions:
- Needed to metabolize protein, fats, and carbohydrates

Sources: eggs, meat, yogurt

B6: Pyridoxine
Functions:
Needed for:
- Amino acid breakdown in the intestines
- Healthy immune system

Sources: chicken, eggs, liver, meat, bananas, carrots

B7: Biotin
Functions:
- Needed for cell growth
- Needed for metabolism of fats and amino acids
- Takes part in the transfer of CO_2 (carbon dioxide)

Sources: egg yolks, liver

B9: Folate
Functions:
Needed for:
- Repair and formation of DNA
- Production of healthy red blood cells

Sources: liver, eggs, dairy, meat, seafood

B12: Cobalamin
Functions:
Needed for:
- Brain and nervous system function
- Blood production
- Metabolism of every cell in the body

Sources: liver, eggs, dairy, meat, seafood

Vitamin C
Functions:
- Needed for growth and repair of tissue
- Supports the immune system

- Protects the body from excess iron
- Antioxidant

Sources: orange juice, peppers, papaya, pineapple, kiwi, watermelon, potatoes

Vitamin D
Functions:
- Needed for proper calcium absorption

Sources: sun, dairy, vitamin D3 supplementation (Carlson's liquid D3)

Vitamin E
Functions:
- Antioxidant
- Opposes estrogen and protects against excess iron Sources: egg yolks, liver

Vitamin K
Functions:
Needed for:
- Proper calcium uptake
- Blood clotting

Sources: foie gras (goose liver), Dutch Gouda cheese, natto, ghee, butter oil, egg yolks, mineral broth (See Chapter 20.)

The Minerals

Calcium
Functions:
- Needed for bone and teeth formation
- Needed for nerve function and muscular contraction
- Regulating heartbeat
- Involved in lowering blood pressure

Sources: dairy, bone broth, eggshell calcium (See Chapter 20.)

Magnesium
Functions:
Needed for:
- Calcium absorption and retention
- Preventing muscle cramping
- Sleep
- Avoiding constipation

Sources: coffee, dark chocolate, fruits, Epsom salt baths, bone broth, mineral broth (See Chapter 20.)

Potassium
Functions:
Needed for:
- Nerve and cell function
- Shuttling sugar into the cell; has insulin-like characteristics
- Low levels are linked to diabetes

Sources: orange juice, fruits, potatoes, bamboo shoots

Sodium
Function(s):
- Increases metabolism
- Helps maintain healthy blood pressure and volume
- Helps with constipation
- Improves immune function
- Suppresses the stress hormones

Sources: white sea salt (Morton's Canning and Pickling salt)

Zinc
Functions:
- Antioxidant properties
- Influences the conversion of T4 to T3
- Needed for proper immune function

Sources: oysters, beef, lamb, shrimp

Copper
Functions:
Needed for:
- Oxidative energy
- Red blood cell production

Sources: oysters, shellfish, liver, potatoes

Selenium
Functions:
- Needed for proper thyroid and liver function

Sources: shellfish, beef, liver, lamb, chicken

Iron
Functions:
Needed for:
- Thyroid conversion
- Hemoglobin production, which transports oxygen from the blood to the tissue
- Too much can be toxic leading to premature aging and oxidation of fats. Age spots are said to be the oxidation of iron, estrogen, and polyunsaturated fats

Sources: beef, liver, dairy, fish, mussels, oysters, chicken

Chapter 14:
What You Need to Know

1. Real food should always be your best source of nutritional supplementation.

2. Salt is an important supplement used to raise metabolic rate, and reduce inflammation and cramping. It helps magnesium absorption, helps relieve constipation, improves sleep, helps decrease stress hormones, and can actually help in lowering blood pressure. Use a clean white source of salt, and salt food to taste.

3. Coffee is a powerful thermogenic and should be consumed with cream, sugar, and/or food to decrease the blood-sugar-lowering effect it will have consumed on its own. Coffee protects the liver from drugs and alcohol. Coffee helps with constipation. Coffee drinkers have lower levels of Parkinson's disease, Alzheimer's disease, diabetes, thyroid disease, and suicide.

4. Eggshell calcium can be made with cooked and ground eggshells from a chicken. Supplementing with eggshell calcium has shown improvements in osteoporosis, blood pressure, weight management, mobility, and joint health. Eggshell calcium is free of additives and is an affordable choice for added calcium.

5. Always establish a strong foundation of health before adding any supplements. This means a good diet, sleep, stress reduction, removing toxins, and the right amount of exercise for you.

Chapter 15
The Importance of Learning to Balance Your Blood Sugar

A well-running metabolism and balanced blood sugar levels go hand in hand. Your metabolism runs best with a constant supply of energy, either from the food you eat or the energy you store. Too much energy will produce energy storage (fat increase), and too little energy will produce a catabolic state (fat, muscle, tissue loss). The trick is to find the right amount of energy input for *you* that will keep your metabolic rate high and your fat storage rate low.

So far you've discovered information about the foods that will support metabolic function (milk, fruit, roots, saturated fats, super proteins, coffee, salt, etc.) and the foods that will hinder metabolic function (legumes, grains, nuts, seeds, polyunsaturated fats, processed foods, alcohol, etc.). You have also learned about using *real* food supplements (coffee, salt, eggshell calcium) to help support a high metabolism. Consuming the right foods and food supplements is a big part of the healing equation, but there is one more *big* part of the food-eating puzzle that must be addressed for you to get optimal results.

What is it?

You want to balance your blood sugar for optimal health results. Learning to balance your blood sugar with the right combinations of macronutrients (fats, carbs, proteins), eating meals the right size for you (not too big and not too small), and the right frequency of meals are equally important to eating the right foods and food supplements when healing the body and metabolism.

First: What Is Blood Sugar?

We have all heard about blood sugar. Most of us know that it goes up when we eat and it goes down when we haven't eaten in a while. Most of us also know if you have a blood sugar issue it can lead to hypoglycemia, insulin resistance, weight gain, or, worse yet, diabetes.

To be more specific, blood sugar concentration is the amount of glucose (sugar) present in the blood of a human or animal. Most of us have ranges between 65mg/dl and 105mg/dl, depending on the day; physical, emotional, and environmental stresses; and what, how much, and when we eat. The body's goal is to keep blood sugar in these desirable ranges to achieve homeostasis so that you can feel energized, alert, and happy, and have an elevated metabolism all day long.

The problems occur when we either let our blood sugar fall too low or when we spike it up too high.

When our blood sugar drops too low, such as when we wait too long to eat, have chronic stress, over-exercise, starve ourselves, diet, or consume too much caffeine or alcohol, our body releases the stress hormones adrenaline, cortisol, and glucagon. These hormones are released to help raise blood sugar by breaking down glycogen stores (glycogenolysis—converting glycogen to glucose) and by breaking down glycerol, amino acids (muscle), lactate, and pyruvate (gluconeogenesis). As you'll remember from Chapter 4, gluconeogenesis is a necessary process for our body to survive under stress. Without the catabolic effect of increased stress hormones, our body would die under stressful situations when food is unavailable. Our stress hormones allow us to survive by using our own resources to maintain blood sugar and provide nutrients to muscles, organs, the brain, and functions of the body.

That being said, although our stress hormones are needed, chronically low blood sugar and chronically elevated stress hormones are not beneficial for long-term health and a high metabolic rate.

On the other hand, if we raise our blood sugar too high (eat too much, eat the wrong ratio of macronutrients or the wrong foods, or eat too fast) we have a whole other set of issues. Once we get a blood sugar spike, our body follows with an insulin (our fat-storing hormone) spike. Insulin is a peptide hormone produced by the beta cells of the pancreas. It is needed to shuttle glucose from the blood into the muscle and fat cells. Glucose is always converted to glycogen first. However, once muscle and liver glycogen levels are full, glucose will be shuttled into the fat cells for storage. To put it simply, chronically spiking blood sugar will lead to fat gain.

What Is Glycogen?

Glycogen is stored sugar (glucose). Stored glycogen is used to provide energy to the brain and red blood cells. Stored glycogen is used as a quick energy source. Glycogen is the first line of energy used under stress to maintain blood sugar (exercise, missed meals, fight or flight).

Glycogen is primarily stored in our muscles and liver but can also be stored in small amounts in the kidneys and intestines. Liver glycogen is used to maintain liver function, and for regulating blood sugar and maintaining metabolic functions of the body. A healthy liver can store about 100–120g of glycogen. A damaged liver will store less glycogen, which can lead to issues regulating blood sugar.

Muscle glycogen is not shared and is only used by the muscles. More muscle mass will allow for more muscle glycogen stores. Muscles may store anywhere from 300 to 600g of glycogen. For every gram of glycogen stored the body will hold up to 3–4 grams of water. Depleting the body of glycogen via starvation, excessive exercise, or a reduction diet can give the illusion of rapid fat loss, when in fact the weight loss is primarily glycogen and water loss. This form of weight loss is not sustainable or healthy.

It is important to maintain blood sugar levels so your body is not under constant stress of blood sugar levels dropping too low or spiking too high. Consistent blood sugar levels will allow your body to heal, give you constant energy, keep stress hormones low, increase thyroid function, help you lose weight, and allow your body to maintain homeostasis.

How to Maintain Your Blood Sugar Levels
Eat the right size meal for you.

What does this mean? Essentially every meal you eat should make you feel good—not stuffed, tired, or hyper. For most people this may be anywhere from 300 to 700 calories. Smaller, less active people will do fine on smaller meals. Larger, more active people will do better on larger meals. You should feel alert, happy, and warm after your meal. Meals that are too large will make you feel sluggish and tired. In addition, larger meals will get stored as glycogen (good) and fat (bad). Meals that are too small will make you hungry in an hour or two. Most meals should be able to sustain hunger for three to four hours.

Limit certain foods.

Recreational drugs, processed foods, alcohol, and calorie-free caffeinated beverages will alter blood sugar levels. I think it's fair to say recreational drugs and processed foods should be completely avoided in times of healing. Recreational drugs create a stress reaction in your body, leading to low blood sugar levels and increased stress hormones. Processed food filled with cheap sugars and unsaturated fats will enter into the body quickly producing blood sugar and insulin spikes, leading to fat gain and metabolic disturbances.

Ingesting alcohol alone will lower blood sugar levels, creating a feeling of hunger or light-headedness. I advise avoiding alcohol while trying to heal. For some people this is not an option; you know who you are. Therefore, to avoid the blood-sugar-lowering effects of alcohol, it's best to consume alcohol with food, or at the very least add a little fruit juice to your alcohol. The fructose in the fruit juice will not only help clear the alcohol quicker from your body, but the additional sugar will help maintain blood sugar levels so you don't experience a blood sugar crash.

Finally, although coffee and tea are thyroid-supporting foods, consuming them black, or without cream or milk and sugar, will drop your blood sugar, setting off a stress reaction. Since caffeine stimulates thyroid and increases metabolic rate, it will increase the body's energy needs. Therefore, sugar will be pulled from the blood to support increased metabolic function. If the coffee or tea you are consuming does not contain any calories, then blood sugar will drop, increasing your stress hormones, cortisol and adrenaline. Cream or milk and sugar will help maintain blood sugar levels. If you feel nauseous, hyper, or anxious after drinking coffee or tea, then more than likely you need to add more sugar and fat to your beverage.

Eat slowly and mindfully.

The five-minute meal, balanced precariously on the dashboard in your car while zooming down the highway, is not the way to maintain healthy blood sugar levels. Slow, conscious, mindful eating is the best way to be aware of how your meal is affecting you. One of the biggest problems with people's eating habits is eating too fast. People are so busy these days they don't have time to sit down and eat at a normal pace. Instead, they grab the quickest, most convenient meal, run out the door, and gobble down the food while driving—and then wonder why they feel like crap, have intestinal issues, and can't lose weight. Take at least 20–30 minutes to finish your meal. You should chew every bite of food at least 10 to 15 times. You should taste and savor your food. Eating slower allows you to be able to listen to your internal cues as to when you are full. Eating quickly overshoots your full feeling, leading to overeating and feeling stuffed.

In addition, eating meals in front of the TV or computer, or while watching a movie or event is more likely to produce mindless eating. Allow your meal to be the center of your attention, *not* the show or event you are watching. Mindless eating will encourage overeating and over-indulging—both of which will lead to unbalanced blood sugar.

Therefore, to support metabolic function eat slowly, mindfully, and without distractions.

The Right Amount of Carbs/Fats/Proteins

When constructing your meals you should keep in mind the functions of each of the macronutrients. Carbohydrates are used for energy and should make up the majority of every meal. Anywhere from 40 to 70 percent of your meal should be carbs. Most people seem to work well with around 50-percent carbs, at least when they start the metabolic healing process. People who are less active and/or more metabolically damaged should start on the lower end of carbohydrate usage. Athletes, young people, and those with a high metabolic rate can afford to eat a higher percentage of carbohydrates. I eat a diet around 55- to 60-percent carbohydrates (more when I am training for an event).

As you begin to heal and/or your activity or stress increase, you will be able to add in more carbohydrates to help increase metabolic rate. Take note that consuming a high amount of carbohydrates too soon will result in weight gain. (Refer back to Chapter 4 for more on carbohydrates.)

Protein is used for repair and metabolic functions. For most people this means eating a diet that contains around 20- to 30-percent protein. Remember: Protein is helpful in slowing the blood sugar rising effects of carbohydrates. Adequate protein with carbohydrates helps maintain meal satiety longer than a carbohydrate-only meal. Yet, too much protein with not enough fat and carbs will increase insulin levels and have a blood-sugar- lowering effect, creating a stress reaction. Start with around 25-percent protein, and adjust up or down depending on the energy needs of your body. (Refer back to Chapter 7 for more on proteins.)

Fat is needed for food to taste good, to transport fat-soluble nutrients, to support hormone balance, and to slow the absorbency of sugars into the blood. Most people do well on a diet that contains 20- to 30-percent fat. My experience tells me people who are more metabolically damaged need a higher percentage of fat, especially women who have hormonal problems (loss of period, infertility, etc.) or who have been on a low-fat diet for a period of time. As the metabolic rate increases and the body begins to heal, fat can be decreased while adding in more carbohydrates.

(Refer back to Chapter 2 and Chapter 3 for more on fats.)

Meal Frequency

How often you eat will depend on how well your liver is storing glycogen. People who cannot store glycogen in the liver very well (hypoglycemic, diabetic, sensitive to sugar) should eat smaller meals more often. These smaller meals will create a constant flow of nutrients and energy, allowing the body to use the energy taken in without storing any of it as fat. Essentially, these small meals will take on the job of what your liver should be doing when you are not eating: maintaining blood sugar. As the liver begins to heal (removing toxins, PUFAs, and estrogenic foods; consuming the right saturated fats, proteins, and carbs), you will be able to store more liver glycogen and meals can become less frequent. If you are experiencing numerous metabolic issues, then eight to 10 small meals may be ideal for you. Most people do well on at least six meals. This may include three larger meals, ranging from 300 to 700 calories, and three smaller meals ranging from 100 to 300 calories.

Tracy's Story

Tracy wanted to lose weight for her son's upcoming wedding—eight months away. Tracy was in her early 60s, a workaholic, and a terrible eater when it came to meal size, meal frequency, and mindful eating. Her daily eating looked something like this: Tracy skipped breakfast or ate something small, ate lunch at her desk (salad or whatever the on-site kitchen made her, which she would eat in less than 10 minutes), then ate a big dinner at home and a sweet snack before bed. Although Tracy was not eating tons of food, her meal size and frequency, and when she was eating, were not allowing her body to lose weight.

Due to Tracy's chaotic schedule, travel, and limited free time, it was a challenge to get her to eat the right foods all the time. However, what Tracy could adjust was how much she ate, her meal frequency, and when she was eating each meal. Slowly, Tracy added more food to her breakfast and lunch, and added a mid-day and evening snack. The size of her breakfast and lunch set the tone for how high her metabolism would run all day. Since Tracy wasn't used to eating breakfast, ate a light lunch, and ate no snacks, her metabolism was running low all day. For her to increase metabolic rate she needed to add more fuel (food) to her early meals.

Slowly Tracy added more food to her early meals so she wouldn't overshoot her current metabolic rate. Making adjustments slowly allowed her metabolic rate to increase without extra fat storage. Imagine adding more wood to a well-burning fire: The more you add, the higher the fire burns. Stop adding fuel and the fire dies out. This is how your metabolism works: When your metabolic rate is high, adding more food throughout the day will keep it running all day. Add too much food, and you can shut down the fire and lead to excess fuel (fat storing), whereas depriving your body of food (fuel) will only kill the metabolic rate (fire).

Over the next eight months, Tracy added a total of 500 daily calories to her diet. All of the additional calories were added before dinner. Tracy also decreased the size of her dinner, made sure she ate a carb, protein, and fat in every meal, and consumed a cup of milk and honey for her nighttime snack. It took a little time, but by month three, Tracy started to lose weight. By month six, Tracy had lost a total of 10 pounds, and by month nine, Tracy had lost close to 20 pounds—all while eating more food, in the right frequencies, size, and ratios.

Tracy learned that starving all day and eating a big dinner is a recipe for disaster when trying to lose weight and maintain a high *metabolic rate. The right food in the right frequencies and ratios is the fuel for a high metabolic rate. You have to eat—period. The key is to eat while your energy needs are high (while you are working, working out, thinking, running around)—and to decrease eating when your energy needs are low (laying around all day, before bed, etc.).*

Take Your Body Temperature and Pulse

In addition to balancing your blood sugar with meal size, macronutrient ratios, and meal frequency, there are other tools you can use to help yourself understand if what you are doing is working for you. In the beginning of this book I talked about the work of Dr. Broda Barnes and Dr. Ray Peat and how they used simple measurements like body temperature and pulse to evaluate metabolic function. Temperatures of 97.8–98.6 degrees Fahrenheit and a pulse of 75–90 bpm are associated with a high metabolic rate. Chronically low body temperature and pulse are signs of a slowing metabolism and decreased cellular function.

In general, a metabolically stimulating meal should be used as fuel, producing ATP (heat), water, and CO_2. Therefore, you should feel warm, content, and happy after eating a supportive meal. Taking your temperature and pulse upon waking, and then 20–30 minutes after each meal will help you understand how well the meal is working for you. In a perfect world, a supportive meal should increase both your temperature and pulse.

However, nothing is completely black and white when it comes to using temperature and pulse to evaluate the success of your meal. Here are some examples of what can happen if you are eating in a stressed or a hypo-metabolic state:

1. Temperature and pulse fall after a meal. This means the increased temp and pulse prior to the meal were due to elevated levels of adrenaline and cortisol, not a high metabolic rate. Since sugar and salt will lower cortisol and adrenaline levels, eating will end up lowering body temperature and pulse if the person is initially warm due to

increased stress hormones.

2. Temperature stays the same after eating. The meal may be too low in calories or the wrong ratio of macronutrients.

3. You already have a high pulse (above 100) and eating increases your pulse even more. This may mean a ratio of too much protein to carbs. Eating eggs by themselves will increase insulin, leading to an increase in adrenaline. This will increase pulse but hinder thyroid function.

4. You have a lower pulse (below 70) and show an increase in pulse after eating. This is a good meal and means thyroid levels may have increased.

5. You have a high pulse (above 100) and low temperature (below 97.8) prior to eating, and food increases temperature and decreases pulse. This is a good meal and means the thyroid is working optimally by lowering stress hormones and increasing heat production.

6. You have low pulse (below 70) and low temperature (below 97.8) before eating, and both rise after eating. This is a good meal. Both increased pulse and increased temperature are supportive to increased metabolic function.

Temperature and pulse are great tools to use to see if your current diet is working for you. Please remember taking temperature and pulse is not an exact science—just feedback for you to use in your healing journey.

Log Your Food-Mood-Poop-Sleep

If there is one single thing everyone should do to help them understand if their current diet is working for them, it is logging their food, mood, poop, and sleep. Recording when you eat, howmuch, the ratio of fats, carbs, and proteins, body temperature and pulse, how you feel after your meals, how you sleep, and a description of your elimination (pooping) will be your own personal guide to understanding your body and how food is affecting your metabolism, health, sleep, etc.

Are You Pooping?

Being able to eliminate at least one time each day is a sign of good health. Chronic constipation is a sign that something is wrong. Constipation is a sign of a sluggish gut and intestine. Constipation is linked to hypothyroidism and a low metabolic rate. Elimination is important so you can remove toxins and bacteria. The longer bacteria and toxins stay in your system the more damage they can do. Your feces are primarily made of dead bacteria, fiber, water, and toxins.

A healthy feces is firm, about 6–8 inches in length, and about an inch in diameter. The color is usually brown, due to the bile from the liver used for fat digestion. Feces can change in color due to the foods you eat. If you are having a hard time eliminating you may be dehydrated and need to add in more minerals (primarily salt), fruit, and water- containing foods to your diet. Increasing saturated fat, especially coconut oil, can help with elimination. Adding a raw carrot or cooked bamboo shoots will help clean out bacterial endotoxins and estrogen from your bowel. Avoiding hard-to-digest foods like nuts, legumes, grains, and raw vegetables will also help with bowel health. Taking an Epsom salts bath or consuming a tablespoon of Epsom salts will help with daily constipation. The herb cascara sagrada is also helpful in relieving constipation.

Using a site like Cronometer (https://cronometer.com) to log your food will give you valuable feedback. Logging will let you know if the size of your meal, your meal frequency, and the macronutrient ratios are supporting a warm body, good digestion, and restful sleep.

So many people think they are eating the right amount of food and the right ratio of macronutrients. However, once they start food logging they learn a completely different story. Many people find they are not eating enough or they are eating far too much. Some find they are eating too much fat, or not enough carbohydrates, or too little or too much protein. Others notice certain foods causing drops in their temperature and pulse, and/or affecting their mood and sleep. The only way you will know what is working for you is by recording your food in an actual food journal. The food log gives you so much usable feedback. Without the log you will be guessing what is working and what is not.

In addition, food logging keeps you accountable for eating the right foods. It is far easier to eat crappy foods when you are not accountable to your food log. Trust me: Logging your food alone will help clean up your diet.

In summary, there is more to optimizing your health and metabolic rate than just eating the right pro-metabolic foods and food supplements, and avoiding the wrong anti-metabolic foods. Balancing your blood sugar through the right ratio of macronutrients, the size of your meal, and the frequency of your meals will help support metabolic function, increased energy, and increased fat loss, and support overall well-being. In addition, receiving valuable feedback by taking temperature and pulse, and logging your food, mood, and poop, will give you valuable information if your new food plan is working. At the end of the day we all are different, are in different states of health, and have different needs. No one food plan is going to work across the board for everyone. Feedback through logging is the only way to individualize your program for you. If you are not logging you will only be guessing.

Chapter 15:
What You Need to Know

1. Balancing your blood sugar through the right macronutrient combinations (fats, carbs, proteins), meal size, and frequency is essential for healing a damaged metabolism.

2. Eating the right size meal means eating a meal that makes you feel good—not stuffed or hungry in an hour. The meal should make you feel warm and energized, not tired.

3. The optimal macronutrient amounts are dependent on the individual's size, age, sex, activity level, and the state of his or her metabolism. A good starting point for most people is to consume a meal with 50-percent carbs, 25-percent fat, and 25-percent protein. These numbers will shift as the person heals.

4. Meal frequency will depend on the person's metabolic rate, activity, and liver health. Healthier or less active people will be able to go longer without food due to the ability of the liver to store more glycogen or use less glycogen stores. Unhealthy or very active people will need to eat more frequently due to their inability to store liver glycogen or their high activity level.

5. Use body temperature, pulse, mood, poop, and sleep to monitor your progress in healing your body. Optimal daily body temperature should be around 98.6 degrees Fahrenheit (or 37 degrees Celsius). Pulse should be 75–90 bpm. Your meals should make you feel good, warm, and happy. Elimination should be daily and sleep should be seven to nine hours without interruption.

Chapter 16
There's More to Healing Than Just Food

Although nutrition and balancing your blood sugar are big players in the healing puzzle, there is more to healing a damaged metabolism than just milk, fruit, eggs, bone broth, liver, coconut oil, coffee, salt, and meal size, frequency, and macronutrient ratios. What you put in your body plays a *huge* role in the healing of your body's systems. Internally, food can be one of the biggest stressors or biggest metabolic stimulators. However, we also face numerous external stressors, which, if not also addressed, will interfere with the healing process. Poor sleep, too much or too intense exercise, too much or not enough water, and even an unhappy life can all affect the health of your metabolism.

Stress and the General Adaptation Syndrome

To begin, let's talk about stress. Stress is how your body reacts to a challenge. Stress can come from something good (winning the lottery, a wedding) or bad (a divorce, a demanding job). Stress is a normal human function, needed to keep us alive. Chronic stress is when stress lasts too long or becomes too hard. Chronic stress is linked to digestive issues, immune disorders, cancer, diabetes, and death.

Endocrinologist Hans Selye is referred to as the father of stress. Selye conducted thousands of studies attempting to understand stress and its effects on the human body. In Selye's decades of work he developed the term "general adaptation syndrome" (GAS) to describe how the body responds to stress. GAS is characterized in three stages:

Alarm

Alarm is an initial phase showing how the body reacts either through shock (non-reactive; i.e., unable to move) or non-shock (fight or flight; i.e., running from a lion) responses.

Resistance

Resistance is characterized as the physiological responses your body has once you understand the stress. Increased lipolysis (fat burning), catabolism (muscle breakdown), and glucose mobilization (used glycogen stores) all occur in the resistance phase. The body is trying to *adapt* to the stressors put upon it. The resistance phase can lead to homeostasis if the body can handle the stress and return back to normal. If the stress continues, the resistance phase can deplete the body's resources very quickly, leading to the next phase.

Exhaustion

This is when the body's resources have been depleted and the body is unable to maintain normal function. Fatigue, depression, weight gain or weight loss, immune and digestive issues, disease, and even death are all a result of the exhaustive phase. In some research this is referred to as "adrenal fatigue." However, as I discussed in Chapter 1, I believe "adrenal fatigue" is just the result of a suppressed thyroid.

In summary, stress cannot be avoided and is a normal function of your body. Stress develops into a problem when it turns chronic and your body's resistance becomes low. This can lead to adrenal exhaustion and thyroid suppression, which will eventually lead to illness, disease and death.

Sleep

The simplest (yet the most challenging for some of us) thing you can do to help heal your metabolism is to get more sleep. We have become a society of "do more and sleep less." With constant stimulation from the moment we wake up until the moment we fall asleep, our sleep quantity and quality have suffered dramatically. In the 1940s the average American was sleeping more than eight hours a night; today that number has dropped to less than seven hours.

Since a reduction of sleep is linked to gaining weight, fatigue, depression, decreased cognitive function, decreased performance, increased stress hormones, and decreased thyroid, it makes sense that our nation has become fatter, more depressed, more stressed out, more infertile, and more ill. Our medical and pharmaceutical industry has responded with more drugs and more procedures, which in most cases are addressing only the symptoms, not the problems. Americans spend more money on health care than any other industrialized nation. If this system was really working, shouldn't we be healthier? Yet we are not.

We already know that all the above symptoms (obesity, depression, libido issues, slow thinking, etc.) are linked to a sluggish thyroid. What you should also know is sleep and metabolism work synergistically with each other. When our metabolism is high we sleep deep and restful; when it is sluggish, we are more inclined to have disrupted sleep. Just like when we sleep less, our metabolism slows down and stress hormones increase. So it only seems logical to work on our sleep so that we can support a well-running metabolism.

Darkness is stressful and catabolic to a human's system. To protect us from the catabolism of darkness, humans are programmed to sleep. This is why we get tired as night approaches; it's our body's way of trying to protect us. Our sleep cycle works on a circadian rhythm (a 24-hour biological process). Ideally, we are awake during the day and sleep during the night. Optimal sleep is deep and lasts seven to nine hours. The problem for most of us (me included) is we like to ignore our bodies signals, and instead of going to sleep we choose to stay up late watching TV, working, surfing the net, or partying. (I'm guilty of all four.) Once we ignore our body's signals, stress hormones rise and thyroid function drops.

Think about this: Have you ever been tired around 9 p.m.,

then had a surge of energy around 10:30 p.m., and then cannot fall asleep? Your stress hormones have kicked in and given you that burst of energy. Some of us may call this our "second wind," but in reality it's just your body reacting to a stressful situation.

What Happens When We Sleep?

A number of repair processes happen when we sleep, most importantly the repair of our cells' mitochondria (cells' power houses). According to nutritional researcher Ray Peat, PhD, "In restful sleep, the oxygen tension is frequently low enough, and the carbon dioxide tension high enough to trigger the multiplication of stem cells and mitochondria." What does this mean? It means sleep helps generate more mitochondria. Remember the cells' mitochondria are where we produce the majority of our energy. More mitochondria result in more energy, which equals a higher metabolic rate. Stress kills mitochondria. Thus lack of sleep and darkness will decrease the amount of mitochondria, slowing metabolic function.

In addition to repairing our very valuable mitochondria, sleep is the safest and best time to burn fat. And who doesn't want to burn more fat, right? At rest your large skeletal muscles and heart muscle prefer to use fat as energy. *But, I thought you said carbohydrates were the ideal source of energy?** Yes, I did—and that is true, especially when you are active, thinking, working, stressing, etc. However, at rest your large muscles and heart prefer to use fat**—so sleeping more and deeper is a great time to utilize fat stores without all the oxidative damage and thyroid-suppressing effects of trying to burn fat while working out.

***While being active, sugar is your best source of energy.** Protein and fat are still utilized while you are awake and busy, but most metabolic processes prefer sugars for optimal energy output and increased CO2 levels.

****While sleeping and resting, fat** *is the ideal source of energy for skeletal and heart muscles.* Sugar and protein are still being utilized while sleeping by organs, repairing tissue, blood, and other metabolic processes, but fat is king when it comes to muscles fuel at night. This is a BIG reason why more muscle is helpful in losing more fat (more on that in the next section).

Better Quality and Quantity of Sleep Equals a Higher Metabolism

Babies and children have a high metabolic rate. They sleep deeper and longer than adults. Thus, a high metabolic rate is associated with good sleep. As we age and damage our metabolism, our sleep becomes disrupted and shorter. Hypothyroid individuals have a hard time falling asleep and they wake up throughout the night. Poor sleep is the result of a stressed body and the inability to regulate blood sugar, all relating to low thyroid function.

As I discussed in Chapter 1, low thyroid will lead to a sluggish liver and the inability of the liver to store glycogen (stored glucose). Once liver glycogen is low, your body cannot regulate blood sugar at night, and this becomes stressful to your body. Remember from the last chapter that low blood sugar will encourage cortisol and adrenaline to increase. A rise in the stress hormones cortisol and adrenaline will lead to a breakdown of your body's tissues (organs, muscle, fat, thymus). The breakdown of tissue through gluconeogenesis will help increase blood sugar levels and keep you alive, but regulating blood sugar this way will come at the expense of you sleeping through the night. Once your stress hormones spike you may wake up or have trouble going to sleep, or, worse, you get insomnia. None of these are helpful for a restful night's sleep.

What Can You Do to Encourage Restful Sleep?

Like I said above, quality sleep supports a high metabolic rate, and a high metabolic rate supports restful sleep. The two work synergistically with each other. If sleep suffers, metabolism suffers, and if metabolism suffers, so will your sleep.

Therefore, anything you can do to increase metabolic rate will help support restful sleep.

How do you do this? Well, let's recap the last 15 chapters of this book:

1. Consume an easy-to-digest pro-metabolic diet including the right carbs, saturated fats, and easy-to-digest proteins.

2. Consume salt and other minerals like calcium, potassium, and magnesium.

3. Remove foods that will lead to digestive upset, such as processed foods, grains, nuts, seeds, PUFAs, legumes, and beans.

4. Decrease toxic load: alcohol, pharmaceutical or recreational drugs, carrageenan, soy lecithin, artificial sweeteners, BPA, fillers, additives, and estrogenic substances (parabens, hormone therapy, plastics).

5. Balance your blood sugar. Eat small regular, balanced meals throughout the day.

6. Reduce external stressors, which may include working less, addressing unhappy relationships, and finding what makes you happy.

Nutrition and diet are vital to a healthy body, but if you continue to work 80 hours a week, stay in an unhealthy relationship, and are unhappy with your life, a good nutritional program will only go so far.

Imagine wearing a bulletproof vest (good nutrition) when you are in the middle of a war (the stress of work, relationships, kids, alcohol, etc.). The vest is only going to do so much. If you really want to save yourself (sleep better), get off the battlefield (reduce all stressors).

Changing your diet and reducing external stressors in your life is going to take a little time, so be patient. But do not fret!

Here are 10 simple things you can do now to encourage a good night's sleep:

1. Consume something sweet and salty an hour to 30 minutes before bed. Sugar and salt lower stress hormones. When blood sugar levels are maintained, stress hormones decrease and getting to sleep becomes easier.

   Examples of *sleepy* nighttime snacks:

   a. Milk, raw honey, and a pinch of salt. The sugar (milk and honey) and salt will bring down stress hormones. In addition, the calcium from the milk is an anti-stress mineral used to decrease parathyroid hormone, a stress hormone.

   b. Pulp-free orange juice, gelatin, and a pinch of salt. The sugar (orange juice) and salt will bring down stress hormones. Gelatin is high in glycine. Glycine has anti-stress properties and has shown improvements in sleep.

   c. Bone broth, salt, and fruit. The sugar (fruit) and salt will bring down stress hormones. Bone broth contains the anti-stress amino acid glycine. Bone broth contains the minerals calcium and magnesium, both of which have anti-stress properties and support relaxation.

   d. Fruit and Parmigiano Reggiano cheese. The sugar (fruit) and salt (cheese) will bring down stress hormones. The calcium in cheese will inhibit PTH.

   Be sure to consume each snack slowly. Eating or drinking too fast can be stressful to the body.

2. Have a salty/sweet drink next to your bed just in case you wake up in the middle of the night. A sweet-salty drink, like orange juice and a pinch of salt, can help bring down adrenaline and cortisol spikes that occur during the night.

Lowering the stress hormones will allow your body to go back to sleep faster.

3. Turn off all electrical devices one to two hours before bedtime. TVs, computers, iPads, and cell phones can stimulate the brain and contribute to poor sleep.

4. Take a warm Epsom salts bath before bed. Warm water can heat the body, producing a thyroid-like effect. In addition, magnesium from the Epsom salts can calm the body and allow it to relax. Make sure the water is not too hot. Very hot water will increase stress hormones.

5. Read a book or listen to soft music. Both of these can help your body and mind relax.

6. Create a relaxing environment. Use a sound machine, turn down the room temperature, and purchase a quality bed. Noises, a lumpy bed, and a hot room can affect your sleep.

7. Stop drinking caffeine four to five hours before bed. Although caffeine is thyroid-supportive, it can disrupt blood sugar levels, leading to sleep issues.

8. Wear socks. Cold hands and feet are signs of hypothyroidism. Simply warming the feet with socks can help the body relax.

9. Consume extra calcium at night. Calcium is an anti-stress mineral. Calcium lowers parathyroid hormone, which rises under stress to raise blood calcium levels by breaking down bone. Bone broth, milk, cheese, and eggshell calcium are beneficial.

10. Journal or meditate before bed. Dumping all your thoughts out on paper before bedtime allows you to get them off your mind. Writing them in a journal helps you from thinking about your issues, problems, and day's activities all night long.

Sleep and metabolism go hand in hand. Even with the best of nutrition plans, if you opt to not sleep, your body is going to suffer. And if your nutrition is poor and your life stressors are high, your sleep will become disrupted and only make your life more stressful. Sleep, as easy as it should be, has become one of the hardest things for people to get more of. We are so busy getting more done, we are sleeping less and stressing more. Sleeping more may be the missing puzzle piece in your healing journey. More sleep is linked to weight loss, happiness, clear thinking, less disease and illness, and a longer life. So before going out and spending thousands of dollars on your next specialist to find out why you are "feeling bad," examine your sleep. Going to bed earlier may be all the medicine you need.

Exercise

Exercise has been a huge part of my life for as long as I can remember, from soccer and tennis as a child and as an adolescent to running, weight lifting, and cycling as an adult. I have always considered myself to be one of the "lucky ones" since I enjoy working out and staying active. Sweat, hard work, competition, and physical challenges were always up my alley.

During most of my teens, my 20s, and even my early 30s, I believed when it came to exercise more was better. In my 20s my workouts were usually two hours every day, weight training one hour and cardio another. In my 30s, I was doing more group and personal training sessions, sometimes teaching one or two classes, weight training with a client, and then training myself for some sort of endurance event, all in one day—craziness. My belief was if one hour of exercise was good, then two or three hours must be better, right? Wrong—so wrong. My excessive exercise was leading to slow healing injuries, low body temperature, digestive issues, sleep issues, hormonal issues, and a very unhealthy relationship to working out. Exercise was no longer supporting my health: It was harming it.

Running a Marathon Suppressed My Metabolism

I decided to run my first marathon in 2009 to raise money for Stand Up for Kids, a charity helping homeless kids. In fact, I decided to run a total of 57 miles for the charity (a 3-mile race, a 6-mile race, a 9-mile race, a 13-mile half-marathon, and a 26-mile marathon) in a six-month period. Every week I added more miles and more time on the road, and every week I became more fit (I could run farther and harder with less exertion).

During this time, my caloric input increased, slightly, to offset some of my caloric output (running), which allowed me to maintain my weight throughout the intense training. I think it is interesting to note that after six months of training, running in six races, and running hundreds of miles I lost zero pounds. I became aerobically fit but not leaner.

The issues started not while I was training, but after my training was over and I resumed my normal pre-training diet. You know what happened? I started to gain weight! The very diet that kept my weight steady before the training was the same diet that allowed me to gain weight after the training.

Why did this happen?

Essentially, all my intense cardio training (lots of stress) had dropped my resting metabolic rate. Although I was burning lots of calories on my one- to three-hour runs, I was beginning to burn fewer calories while not working out the remaining 21–23 hours a day. So when the running decreased and I resumed normal eating, my metabolism was now suppressed, resulting in weight gain.

When this happened to me, I had no idea metabolic slowing is what was going on. So instead of resting and allowing my metabolism to recover, I pushed myself more. This was the start of my metabolic downfall.

As you know from my initial story earlier in the book, my metabolic breakdown was a big turning point for me. I finally realized the very things I thought should be helping me (lots of exercise and a low-carb/high-protein diet) were only making things worse. For the first time in my life, I took time off from working out. I rested more, reduced workout times and intensity, and allowed my body to heal. Who knew resting could be so metabolically stimulating?

Intense Exercise Suppresses Thyroid Function

Most people are led to believe that exercise increases basal (resting) metabolic rate (BMR). Yet, this couldn't be further from the truth. In numerous studies conducted on athletes, strenuous exercise (cardiovascular and weight training) from as little as one week up to as long as one year had a negative correlation to thyroid function. Many of us know long-duration cardio can suppress metabolism, yet most are unaware that intense weight training can lower thyroid levels as well. I know this is going to upset most personal trainers, but high intensity interval training, Cross-fit, or high intensity strength training does not increase metabolic rate (thyroid levels).

We have been led to believe if we are burning more daily calories that our metabolism has increased, but this has nothing to do with an increased resting metabolic rate. It only has to do with increased energy expenditure from more work (exercise) and an increase in stress hormones.

Yes, you may burn a load of calories during these intense exercise plans, but this is in response to a stressful activity and increased adrenaline and cortisol, not because your thyroid levels are increasing. Thyroid levels recover to normal levels *only* when cortisol levels have decreased.

Note: In a healthy person, thyroid levels can return very quickly post-workout, especially with the aid of sugar and minerals (salt, magnesium calcium, potassium). In someone with a damaged metabolism, thyroid levels will remain suppressed, leading to more damage.

Has Exercise Suppressed Your Metabolism?

Want to know if exercise has suppressed your metabolism? Check your body temperature and pulse. Most endurance athletes run a cool 96 degrees Fahrenheit and have a pulse around 50 beats per minute (bpm). Low body temperature and pulse are *not* supportive of a high running metabolic rate. Yet, these factors are needed for long endurance activity. This is an adaptive measure to allow the body to perform at a high level for a long time. This stress adaptation makes your body more efficient, allowing the athlete to use less fuel to go harder and longer. However, although this works well for the athlete's performance, it actually slows his or her metabolism at rest. The lower metabolic rate can lead to suppressed digestive, detox, and immune systems.

World-class endurance athletes have heart rates around 45–50 bpm and low body temperature (95–96 degrees Farenheit). In fact, every long-distance athlete I know seems to be freezing all the time. Many of them have horrible digestion, hormonal issues, hair loss, premature aging, and chronic colds and illness.

Yes, they may be lean and great at their sport, but this does not mean they are healthy. It just means their body has become very efficient at conserving fuel by lowering immune function, lowering body temperature and pulse, decreasing hormonal and digestive function, and decreasing hair and skin growth.

Now, this does not mean you should never engage in intense exercise.

Intense exercise has its place when you want to drop fat, increase strength and power, and increase athletic performance, but not when you are trying to heal a damaged metabolism. All of these types of activities need to be done when the body is healthy, not when you are suffering from lack of sleep, an 80-hour workweek, digestive-upset, no sex drive, and/or a cold.

A Stressed-Out Body Should *Not* Be Doing a Stressful Workout

If you are healthy, intense exercise like heavy lifting, sprinting, or high-intensity training can be done successfully with good results. Still, all intense exercise should be done in moderation, with enough recovery and rest to restore metabolic function without long-term damage. This means no more than two to three intense sessions a week. At my peak, I was working hard and long five or seven days a week. Intense workouts five to seven days a week will lead to overtraining and a depressed thyroid. Overtraining can lead to sleep issues, slow recovery, muscle breakdown, injury, and digestive and hormonal issues. All were true for me.

Please note: I am not against participating in any of these activities—as long as you are healthy. I still participate in endurance events (one each year), and I love high-intensity training and weight training. I do them because I enjoy the challenge and social aspects. I am also in a healthy state, am aware of my limits, and now give myself ample rest and recovery, all while eating a very supportive diet. When you have a strong foundation (good diet and health) intense exercise can be very beneficial, but for someone with a weak foundation (hypo-thyroid and poor diet and sleep) intense exercise will just exacerbate the issues.

Exercise and Healing

The right amount of exercise has many positive qualities: increased muscle mass, better mood, more energy, and increased bone density, coordination, agility, balance, heart strength, and endurance. When people are healthy they will benefit from exercise, even from intense exercise. However, when you are metabolically damaged the rules change, and sometimes that means very little exercise or no exercise at all. In a stressed body with a damaged metabolism, exercise can cause more harm than good. We have to remember: Exercise is stress. If your body is already overloaded with too much work, a poor diet, and a lack of sleep, adding exercise will only contribute to more stress, and this will inhibit the healing process.

This makes you wonder:

Should you exercise while healing?

For most this answer is yes, but for some people, especially those with very low body temperature and pulse, and a series of health issues (poor digestion, hormone issues, depression, sleep issues), exercise should be decreased or even stopped, at least until symptoms have improved with a supportive diet, rest, and the removal of stressors in their life.

For others, some exercise can be beneficial as long as it is light to moderate. This may include gentle yoga (not hot or Bikram yoga), walking, easy swimming, tai chi, lightweight training, or anything that feels stress-free versus stressful. Exercise in a well-lit room, with natural light, that is kept cool. Dark rooms and heat are stressors to the body. Most workouts should last no longer than 30–45 minutes and should keep your heart rate under 100 bpm. Intense hiking, running, high-intensity intervals, and intense weight training are very stressful activities and will not be supportive to a healing metabolism. A low-stress workout should make you feel better throughout your day, not more exhausted. If you feel more drained an hour or two after your workout, then you have pushed too hard and need to back down.

For many, including me, resting is a challenging concept, especially since I work in the fitness industry. Yet, working out less and sleeping more were just what my body needed. My two-hour workouts turned into two-hour naps. I slept more, ate more, and moved less. A far cry from what I was used to, but for the first few months, this was exactly what I needed. With the support of proper nutrition, more sleep, and not stressing about perfection, I slowly started to recover from my 20 years of metabolic destruction.

The *Right Amount* of Weight Training Can Support the Healing Process

Once my body began to heal (more energy, better sleep, improved digestion), I started to incorporate a more vigorous weight-training program. Moderate weight lifting is an excellent way to strengthen your body and increase fat burning by adding more muscle without excessive stress. More muscle equals increased *safe* fat-burning at night and while resting throughout the day. Remember: At rest, your heart and skeletal muscles prefer fat as fuel. However, while you are exercising, thinking, and working all day long your muscles will use a combination of macronutrients (fats, carbs, proteins) but primarily carbs (sugars).

Although I was feeling better with more food and more sleep, I did add a few pounds (which is normal) when trying to heal my body. Working as a personal trainer, I was eager to regain my body, yet cautious about overdoing my exercise program. My workouts were no longer than 45 minutes, and I decreased the number of workouts to four to five times each week (versus one to two times each day, five to seven days a week). The shorter workouts kept me sane, while not pushing me too hard.

Here are some quick guidelines to follow when starting your weight-training program:

- Work out in the morning or midday. Nighttime workouts tend to keep you awake.

- Start slow with a 30-minute session one to two times each week.

- Gradually add workout days, but do not to exceed four to five days per week.

- Allow for a rest day every two to three days.
- Increase workout time, but do not exceed 60 minutes (warm up and cool down included).
- Rest one to three minutes between sets.
- Perform two to five sets of each exercise.
- Perform 12–20 reps of each set.
- Start with light weights but aim to eventually lift heavy weights; 3- to 5-pound weights are not going to add muscle.
- Work large muscles: legs, chest, back, and shoulders.
- Best exercises include:

  Legs: squats, lunges, step-ups, deadlifts.

  Chest: push-ups, chest press, bench press, pec fly.

  Back: pull-ups, pull downs, cable rows, dumbbell rows.

  Shoulders: shoulder press, lateral raises, upright rows.

Eat Supportively While Working Out

For maximum weight-training results make sure you eat a supportive diet and get enough sleep. Being properly fueled and rested is imperative for the additional exercise stress you will be placing on your body. In addition, what you eat before, during, and after your workout is very important to building fat-burning muscle.

Pre-Workout: Your pre-workout meal is essential so that your body has enough fuel for the increased energy demands you are about to put upon it. Too much food or too little food will hinder performance. For a 30–60 minute workout, 200–400 calories prior to the workout should be adequate. Individuals who work out on an empty stomach, to increase fat burning, are just stressing their bodies by increasing cortisol and decreasing thyroid. According to Ray Peat, PhD, "Men who went for a run before breakfast were found to have broken chromosomes in their blood cells, but if they ate breakfast before running, their chromosomes weren't damaged."

Bottom line: Eat something prior to exercise to decrease cellular damage.

Good examples are eggs and OJ, fruit and cheese, or a milk smoothie.

During Workout: It is not necessary to consume calories during a workout, especially if you have consumed adequate calories prior to exercise, to gain muscle. However, for many, a constant flow of easy to digest carbohydrates (sugars) while exercising will maintain blood sugar levels and help to decrease stress hormones, which is supportive to increasing thyroid levels.

I like to use Kate's Miracle Drink. (See Chapter 20.) This drink contains healthy carbs, proteins, and minerals (salt, magnesium, calcium, and potassium) to help support the body under stress. This beverage can also be consumed between meals to help maintain blood sugar levels.

Post-Workout: If you are looking to add muscle, your post-workout meal or drink is very important. For up to two hours post-exercise your muscle cells are more sensitive to insulin. Increased insulin sensitivity will allow for more carbohydrates and protein to be shuttled into the muscle cells. Carbohydrates decrease the catabolism of tissue under stress and allow for used muscle glycogen stores to be replenished. Protein is needed for growth and repair. If a full meal is not in your future, then any one of the below milk-based drinks can elicit the desired effect.

Good examples are homemade chocolate milk; milk, raw honey, and salt; and an orange-creamsicle smoothie. (All recipes are found in Chapter 20.)

We must remember exercise is stress, and an excess of stress can lead to a suppressed metabolism. Your current lifestyle, including diet, sleep habits, and daily stressors (work, family, relationships), should be considered before starting an exercise program. If your life is already incredibly stressful, focus should be on reducing stress and participating in exercise that is low to moderate in intensity, like yoga, light swimming, lightweight training, and walking. Doing an intense exercise program in a stressed state will only lead to more dysfunction long-term.

While you are healing, emphasis should be placed on mood, energy, digestion, sleep, and immune and hormonal function, and not on weight loss. Exercise should support thyroid health and low stress until the body begins to heal. Once you begin to feel better, with more energy and fewer health issues, a more intense exercise program can be implemented to help support weight loss. Exercise can be a great tool in helping you regain your health and keeping you lean—as long it is used properly. Too much exercise can lead to muscle catabolism, sleep issues, heart issues, anxiety, hormonal issues, and depression—just as too little exercise can lead to the same. Know and understand your limits. Moderation is key!

Water

The water craze has been going on for years and years. Health-conscious people cannot leave their homes without a BPA-free bottle filled with water. Health, nutrition, and fitness professionals are constantly promoting the importance of drinking tons of water. The health industry tells us to drink anywhere from eight 8 oz. glasses/ day to 1 gallon/day to half our body weight in ounces of water/day. The question is: Should we be doing this? Should we be drinking tons of water, just because we read in *Shape* or *Fitness* magazine that it will solve all our weight-loss woes? Should we be drinking tons of water even if we are not thirsty? Should we be drinking tons of water if we are consuming fruits and vegetables and other water- filled foods? Should we be drinking tons of water if we are peeing every 20 minutes? The answer, on all accounts, is *no!* But many of us are drinking liters and liters of water because we believe it is healthy—when, in fact, we may be overhydrating, diluting our cells, and causing additional stress to our bodies.

I am not saying drinking water is bad; you definitely need

water. I am just saying to follow a generalized guide like "drink 64 ounces of water a day" makes *no* physiological sense. Telling everyone they need to drink eight glasses of water a day, without taking into consideration their metabolic rate and their activity, and without understanding their diet and the current temperature and humidity, is like telling everyone they should eat 1,200 calories and work out two hours a day to lose weight. Wait, we do that too—maybe not the greatest example. My point is: There are many myths surrounding the health and fitness world that make no physiological sense, yet we continue to follow them, because someone (your trainer, your nutritionist, your doctor, Dr. Oz) told us it was a good idea. I am here to tell you it may not be. Why? One word: hyperhydration.

Hyperhydration

Hyperhydration, water intoxication or over-hydrating, occurs when someone drinks too much water, creating an electrolyte imbalance. This usually occurs when they are trying to prevent dehydration. Once this imbalance occurs your cells swell, including those of your brain, to try to balance the concentration of solutes (water) to solvents (salt). This can lead to headaches, confusion, weight gain, vomiting, cramping, twitching, and even death. Basically too much water without enough electrolytes, especially salt, will lead to overhydration (swelling) of the cells—which is bad, just in case you were wondering.

Many health-conscious people, even health and fitness professionals, are walking around carrying liters or even gallon water jugs, chugging them all day long and wondering why they feel so crappy—all in the name of health. These are the same people on a low-sodium diet, scared to drink juice and milk, and avoiding high-mineral foods like fruits because they contain too much sugar. The truth is, the only thing these people are creating is a body deficient of minerals and good sugars, and an overload of water in the cells.

Funny story: Last year, I was traveling with my good friend Shari, who is also in the health and fitness industry. Although Shari and I are both in the industry, we definitely hold different beliefs when it comes to diet and nutrition. When I met up with Shari, she told me she was attempting to super-hydrate herself by drinking 1–2 liters of water a day for the next seven days. She also told me she was peeing about every hour, and felt bloated and heavy. Her sleep was interrupted from waking up to pee, and her urine was completely clear.

After noticing how little water I was drinking and that I was only peeing five to six times a day (versus her 20 times), Shari asked my thoughts about her super-hydrating. Basically, I told her she wasn't doing herself any favors forcing water down her throat even if she was not thirsty. I told her that her increased water, without adequate mineral intake, was diluting the minerals in her body, leading to cramping, fatigue, sleep issues, nausea, and bloating.

A little perplexed, Shari decided to stop her crazy water goal while she was on our trip. You want to know what happened? Within one day, she felt lighter, her bloating went away, she started to pee less, she felt warmer, and she slept better. All by drinking less water. I truly love fitness professionals, but the industry has created a lot of "healthy rules" that quite honestly have no physiological backing and are creating unhealthy teachings. Understanding your body and listening to your own thirst mechanism is your best way to judge when and how much water you should drink.

How Do You Know if You Are Overhydrating?

Here are five symptoms that may happen if you are consuming too much water:

1. You pee every hour or more than five times a day. You should pee about four or five times a day, and you should be able to sleep through the night without getting up to pee.

2. Your pee is clear. Clear pee is *not* a sign of health. Clear pee is a sign you are diluting your electrolytes. Pee should be yellow. Pale or light yellow urine is a sign of overhydration.

3. You have sleep issues due to getting up in the middle of the night to pee.

4. You are cold. Your hands and feet are cold.

5. You feel thirsty all the time. Sometimes over-hydration increases thirst, which makes you drink even more and exacerbates the issue. This usually means you need more salt and sugar in the diet, not more water. Exchange your water for Kate's Miracle Drink, bone broth, orange juice, and milk to help the electrolyte imbalance.

In addition, if you are suffering from a low metabolism, excessive water drinking may be putting additional strain on your already-compromised metabolism. Excess water can be stressful to the body. Diluting electrolytes makes nerve connection and signaling more challenging. In addition, the kidneys have to work harder to excrete all the additional liquid. Therefore, high amounts of water will produce a stress response in the body. And as you know, stress reduces thyroid function. Therefore, excessive water drinking can suppress your already-suppressed thyroid, which will lower your metabolic rate even more.

Please understand: I am not trying to scare you away from drinking water. Once again, you *need* water. However, what you should understand is that your body not only receives water from the water you drink, but also through the foods you eat and through cellular respiration. Fruits and vegetables are about 70-percent water. Coffee, bone broth, orange juice, and milk all have a high water content. To be honest, all foods have a percentage of water, so there is really no real need to drink half your body weight in water—unless you love hanging out in your bathroom. In addition, your cells produce water through cellular respiration (metabolism). Water is an end product along with CO_2 and ATP (energy).

How Much Water should You Drink?

Well, like everything else in this book, the answer is based on the person. Water consumption can depend on the person's metabolic rate, current diet, the temperature and the humidity outside, and the person's activity level. If you have a high metabolic rate, you are highly active, and the temperatures outside are warmer, you will need to consume more water, but not more than your body is telling you. Remember to listen to your thirst. In addition, you will also need to consume more salt *and* other electrolytes like magnesium, calcium, and potassium. When you sweat more you release more salt. Replacing the lost water and not the salt can result in hyponatremia. Hyponatremia is when sodium levels become dangerously low. This can be seen in many endurance athletes who only hydrate with water. A study on runners in the Boston Marathon found that 13 percent of runners had hyponatremia by the end of the race. The hyponatremia resulted from consumption of more than 3 liters of fluid throughout the race and a race time of four hours. Hyponatremia can result in weight gain, gait disturbances, mental fatigue, and even bone fractures.

Think about this: When you go to the hospital and you are dehydrated, the hospital *never* gives you an IV of only water. Right? The IV usually contains a combination of both water and salt, and sometimes glucose. Proper hydration does not come from water only. An IV of water only could kill you. An IV of water and salt will bring you back to life. Making sense yet?

Moral of the story: If you are going to drink more fluids due to heat, humidity, or excess exercise, consume adequate amounts of salt and sugars to help support electrolyte levels and metabolic health.

Basic guidelines for water consumption

1. Drink when you are thirsty.

2. Drink more in dry, hot, or humid weather. Add additional salt and sugar to fluids.

3. Consume more fluids with salt, additional minerals, and sugar. Milk, orange juice, bone broth, and Kate's Miracle Drink are all good options.

4. Consume foods that contain water, especially fruits—and add salt.

5. If you are cold, tired, low energy, and hypo-metabolic, eat more calorie-rich, salty-sweet foods (like cheese and fruit) and drink less water.

To sum it up, you need water; you just don't need to be forcing it down your throat in the name of health. Too much water can be stress on the body, leading to over-hydration and hyponatremia. In extreme cases too much water can lead to vomiting, cramping, fainting, and even death. The right amount of water for you should be based on your metabolic rate, current diet, and activity level, and the temperature and humidity of the outside. Listening to your body's thirst mechanism is the best way to determine when and how much you should drink.

Chapter 16
What You Need to Know

1. Deep, quality sleep goes hand-in-hand with a high metabolic rate. Good sleep supports metabolism. A healthy metabolism will support good sleep. Sleep helps generate more cellular mitochondria (the cells' energy source). Sleep allows muscles to burn fat with less oxidative stress. Optimal sleep is uninterrupted for seven to nine hours. Consume something sweet and salty before bed to help with sleep.

2. Exercise is stress and can lower thyroid function. A healthy person can handle intense, stressful exercise. A hypo-metabolic person should refrain from intense exercise until he or she shows improvements in symptoms. Weight training, due to its muscle-increasing results, is the best form of exercise for body composition changes.

3. Eat supportively before, during, and after a workout to support thyroid function. The more intense and longer your workout, the more you need to eat.

4. Water consumption should be based on thirst, not a set amount, like 64 ounces or eight glasses of water a day. Warmer weather, a high metabolic rate, and more activity will require more water—and more minerals. Water is obtained by not only water drinking but also by the food we eat, and our body produces water through energy production.

5. If you are going to drink more fluids due to heat, humidity, or excess exercise, consume adequate amounts of salt and sugars to help support electrolyte levels and metabolic health.

Chapter 17
Be Happy

There is one more important ingredient to health, well-being, and obtaining a high metabolic rate, and that is happiness.

Being unhappy is incredibly stressful to your body. Being happy should seem simple, but in today's society, trying to "get happy" seems to be impossible for some people. Why is it so hard for people to be happy in today's world? I think the answer comes down to personal choice and what you believe you deserve out of life.

You have to understand you are the master of your own destiny. You make choices every day: what you put in your body, how much you exercise, who you spend time with, where you go to work, how hard you work, how much you sleep, what you do with your free time, how you react to certain situations, etc. I believe you choose your life, and you can choose to change it (for better or worse) if you desire.

When my life became out of control with drugs, alcohol, and partying, I made a *huge* life decision that I didn't want to live that life anymore. I *chose* to change my situation because I *believed* I *deserved* something better. Years later I chose to follow a different nutritional philosophy because my path was no longer working. When my situation was no longer making me happy or healthy, I chose a different path so that I could find both. Was this decision easy?

You would think the answer would have been yes—especially

since my happiness and health dramatically improved in both situations! Yet making these huge life changes was hard, even when my situation was making me unhappy, unhealthy, and just plain miserable. I knew for me to be successful and find happiness I needed to remove myself from my situation, which included where I worked, who I hung out with, what I was doing with my free time, and even where I lived. This choice was very hard, but I knew the other choice—to keep doing what I was doing (partying)—was only going to create more unhealthy habits and more unhappiness long-term. What I realized was that the short-term gratifications of partying did not result in a long-term happy life, just like short-term weight-loss tactics do not result in a long-term thin and healthy body.

A stressful, lonely, unhappy life will create more disease and a shorter life. In the book *The Blue Zones,* Dan Buettner discusses seven cities throughout the world that have significantly higher life spans than the rest of the world. Two of the few things that *all* the cities had in common were a low-stress lifestyle and a strong community. These communities had strong personal connections and were happy, and life was about living, not "working" and "doing." Jeanne Calment, a French woman and the oldest documented living person, who made it to 122 years old, credited her long life to laughing a lot and not getting stressed out. We can conclude that laughing, happiness, community, and low stress will support your health and longevity.

If the journey to health and happiness seems too challenging or creates more stress than just staying comfortable in your life, then ask yourself: Do I truly want to change? If you really want to change, you will find a way. If you don't want to really change (many don't), you won't. It's as easy as that. For many it is easier to stay in their comfort zone and be unhappy than to change (which brings discomfort) and find a way to become happy.

It has been almost 12 years since I moved across the country and changed everything about my life. I left a life of destruction and chose a life of freedom and happiness. It certainly has not been flowers and rose petals the entire journey, but I am a far happier and healthier person than I was 12 years ago. Had I not changed, I'm sure life would be very different for me right now.

My Top-10 Tips to Find Happiness

1. Write everything down you want to improve upon.

2. Change one thing at a time. Too many changes at once can become overwhelming and can lead to doing nothing.

3. Make slow, yet continual changes. Slow, continuous changes bring about new habits.

4. Get help if you need it—from a health practitioner, therapist, doctor, etc. If you find you cannot make changes by yourself, get the help you need.

5. Trust in the journey. You have to trust that your new changes will create a better life—even if it seems hard in the beginning.

6. Do the work. Wishing and hoping for change is not enough; you have to do the work to make life shift.

7. Allow your life to shift. You have to stop resisting the shift if you want to find happiness.

8. Believe in yourself. Don't allow your fears to get in the way of you becoming happy.

9. Stop worrying about what others are doing, saying, wearing, eating, etc. Doing this alone will make your life so much easier and happier.

10. Be authentic. Being yourself will support your happiness. Trying to be someone you are not will create nothing but stress.

I'm not going to lie: Health and happiness take some work. Yet, you do deserve it. You just have to *believe* you deserve it. Once you *choose* health and happiness, the journey to get there will be created for you. You just have to choose to take it.

If your current job, relationship, or life is stressing you more than making you smile, you may need to make a shift. Remember: A happy healthy life brings increased vitality and longevity. And isn't that what we all want: a long, vital, happy, healthy life?

I know I do.

I hope after reading this book you have some more insight on how the right foods, nutrients, exercise, water, sleep, supplements, and finding your happiness can support and help heal your metabolism. What must be understood is there is just not "one thing" that is going to kick-start your metabolism and improve your health. A combination of all aspects of health is what is going to allow you to improve your metabolic rate, your health, and your life span.

The journey to increasing my metabolic rate, my health, and my happiness has been just that—a journey. There is no end destination to health and happiness. Finding health and happiness is an ongoing journey that will shift and change as your life changes. I hope this book can support you in your journey as it has supported me.

Chapter 17
What you Need to Know

1. Become happy to improve your metabolic rate. Living a life that is authentic and makes you happy improves metabolic function and decreases stress in your life. Lower stress supports thyroid function.

2. Create the life you *believe* you *deserve* you should have and happiness is sure to follow.

3. Be willing to make slow continual changes to create the life you want. Do the work. Believe in yourself. Allow the shift. And welcome your new life.

4. Always be authentic. And stop caring what other people think

5. Creating the life you want and being a happy person is an ongoing journey—be sure to enjoy the ride.

Chapter 18
What a Metabolically Supportive Diet Looks Like

The below five-day eating plan is an example of a typical week of eating for me. Please understand this is only an example and not a diet to follow. My diet has gone through many shifts while healing. Currently, to maintain my weight at 120 pounds, I eat anywhere from 1,750 to 2,200 kcal daily. I will consume more on intense or longer training days.

On workout days I eat anywhere from 2,000 to 2,200 kcal. More if I am training for an event. On non-workout days, calories will drop to 1,750 to 1,900 kcal. At least once a week I try to consume more high-nutrient-rich foods, which will include organ meats like liver (high in vitamins A and B, and selenium) and some type of shellfish like oysters (high in zinc, copper, and selenium). I will usually consume more milk and OJ on high nutrient days (for added calcium, magnesium, potassium).

Day 1 = No Workout

*recipes provided

Breakfast	Snack	Lunch
2 Eggs 1 tsp. Coconut Oil *1 c. Cooked Fruit 4 oz. OJ + 1 T. Gelatin 8 oz. Coffee + 2 oz. Milk + 1 T. Sugar	8 oz. OJ +1 T. Gelatin ½ c. Cottage Cheese 1 raw Carrot	4 oz. Cod 1 tsp. Coconut Oil ½ med. Sweet Potato + 1 tsp. Butter 1 c. Fruit
C=45g/P=21g/ F=14g **Calories = 390**	**C=35g/P=19g/ F=3g** **Calories = 264**	**C=45/P=26/F=12** **Calories = 392**
Snack	**Dinner**	**Bedtime Snack**
8 oz. 2% milk 8 oz. Orange Juice 1 T. Gelatin + Salt	4 grilled shrimp 1 c. cooked Squash + 1 tsp. Butter 1 c. fresh Fruit 1 small Salad w/ Olive Oil and Vinegar Dressing	(if needed) 8 oz. Milk 1 T. Honey + Salt
C=39g/P=14g/ F=5g **Calories = 257**	**C=50g/P=25g/ F=10g** **Calories = 390**	**C=25/P=8/F=5** **Calories = 177**

Day 1 Daily Totals:

C =239 g/P=113g/F= 49g
Calories= 1,870

Day 2 = Normal Day with Added Workout

Breakfast	Snack	During Workout
*Sweet Potato/ Banana Pancakes ½ T. Coconut Oil 1 T. Raisins 8 oz. Tea + 2 oz. Milk + 1 T. Sugar	1 c. Cooked Fruit 1 oz. Parmigiano Reggiano Cheese 1 raw Carrot 4 oz. 2% Milk	*Kate's Miracle Drink **C=16/P=6/F=0** Calories = 88
		Post Workout 8 oz. Milk + 1 T. Sugar + 1 T. Cacao (Chocolate Milk)
C=60g/P=22g/ F=16g Calories = 472	**C=39g/P=10g/ F=9g** Calories = 278	**C=24g/P=11g/ F=9g** Calories = 221
Late Lunch 3 oz. Grass-Fed Beef Patty 8 oz. *Bone Broth 1 c. Mashed Potatoes + 1 tsp. Butter 1 c. Cooked Fruit	**Snack** 8 oz. Milk 4 oz. Orange Juice 1 T. Gelatin	**Dinner** *2 c. Spaghetti Squash w/Seafood Marinara 1 c. Watermelon + Salt 4 oz. Orange Juice
C=55g/P=30g/ F=10g Calories = 430	**C=25g/P=14g/ F=5g** Calories = 201	**C=53g/P=25g/ F=6g** Calories = 366

Snack
(if needed) ½ c. Fruit ½ oz. Cheese
C=15g/P=4g/F=4g Calories = 112

Day 2 Daily Totals:
C =280g/P=122g/F= 59g
Calories= 2,167

Day 3 = High-Nutrient Day

Breakfast	Snack	Lunch
*3 oz. Grilled Liver + Onions ¼ c. Marinara 1 Egg 1 c. Cooked Fruit 8 oz. Coffee + 2 oz. Milk + 1 T. Sugar	8 oz. Milk 8 oz. Orange Juice + 1 T. Gelatin	*16 oz. Bone Broth + Salt ½ c. Potatoes + 1 tsp. Coconut Oil 1 oz. Parmesan Cheese ½ c. Cottage Cheese 1 c. Cucumber/Tomato/Carrot Salad
C=57g/P=25g/F=13g Calories = 445	C=39g/P=14g/F=5g Calories = 257	C=52g/P=37g/F=13g Calories = 473
Snack 8 oz. Milk 8 oz. Orange Juice 1 T. Gelatin	**Dinner** 5 oz. steamed Oysters + Tomato Sauce 1 c. cooked Squash + 1 tsp. Butter 1 c. cooked Fruit 8 oz. Coffee w/Milk + 1 T. Gelatin + 1 T. Sugar	**Bedtime Snack** (if needed) 8 oz. Milk 1 T. Honey + Salt
C=39g/P=14g/F=5g Calories = 257	C=56g/P=18g/F=11g Calories = 395	C=25g/P=8g/F=5g Calories = 177

Day 3 Daily Totals:
C =268 g/P=116g/F= 52g
Calories= 2,004
High levels of vitamins A, B, C, D, and minerals zinc, selenium, calcium, potassium, magnesium, and sodium are included in this day.

Day 4 = Workout Day

Breakfast	Snack	During Workout
*Veggie Spaghetti Squash Quiche 1 c. cooked Fruit 8 oz. Coffee + 1. T Gelatin + 2 oz. Milk + 1 T. Sugar	*Raw Carrot Salad ½ c. Cottage Cheese 8 oz. Orange Juice	*Kate's Miracle Drink C=16g/P=6g/F=0g Calories = 88 **Post Workout** 8 oz. Milk + 1 T. Sugar + 1 T. Cacao (Chocolate Milk)
C=55g/P=22g/ F=13g Calories = 425	C=31g/P=13g/ F=7g Calories = 192	C=24g/P=11g/ F=9g Calories = 221
Late Lunch 4 oz. Sautéd Sole in 2 tsp. Butter 1 c. Cooked Vegetables 8 oz. Orange Juice 2 pieces Soy-Free Dark Chocolate	**Snack** 1 c. Fruit 4 oz. Fage Yogurt	**Dinner** *Potato-Butternut Squash Soup ½ c. Fruit
C=48g/P=27g/ F=19g Calories = 471	C=29g/P=13g/ F=2g Calories = 186	C=47g/P=16g/ F=8g Calories = 324

Bedtime Snack
4 oz. Milk 4 oz. Orange Juice ½ T. Gelatin + Salt
C=20g/P=7g/ F=2.5g Calories = 130.5

Day 4 Daily Totals:

**C =270 g/P=115g/F= 60.5g
Calories= 2,084.5**

Day 5 = Non Workout Day

Breakfast	Snack	Lunch
*Breakfast Smoothie 8 oz. Coffee + 2 oz. Milk + 1 T. Sugar	1 c. Fruit ½ c. Cottage Cheese 1 T. Gelatin	4 oz. Tuna ½ T. Coconut Oil and Vinegar 1 raw Carrot 1 cup Cucumber, Onion, Tomato 1 c. cooked Fruit
C=43g/P=22g/F=10g Calories = 360	C=27g/P=19g/F=6g Calories = 238	C=50/P=26/F=8 Calories = 376
Snack 1 Hard-Boiled Egg 8 oz. Orange Juice + 1 T. Gelatin	**Dinner** *Cod with Coconut Sauce ½ c. Mashed Potato + 1 tsp. Butter 1 c. Fruit	**Bedtime Snack** 8 oz. Milk 1 T. Honey + Salt
C=26g/P=13g/F=4g Calories = 192	C=45g/P=30g/F=18g Calories = 462	C=25/P=8/F=5 Calories = 177

Day 5 Daily Totals:

C =216g/P=118g/F= 51g
Calories= 1,795

*See Recipes Provided

Chapter 19
Frequently Asked Questions (and Answers)

1. Will I gain weight?

   Every person is different. Some lose weight, some stay the same, and some gain weight. If you are coming from a low-carb/low-fat/high-protein/low-calorie diet and/or over-exercising you may initially gain weight. Initially eating more and working out less may result in a weight gain. This is why making changes slowly is important. Slow, gradual changes will create less of a weight gain. Adding in too much food too quickly, although it can support the healing process, will result in more of a weight gain.

2. How long will the healing journey/process take?

   Depending on the person, the damage to his or her metabolism, and how quickly the person is able to make shifts, the journey may take anywhere from three months to several years.

3. How will I know when my metabolism is healed?

   Healing your metabolism is not a destination. It is a constant journey, since you will always encounter stressors that will affect your health and metabolism negatively. However, you will show improvements in energy, body temperature (98–99 degrees Fahrenheit), pulse rate (75–90 bpm), sleep quality (seven to nine uninterrupted hours), bowel movements (one to three per day), mood, hormones, digestion, and immune function along the way.

4. This is a lot to change! Should I implement all these changes at once?

The key to success is to go at a pace that makes you feel comfortable. For most, making one or two changes at a time works best. Make slow changes until you have established new habits, and then add in another shift. Making too many changes at once usually results in hormonal chaos, feeling overwhelmed, frustration, and stopping the program altogether.

5. If my temperature and pulse continue to run low, should I go ahead and eat more to increase it?

Possibly. Eating more will increase heat production as long as the food is being used as energy and not stored as fat. This is why it is important to add more food in slowly. Increasing salt intake will also add to heat production.

6. I tend to drink a lot of water and find I am frequently thirsty. What compromise, if any, to alleviate thirst without drowning my body with too much water?

Many so called "healthy people" seem to be over-hydrating. Slowly add in mineral filled beverages like milk, bone broth, and orange juice, and decrease water intake. The increase in mineral-to-water ratio should help alleviate thirst and decrease trips to the bathroom.

7. How do I make my own calcium, naturally?

Refer to Eggshell Calcium recipe in Chapter 20.

8. How much bone broth is recommended to be consumed daily?

Depending on the person, 1–2 cups a day. I recommend 1 cup of bone broth to be consumed with all muscle meats. For someone with very poor digestion, up to 50 percent of protein can come from bone broth and gelatin.

9. What is the nutritional content in the bone broth (e.g., how do I count this in my food log)?

One cup of bone broth has about 8 grams of protein.

10. Why do you recommend I consume bone broth with muscle meats?

Since bone broth lacks in tryptophan, cysteine, and methionine, bone broth balances the inflammatory amino acid profile of muscle meats, which are high in these amino acids. Bone broth can also help break down muscle meat, making it easier to digest.

11. I took my temperature and pulse after a workout, and both have dropped dramatically! What does this signify and how do I avoid this happening?

Essentially a drop in temperature and pulse post-workout means your thyroid has been suppressed. Remember: Exercise suppresses thyroid function. Essentially the workout was too long, too hard, or too intense, or a combination of all three. To avoid this from happening decrease workout time, increase rest time, and/or decrease intensity.

12. To lose weight, don't I want to burn fat as fuel?

The concept of becoming a "fat burner" to lose weight and gain health is false. At all moments in time we are using glucose, fat, and even protein as energy. However, the majority of energy used should come from glucose oxidation because it produces the greatest amount of heat and CO_2. Becoming primarily a "fat burner" makes the body more efficient, slows down metabolic rate, and blocks proper glucose metabolism.

However, at rest the heart and muscle prefer fat as fuel. This is why sleep and increasing muscle mass will support a high running metabolism and lean body.

13. Can I eat out on this program?

Of course, but beware many restaurants use cheap and low-quality meats, vegetables, fruits, and fats. The majority of restaurants use vegetable, seed, and nut oils to cook in. Ask the restaurant to have your food cooked in butter or olive oil. Ask for grass-fed meats and organic produce when available. Limit out-to-eat experiences to once or twice per week (versus one to two times per day). Health will not be regained by eating out all the time. Food shopping, preparing your own food, and cooking will be keys to increase metabolic function.

14. **I thought drinking orange juice was bad for me. Isn't that too much sugar?**

    Consuming the right sugars supports a high running metabolism. Fruit juice, especially orange juice, provides the body with a good amount of healthy sugars, vitamins, and minerals. Unless you already have a high metabolic rate, juice should be combined with a fat and protein to slow the sugars' absorbency into the blood. This will help maintain a balanced blood sugar.

    It's important to note if you have not been consuming juice and sugars you should add them in slowly. Too much sugar, added in too quickly, will result in weight gain, hormone issues, a rise in cholesterol, and blood sugar issues.

15. **Why should I consume pulp-free juice?**

    Using pulp-free juices eliminates the fibers that help feed bacteria in the stomach. Juice is best if it is freshly squeezed and run through a cheesecloth.

16. **I am having recurring headaches. Is there something nutritionally I can do to alleviate?**

    For many, just balancing your blood sugar can alleviate headaches. Headaches can also be caused by a lack of good sugars and not eating enough. Try eating many, small, balanced meals to help balance your blood sugar and keep headaches at bay.

17. **Although potatoes are a below-ground vegetable, they are also a starch. Should I limit the amount I consume?**

    Some people are able to consume potatoes at every meal with few problems. However, for the individual who is looking to gain gut health or lose fat, potato consumption should be limited to no more than once per day. Potatoes should be washed and drained to help remove the starch, cooked thoroughly, and consumed with a fat to help digestibility. For gut health and improved fat loss, the preferred time to eat potatoes is breakfast or lunch.

18. If I do drink alcohol, are there steps I can take to minimize the effect on my metabolism?

Consuming alcoholic beverages with food will decrease the blood-sugar-lowering effects of alcohol. In addition, consuming alcohol with fruit juice (fructose) will help clear the alcohol from the liver 80-percent faster.

19. This journey is so contrary to everything I've been told or read, and is overwhelming in detail! How can I possibly proceed to ensure success?

The best advice I can give to ensure success is to make slow, constant changes. Read this book not once, but three or four times. In addition to reading this book, do your own research, get help from a health practitioner, ask your doctor and health care provider tons of questions, draw your own conclusions, and from there make changes that feel right to you.

20. Where can I go to get more personal nutritional coaching?

I can be reached through my website at Kate@KateDeering.com. Information about all nutritional coaching programs is located at https://katedeering.com/services/nutritional-coaching/.

Chapter 20
Recipes

Breakfast

Spaghetti Squash Veggie Quiche

C = 20g P = 25g F = 20g
360 calories per serving (does not include added fruit)
Serves = 4

Ingredients:

3 c. cooked spaghetti squash (1 medium spaghetti squash)
1 T. coconut oil
1 c. red peppers, chopped
1 c. zucchini, chopped
½ c. onion, chopped
8 oz. (1 c.) Parmigiano Reggiano cheese, shredded
5 pastured, farm-fresh eggs
½ tsp. sea salt
¼ tsp. black pepper
Ground nutmeg, to taste
2 cloves garlic
1 c. 2% organic milk

Directions:

1. Preheat oven to 350°F.
2. Spread ½ T. coconut oil in bottom of 9-inch baking dish.
3. Press cooked spaghetti squash on sides and bottom of baking dish, forming an even crust.
4. Place other ½ T. coconut oil, garlic, and onions into pan. Cook until soft. Add peppers and zucchini. Cook for another 2–3 minutes.
5. Layer the veggies on top of the spaghetti squash and add 6oz. shredded cheese.
6. Beat eggs, milk, salt, pepper, and nutmeg in medium bowl.
7. Pour over veggies and cheese.
8. Bake 30 minutes; remove from oven and sprinkle with remaining 2 oz. cheese.
9. Return to oven and bake 10–20 minutes longer, or until egg mix is set and top is slightly brown.
10. Remove from oven and let stand 5 minutes before serving.
11. Serve with a side of fruit.

Banana–Sweet Potato–Raisin Cakes

C = 55 g F =21 P =14g
Calories = 430
Serves = 1
(does not include topping)

Ingredients for Pancakes:

2 pastured eggs
1/2 very ripe and soft banana
½ large cooked and cooled yellow sweet potato
1/2 tsp. baking soda
1 T. hydrolyzed collagen
¼ tsp. cinnamon
½ T. sugar
1/2 T. ghee or coconut oil for cooking pan
20 raisins

Ingredients for Extra Topping:

1 scoop Fage Greek Yogurt
1 tsp. powdered sugar
1 T. maple syrup

Directions:

1. Mash up bananas and sweet potato in bowl with a fork.
2. Add eggs, baking soda, cinnamon, hydrolyzed collagen, and sugar.
3. Mix well until batter is a smooth consistency.
4. Using medium heat, warm skillet.
5. Melt coconut oil in pan. (You may use a non-stick pan. Just make sure it is not chipped.)
6. In heaping 1 T. servings make small pancakes.
7. While cakes are in pan, add 2 raisins per pancake.
8. Flip pancakes when they begin to bubble on top.
9. Add desired topping before serving.

This recipe should make between 10 and 12 small pancakes.

Breakfast Smoothie

C = 35g P = 21g F = 9g
315 calories per serving
Serves = 1

Ingredients:

1 c. 2% milk	1 T. hydrolyzed collagen
¾ c. frozen fruit	1 T. sugar or honey
1 raw pastured egg	Pinch of white sea salt

Directions:

1. Place all ingredients in a Vitamix or blender. Blend until smooth.

Snacks

Baked Apples/Peaches/Pears/Nectarines

C= 22   P= 8   F= 8
200 calories per serving
Serves = 10

Ingredients:

4 medium apples	2 T. organic butter
4 medium pears	1 T. cinnamon
3 medium peaches (if not in season, add 3 different types of apples or pears)	10 oz. shaved Parmigiano Reggiano cheese (no additives)

Directions:

1. Preheat oven to 350 degrees.
2. Cut apples, peaches, and pears into bite-sized pieces.
3. Place all fruit along with butter and cinnamon into a glass cooking dish.
4. Bake 45–55 minutes or until soft.
5. Stir fruit every 10 to 15 minutes.
6. Allow fruit to cool or eat warm.
7. Add 1 oz. (about 3 level T.) of graded Parmesan Reggiano cheese to each 1-cup serving.
8. Place rest of fruit in glass containers. Only add cheese once you are ready to serve.

*You may substitute ¼ cup organic ricotta cheese or add ½ cup milk.

Raw Carrot Salad

C =7   P = 0   F = 3
55 calories per serving
Serves = 2

Ingredients:

2 raw medium carrots
½ T. melted coconut oil
½ T. white vinegar
Salt to taste

Directions:

1. Grate carrots, length-wise, in a small bowl.
2. Mix in melted coconut oil and vinegar.
3. Add salt.

Consume with cottage cheese or added Parmesan cheese for added fat and protein.

Kate's Miracle Drink

C = 16 g   P = 6g   F = 0
Calories: 88
Serves = 1

Ingredients:

4 oz. pulp-free organic orange juice

2 oz. organic, pulp-free coconut water (optional)

1 T. hydrolyzed gelatin protein

1/8 tsp. white sea salt (you can add more if needed)

Ice

6—10 oz. carbonated (CO_2) or filtered water (whatever fills up bottle)

Directions:
1. Add OJ, coconut water, salt, and gelatin to a 20-ounce bottle. Shake or blend together well.
2. Add ice and shake. *Do not blend.*
3. Add CO_2 water or filtered water. Shake bottle lightly or the CO_2 water will make the drink fizz over.
4. Sip throughout the day and/or while working out.

This drink is *not* meant to be gulped down in a two-minute sitting. Sip slowly! Please note the coconut water is optional when it comes to making this drink. Some of my clients love it, while others could live without it. If you choose to remove the coconut water you may add in 2 more ounces of pulp-free orange juice.

Post-Workout Smoothies

Homemade Chocolate Milk

C = 32   P = 21   F = 12
Calories = 320
Serves = 1

Ingredients:

1.5 c. 2% organic milk
1 T. raw cacao chocolate
1 T. sugar or raw honey
1 T. hydrolyzed collagen
1 pinch salt

Directions:

1. Blend all ingredients in blender or shake bottle. Sip-post workout.

Add ice for a thicker, cooler smoothie.

Orange Creamsicle Smoothie

C = 25 P = 14   F = 5
Calories = 201
Serves = 1

Ingredients:

1/2 c. pulp free orange juice (fresh squeezed is best)
1 c. 2% organic milk
1 T. hydrolyzed collagen
1 pinch salt

Directions:

1. Blend all ingredients in blender or shake bottle. Sip post-workout.

Add ice for a thicker, cooler smoothie. You may also add ½ cup Häagen-Dazs vanilla ice cream for increased texture and taste.

Milk and Honey

C = 32   P = 14   F = 5
Calories = 229
Serves = 1

Ingredients:

1.5 c. 2% organic milk	1 T. raw honey
1 T. hydrolyzed collagen	1 pinch salt

Directions:

1. Blend all ingredients in blender or shake bottle. Sip post-workout.

Add ice for a thicker, cooler smoothie. You may also add ½ cup Häagen-Dazs vanilla ice cream for increased texture and taste.

Lunch and Dinner

Liver and Onions

C = 10 g P = 22g F = 10g
220 calories per serving
Serves = 5

Ingredients:

1 lb. grass-fed beef liver cut in ¼- to ½-inch thickness
3 T, butter
1 medium onion, diced
2 T. white sugar
1 c. milk
½ c. coconut flour

Directions:

1. Before cooking soak liver in 1 cup milk overnight.
2. Caramelize onions: Melt 2 T. butter in medium saucepan, and add diced onion and sugar. Set aside.
3. Coat liver in coconut flour.
4. Melt 1 T. butter in saucepan.
5. Fry liver slices 1–2 minutes per side.
6. Cover with onions and serve.

Homemade Marinara and Spaghetti Squash

C = 25 P = 5 F = 6
Calories = 175 (Does not include added meat of fish)
Servings = 6 (1/2 cup each)

Ingredients:

2 medium spaghetti squash
1 can organic whole peeled tomatoes (Bionature is a good brand)
2 T. refined coconut oil
2 T. hydrolyzed gelatin (optional)
1 T. organic Italian herbs (basil, oregano, thyme, rosemary)
2 cloves garlic, diced
1/3 large onion diced
1 medium grated carrot
½ T. sugar
Salt and pepper to taste
½ c. Parmesan cheese
*May add 1lb. of ground beef, lamb, or shrimp to sauce

Instructions:

1. Heat oven to 350 degrees.
2. Cut spaghetti squashes in half and scoop out seeds.
3. Place each half on a baking dish upside down.
4. Bake 35–45 minutes or until squash pulls out easily.
5. In a large saucepan, over medium heat, place coconut oil, onion, and garlic.
6. Cook until soft, about 8–10 minutes.
7. Add in carrots, salt, and pepper, and cook another 3–5 minutes.
8. Mash up whole tomatoes, and add tomatoes and juices to saucepan.
9. Stir in herbs, sugar, gelatin, and more salt and pepper to taste.
10. Allow sauce to simmer 20–30 minutes.
11. Pull out 2 cups spaghetti squash, add ½ cup sauce, and sprinkle 1 T. Parmesan on top.

Serve fresh. Store in refrigerator for one week or store in freezer for six months.

Potato-Butternut Squash Soup

C = 45g P = 15g F = 7g.
Calories = 302
Serves = 8

Ingredients:

2 lbs. golden yellow potatoes	Pepper to taste
2 lbs. butternut squash	3 T. butter
2 medium apples	2 c. 1 or 2 % milk
2 medium yellow onions	1–2 c. organic vegetable broth
1/8 tsp. cumin	(or homemade vegetable broth)
1/8 tsp. curry	½ c. ricotta cheese
1/8 tsp. cinnamon	12 T. hydrolyzed collagen
Salt to taste	

Directions:

1. Heat oven to 425 degrees.
2. Remove skin from potatoes, apples, butternut squash, and onions. Cut into 1-inch pieces and place into cooking dishes. (Using two dishes will allow for more even cooking.)
3. Place 1 1/2 T. butter into each cooking dish. Place into oven and cook for 45 minutes or until tender. Stir occasionally.
4. Once potatoes, butternut squash, apples, and onions are soft, remove from oven and place in Vitamix or food processor. Add milk, broth, cumin, curry, cinnamon, salt, and pepper (you may have to mix 2 separate batches).
5. Once you create a consistency you like (add more vegetable broth for thinner soup) place all contents in a 2-quart pan. Stir in hydrolyzed collagen.

Serve with a 1 T. ricotta on each 8-ounce serving.

Cod with Coconut Sauce

C = 2g P = 30g F = 12g
250 calories per serving
Serves = 8

Ingredients
Sauce:

1 can light coconut milk
1 c. coconut flakes
1 T. chili sauce
1 T. sugar
1 T. minced fresh parsley

1 T. tomato paste
1 T. white sea salt
Juice of 6 limes
2 T. butter, softened

Fish:

2 lb. fresh cod, divided into 8 four-ounce portions
Salt and freshly ground black pepper
1 tsp. ground coriander

Sauce Directions:
1. In a bowl, blend the coconut milk, coconut flakes, chili sauce, sugar, parsley, tomato paste, salt, and lime juice, and allow to marinate for 30 minutes.
2. Pour through a strainer into a saucepan. Heat over low heat until warmed.
3. Whisk in the butter off the heat before serving.

Fish Directions:
1. Preheat grill to 350 degrees F or a grill pan over high heat.
2. Sprinkle fish with salt, pepper, and coriander.
3. Cook fish on both sides until medium-well in temperature, 5–6 minutes per side.
4. Once cooked, remove from the heat and rest for 2 to 3 minutes.
5. Finish with the sauce.

Serve with mashed potatoes, white rice, and/or baked fruit
*This recipe has been altered from Robert Irvine of the Food Network.

Beef Bone Broth

$C = 0 \quad P = 8g \quad F = 0$
Calories: 36/cup

Ingredients:

4 lb. raw grass-fed beef bones: knuckle, oxtail, neck, shank
1–2 chicken feet (makes broth more gelatinous)
2 T. vinegar or lemon juice
2 T. orange juice
1 T. salt

Enough water to cover the bones

Chopped vegetables:
2 carrots
2 celery stocks
1 small onion

Directions:

1. Place raw bones in a roasting pan and roast 40–50 minutes at 350 degrees F.
2. Add cooled bones to a pot of cold filtered water.
3. Allow bones to sit in cold water for 30 minutes.
4. Add vinegar or lemon juice and/or orange juice and salt.
5. Bring the pot to a boil and then bring down to simmer.
6. Every 20 minutes for the first few hours, skim the top of the broth to remove any impurities.
7. Allow bone broth to cook for at least 4 hours.
8. In the last three hours of cooking, add the vegetables.
9. Once broth is done, allow it to cool, and then place in the refrigerator.
10. By the next day, the fat will rise to the top and can be skimmed off.

Store your broth in glass or BPA-free plastic containers in the refrigerator and freezer. Broth will last up to 5 days in the refrigerator and 2-3 months in the freezer.

Mineral Broth

0 = C   0 = F   0 = P
0 calories per serving

Ingredients:

½ lb. kale
½ lb. spinach
½ lb. chard

2 cloves garlic
1 T. salt
1 gallon filtered water

Directions:

1. Add all ingredients to a pot of boiling water.
2. Submerge vegetables in boiling water.
3. Reduce heat and allow vegetables to cook 45 minutes.
4. Remove all ingredients from pot. Liquid should look light green in color and have a vegetable-like smell.

Store liquid in glass containers for up to 2 weeks.

Every day drink 1–2 shots of mineral broth for a magnesium, vitamin K, and B vitamin supplement.

Eggshell Calcium

0 = C   0 = F   0 = P
0 calories per serving

Ingredients:
12–24 eggshells from pastured organic chickens

Directions:
1. Fill a large cooking pot with water and bring to a boil.
2. Add eggshells and turn down heat.
3. Allow eggshells to disinfect in boiling water about 10–15 minutes.
4. Remove eggshells and place on a cookie sheet.
5. Place eggshells in oven 10–15 minutes at 275 degrees F.
6. Cook until, dry not browned or burned.
7. Remove eggshells and allow them to cool.
8. Place dried eggshells in a Vitamix blender or coffee grinder.
9. Blend until eggshells produce a fine powder.

Store eggshell powder in a sealed tight glass container.

½ tsp. = 400mg calcium carbonate

Best if consumed with food or orange juice, as calcium alone may be irritating on an empty stomach.

Appendix A
Optimal Carbohydrates

(All are best if organic)

Fruits:

Pulp-free orange juice
Watermelon
Papaya
Kiwi
Cooked apples/apple sauce
Cooked pears
Ripe, mushy, *or* cooked bananas
Cooked peaches
Nectarines
Pineapple
Prunes
Sapote
Orange
Cherry
Apricots
Dates
Plums
Raisins
Lemons
Limes
Grapes
Coconut water
Lychees
Pawpaw

Vegetables:

*Russet potatoes
*Sweet potatoes (light colored)
Raw carrots
Beets
Cucumbers
Squash
Zucchini
Pumpkin
Onion
Red, green, yellow peppers
Bamboo shoots

*A fat should always be added to starches to increase digestibility. All other vegetables should be *used in moderation* and best if well cooked and eaten with a fat.

Dairy:
*Cow's milk: 1%, 2%, whole
*Goat's milk
*Raw milk
*Organic, pastured milk is best

Milk is a complete food, so it can be listed under sugars, proteins. and fats.

Grains:
Organic white or jasmine rice
Organic slow-cooked oatmeal
Organic sourdough bread
Organic masa harina
*All grains should be *used in moderation* and with good gut health. A fat should always be added to the grains to increase digestibility.

Other:
Raw honey
White sugar

Appendix B
Best Proteins

List of Super Proteins

Dairy: (consume daily 2–6 servings)
*Milk:
Cow's milk: 1%, 2 %, whole
Goat's milk
Sheep's milk
*Organic is best
Milk is a complete food, so it can be listed under sugars, proteins, and fats.

Cheese:
Parmigiano Reggiano (no fillers)
Ricotta (organic, no additives)

Eggs: (consume up to 2 day as long as from a good source)
Best are pastured, organic, no soy or corn fed.

Grass-fed beef liver (1 time per week, 3–6 oz.)

Shellfish: (1–3 times per week)

Lobster	Oysters
Shrimp	Clams
Scallops	Crab
Mussels	

Warm-water fish: (2–4 times per week)

Sole	Tilapia
Cod	Flounder
White fish	Catfish

Potato Protein
Beef Bone broth (daily 1–3 c.)
Powdered gelatin (daily 1–6 T.) (Great Lakes Gelatin)

Proteins to be consumed in moderation:

Muscle meats (1 time per week or less if person is severely inflamed)
Grass-fed beef
Grass-fed bison
Grass-fed lamb
*Pastured chicken
*Pastured turkey
*Pastured pork

*All are non-ruminant animals so they contain a higher PUFA level. Avoid all meats fed corn and soy. They contain antibiotics and hormones.
Can be consumed 1–2 times per month, if tolerated.

*Nuts:
Macadamia
Hazel nuts
Cashews
*Lightly roasted, soaked, and sprouted are best. Consume 1–2 times per month if desired. May consume more with good gut health.

Appendix C
Best Fats

*Saturated fats:
Organic expeller pressed coconut oil (refined coconut oil)
Ghee
Grass-fed butter
Raw cacao
Beef lard
*Use for cooking and baking

Moderate fats:
**Monounsaturated fats
Extra-virgin organic olive oil
**Use as a dressing. Do not cook with olive oil.

Appendix D
PUFA Oils to Be Avoided

(% is the amount of Omega-6 polyunsaturated fat in each oil.)

Grapeseed oil 70.6%
Corn oil 54.5%
Walnut oil is 53.9%
Cottonseed oil 52.4%
Soybean oil 51.4%
Sesame oil 42.0%
Peanut oil 33.5%
Margarine 27.9%
Chicken fat 19.5%
Almond oils 19.1%
Canola oil 19.0%
Flaxseed oil 12.9%

References:

(References are listed in the order they are appear in each chapter.)

Chapter 1

1. Frank P. Grad, "The Preamble of the Constitution of the World Health Organization," www.who.int/bulletin/archives/80(12)981.pdf.

2. "What Is Health? The Ability to Adapt," *The Lancet, Volume 373, Issue 9666,* Page 781, March 7, 2009.

3. Dr. Broda Barnes, MD, and Lawrence Galton, *Hypothyroidism: The Unsuspected Illness,* Harper and Row Publishing, 1976.

4. Constance R. Martin, "Endocrine Physiology," Oxford University Press, 1985, pp. 50–52, 67, 745–747, 754, 770, 773–775, 777.

5. L. Landsberg, JB Young, WR Leonard, RA Linsenmeier, and FW Turek, "Is Obesity Associated with Lower Body Temperatures? Core Temperature: A Forgotten Variable in Energy Balance," *Metabolism,* June 2009, 58(6):871–6.

6. Dr. Ray Peat, "TSH, Temperature, Pulse Rate, and Other Indicators in Hypothyroidism." www.raypeat.com

7. "Important Derivatives of Cholesterol Include Bile Salts and Steroid Hormones," Section 26.4, *Biochemistry,* 5th edition, www.ncbi.nlm.nih.gov/books/NBK22339/.

8. P. De Vito, S. Incerpi, JZ Pedersen, P. Luly, FB Davis, and PJ Davis, "Thyroid Hormones as Modulators of Immune Activities at the Cellular Level," *Thyroid,* August 2011, 21(8):879–90. doi: 10.1089/thy.2010.0429. Epub July 11, 2011.

9. CF Hodkinson, EE Simpson, JH Beattie, JM O'Connor, DJ Campbell, JJ Strain, and JM Wallace, "Preliminary Evidence of Immune Function Modulation by Thyroid Hormones in Healthy Men and Women Aged 55–70 Years," *Journal of Endocrinology,* July 2009, 202(1):55–63. doi: 10.1677/JOE-08-0488. Epub April 27, 2009.

10. Janie A. Bowthorpe, M.Ed. "Stop the Thyroid Madness". Laughing Grape Publishing. 2008.

11. "Baby Business: (Infertility Services) Worth $4 Billion," Tampa Fla., 2009, www.prweb.com/releases/2009/08/prweb2750574.htm.

12. "The Relationship Between the Thyroid Gland and the Liver," *Oxford Journal, V95, Issue 9,* pp. 559–569.

13. Jonathan V. Wright, MD, and Lance Lenard, PhD, "Why Stomach Acid Is Good for You," M Evans Publishing, 2001.

14. Carsten Kirkegaard and Jens Faber, "The Role of Thyroid Hormones in Depression," *European Journal of Endocrinology* (1998) 138:1–9.

15. H. Engler, WF Riesen, and B. Keller, "Anti-Thyroid Peroxidase (anti-TPO) Antibodies in Thyroid Diseases, Non-Thyroidal Illness and Controls: Clinical Validity of a New Commercial Method for Detection of Anti-TPO (Thyroid Microsomal) Autoantibodies," *Clin Chim Acta,* March 1994, 225(2):123–36.

16. Vahab Fatourechi, MD, "Subclinical Hypothyroidism: An Update for Primary Care Physicians." *Mayo Clinic Proceedings.* 2009 Jan; 84(1): 65–71.

17. Kent Holtorf, MD, "Deiodinases: Understanding Local Control of Thyroid Hormones(Deiodinases Function and Activity)," National Acadamy of Hypothyroidism.

18. BM Nabishah, BA Khalid, PB Morat, and A. Zanariyah, "Regeneration of Adrenal cortical Tissue After Adrenal Autotransplantation," *Exp Clin Endocrinol Diabetes,* 1998, 106(5):419–24.

Chapter 2

1. AA Nanji, SM Sadrzadeh, EK Yang, F. Fogt, M. Meydani, and AJ Dannenberg, "Dietary Saturdated Fatty Acids: A Novel Treatment for Alcoholic Liver Disease," *Gastroenterology,* August 1995, 109(2):547–54.

2. R. Gupta and H. Prakash, "Association of Dietary Ghee Intake with Coronary Heart Disease and Risk Factor Prevalence in Rural Males," J Indian Med Assoc, March 1997. 95(3):67–9, 83.

3. AA Nanji, EK Yang, F. Fogt, SM Sadrzadeh, and AJ Dannenberg, "Medium Chain Triglycerides and Vitamin E Reduce the Severity of Established Alcoholic Liver Disease," J Pharmacol Exp Ther., June 1996, 277(3):1694–700.

4. AA Nanji, D. Zakim, A. Rahemtulla, T. Daly, L. Miao, S. Zhao, S. Khwaja, SR Tahan, and AJ Dannenberg. "Dietary Saturated Fatty Acids Down-Regulate Cyclooxygenase-2 and Tumor Necrosis Factor Alfa and Reverse Fibrosis in Alcohol-Induced Liver Disease in the Rat." *Hepatology,* December 1997, 26(6):1538–45.

5. R. Micha and D. Mozaffarian. "Saturated Fat and Cardiometabolic Risk Factors, Coronary Heart Disease, Stroke, and Diabetes: A Fresh Look at the Evidence." *Lipids*, 2010, 45:893–905.

6. PW Siri-Tarino, Q. Sun, FB Hu, and RM Krauss, "Meta-Analysis of Prospective Cohort Studies Evaluating the Association of Saturated Fat with Cardiovascular Disease," *American Journal of Clinical Nutrition,* 2010, 91:535–46.

7. St-Onge MP, Bourque C, Jones PJ, Ross R, Parsons WE, "Medium- Versus Long-Chain Triglycerides for 27 Days Increases Fat Oxidation and Energy Expenditure Without Resulting in Changes in Body Composition in Overweight Women, *Int J Obes Relat Metab Disord,* January 2003, 27(1):95–102.

8. Kasai M1, Nosaka N, Maki H, Suzuki Y, Takeuchi H, Aoyama T, Ohra A, Harada Y, Okazaki M, Kondo K., "Comparison of Diet-Induced Thermogenesis of Foods Containing Medium- Versus Long-chain Triacylglycerols," *J Nutr Sci Vitaminol* (Tokyo), December 2002, 48(6):536–40.

9. Hill JO1, Peters JC, Yang D, Sharp T, Kaler M, Abumrad NN, Greene HL., "Thermogenesis in Humans During Overfeeding with Medium-Chain Triglycerides," *Metabolism,* July 1989, 38(7):641–8.

10. Baba N, Bracco EF, Hashim SA., "Role of Brown Adipose Tissue in Thermogenesis Induced by Overfeeding a Diet Containing Medium Chain Triglyceride," *Lipids,* June 1987, 22(6):442–4.

11. T B Seaton, S L Welle, M K Warenko, and R G Campbell, "Thermic Effect of Medium-Chain and Long-Chain Triglycerides in Man," *American Journal of Clinical Nutrition,* November 1986, 44(5):630–4.

12. Baba N, Bracco EF, Hashim SA., "Enhanced Thermogenesis and Diminished Deposition of Fat in Response to Overfeeding with Diet Containing Medium Chain Triglyceride," *American Journal of Clinical Nutrition,* April 1982, 35(4):678–82.

13. Weston A. Price, "Nutrition and Physical Degeneration," Published by The Price-Pottenger Nutrition Foundation, Inc., 1945.

14. Takeuchi H1, Sekine S, Kojima K, Aoyama T., "The Application of Medium-Chain Fatty Acids: Edible Oil with a Suppressing Effect on Body Fat Accumulation," *Asia Pac J Clin Nutr,* 2008, 17 Suppl 1:320–3.

15. Hiroshi Kono, Hideki Fujii, Masayjki Yamamoto, Masanori Matsuda, Masami Asakawa, Akira Maki. "Protective Effects of Medium-Chain Triglycerides on the Liver and Gut in Rats Administered Endotoxin," *Ann Surg,* February 2003, 237(2):246–55.

16. Cha, Y. S. and Sachan, D. S., "Opposite Effects of Dietary Saturated and Unsaturated Fatty Acids on Ethanol-Pharmacokinetics, Triglycerides and Carnitines," *J Am Coll Nutr*, August 1994, 13(4):338–43.

17. "The Effect of Medium-Chain Triglyceride on 47 Calcium Absorption in Patients with Primary Biliary Cirrhosis," *Gut,* August 1973, 14(8):653–6.

18. Lemieux H, Bulteau AL, Friguet B, Tardif JC, Blier PU. "Dietary Fatty Acids and Oxidative Stress in the Heart Mitochondria," *Mitochondrion,* January 2011, 11(1):97–103. Epub August 5, 2010.

19. Renata Micha and Dariush Mozaffarian "Saturated Fat and Cardiometabolic Risk Factors, Coronary Heart Disease, Stroke, and Diabetes: A Fresh Look at the Evidence," *Lipids,* October 2010, 45(10):893–905. Epub March 31, 2010.

20. Mary A. Zimmerman, Nagendra Singh, Pamela M. Martin, Muthusamy Thangaraju, Vadivel Ganapathy, Jennifer L. Waller, Huidong Shi, Keith D. Robertson, David H. Munn, and Kebin Liu, "Butyrate Suppresses Colonic Inflammation Through HDAC1-Dependent Fas Upregulation and Fas-Mediated Apoptosis of T Cells," *Am J Physiol Gastrointest Liver Physiol,* 2012, 302: G1405–G1415.

21. C. Dwivedi, AE Crosser, VV Mistry, and HM Sharma. "Effects of Dietary Ghee (Clarified Butter) on Serum Lipids in Rats," *J Appl Nutr,* 2002, 52:65–8.

22. S. Couvreur, C. Hurtaud, C. Lopez, L. Delaby, and JL Peyraud, "The Linear Relationship Between the Proportion of Fresh Grass in the Cow Diet, Milk Fatty Acid Composition, and Butter Properties," *J Dairy Sci,* June 2006, 89(6):1956–69.

23. C. Vermeer and E. Theuwissen, "Vitamin K, Osteoporosis and Degenerative Diseases of Aging," *Menopause Int.,* March 2011, 17(1):19–23.

24. Chris Masterjohn, On the Trail of the Exclusive X factor: A 60 Year Old Mystery Finally Solved, Feb. 14, 2008.

25. J. Edward Hunter, Jun Zhang, and Penny M. Kris-Etherton, "Cardiovascular Disease Risk of Dietary Stearic Acid Compared with Trans, Other Saturated, and Unsaturated Fatty Acids: A Systematic Review," *American Journal of Clinical Nutrition* (American Society for Nutrition), January 2010, 91 (1): 46–63.

26. Dr. Ray Peat, "Suitable Fats, Unsuitable Fats: Issues in Nutrition," www.raypeat.com

27. Dr Ray Peat, "Unsaturated Vegetable Oil: Toxic", www.raypeat.com

28. Dr. Mary Enig and Sally Fallon, "Eat Fat, Lose Fat." Penguin Group Pusblishing, 2005.

29. Ancel Keys, *Seven Countries: A multivariable Analysis or Death and Coronary Heart Disease.* Commonwealth Fund Publications. 1980.

30. Uffe Ravnskov, "The Cholesterol Myths, Exposing the Fallacy that Saturated Fat and Cholesterol Cause Heart Disease" Oct. 2000

31. H. Lindmark Månsson, "Composition of Swedish Dairy Milk 2001," Swedish Dairy Association, 2003, Report Nr 7025-P (in Swedish).

32. Dr. Broda Barnes and Lawrence Galton, "Hypothyroidism: The Unsuspected Illness." Harpler and Row Publishers, 1976.

33. DK Houston, J. Ding, JS Lee, M. Garcia, AM Kanaya, FA Tylavsky, AB Newman, M. Visser, and SB Kritchevsky. "Dietary Fat and Cholesterol and Risk of Cardiovascular Disease in Older Adults: The Health ABC Study," *Nutr Metab Cardiovasc Dis,* June 2011, 21(6):430–7.

34. Dr. Ray Peat, "Cholesterol, longevity, intelligence, and health." www.raypeat.com

35. CN Blesso, CJ Andersen, J. Barona, JS Volek, and ML Fernandez, "Whole Egg Consumption Improves Lipoprotein Profiles and Insulin Sensitivity to a Greater Extent than Yolk-Free Egg Substitute in Individuals with Metabolic Syndrome," *Metabolism,* March 2013, 62(3):400–10.

36. LL Smith, "Another Cholesterol Hypothesis: Cholesterol as Antioxidant," *Free Radic. Biol. Med.,* 1991, 11 (1): 47–56.

37. IA Prior, F. Davidson, CE Salmond, and Z. Czochanska, "Cholesterol, Coconuts, and Diet on Polynesian Atolls: A Natural Experiment: The Pukapuka and Tokelau Island Studies," *American Journal of Clinical Nutrition,* August 1981, 34(8):1552–61.

Chapter 3

1. M. Orchin, RS Macomber, A. Pinhas, and RM Wilson, editors, *The Vocabulary and Concepts of Organic Chemistry,* 2nd ed., John Wiley & Sons, 2005.

2. M. Erbas and H. Sekerci, "Importance of Free Radicals and Occurring During Food Processing," SERBEST RADİKALLERİN ONEMİ VE GIDA İSLEME SIRASINDA OLUSUMU, 2011, 36(6):349–56.

3. JR Speakman and C. Selman, "The Free-Radical Damage Theory: Accumulating Evidence Against a Simple Link of Oxidative Stress to Ageing and Lifespan," *BioEssays,* 2011, 33(4):255–9.

4. G. O. Burr, M. M. Burr "A New Deficiency Disease Produced by the Rigid Exclusion of Fat from the Diet." *J. Biol. Chem.* 1929 82, 345–367

5. G. O. Burr, M. M. Burr. "On the Nature and Role of the Fatty Acids Essential in Nutrition." *J. Biol. Chem.* 1930 86, 587–621

6. S. Miura, H. Imaeda, H. Shiozaki, N. Ohkubo, H. Tashiro, H. Serizawa, M. Tsuchiya, and P. Tso, "Increased Proliferative Response of Lymphocytes from Intestinal Lymph During Long Chain Fatty Acid Absorption, *Immmunolity*, January 1993 volume 78.

7. A. Abbasi, AR Bhutto, N. Butt, K. Lal, and SM Munir, "Serum Cholesterol: Could it Be a Sixth Parameter of Child-Pugh Scoring System in Cirrhotics due to Viral Hepatitis?" *Coll Physicians Surg Pak,* August 2012 , 22(8):484–7.

8. A. D'Arienzo, F. Manguso, G. Scaglione, G. Vicinanza, R. Bennato, and G. Mazzacca, "Prognostic Value of Progressive Decrease in Serum Cholesterol in Predicting Survival in Child-Pugh C Viral Cirrhosis," *Scand J Gastroenterol,* November 1998, 33(11):1213–8.

9. Morton Lee Pearce and Seymour Dayton, "Incidence of Cancer in Men on a Diet High in Polyunsataurated Fat, *The Lancet,* Volume 297, Issue 7697, pp 464–467, March 6, 1971.

10. LA Sauer and RT Dauchy, "Identification of Linoleic and Arachidonic Acids as the Factors in Hyperlipemic Blood that Increase [3H]Thymidine Incorporation in Hepatoma 7288CTC Perfused in Situ," *Cancer Res,* June 1, 1988, 48(11):3106–11.

11. "Use of Dietary Linoleic Acid for Secondary Prevention of Coronary Heart Disease and Death: Evaluation of Recovered Data from the Sydney Diet Heart Study and Updated Meta-Analysis," BMJ 2013, 346, published Febuary 5, 2013. doi: http://dx.doi.org/10.1136/bmj.e8707.

12. Sang Mi Kwak, MD; Seung-Kwon Myung, MD; Young Jae Lee, MD, MS; and Hong Gwan Seo, MD, PhD, for the Korean Meta-analysis Study Group, "Efficacy of

Omega-3 Fatty Acid Supplements (Eicosapentaenoic Acid and Docosahexaenoic Acid) in the Secondary Prevention of Cardiovascular Disease Meta-analysis of Randomized, Double-blind, Placebo-Controlled Trials," *Arch Intern Med,* 2012, 172(9):686–694REE.

13. Michel Lucas, Fariba Mirzaei, Eilis J. O'Reilly, An Pan, Walter C. Willett, Ichiro Kawachi, Karestan Koenen, and Alberto Ascherio, "Dietary Intake of n–3 and n–6 Fatty Acids and the Risk of Clinical Depression in Women: A 10-y Prospective Follow-Up Study," American Society for Nutrition, 2011.

14. EC Rizos, EE Ntzani, E. Bika, MS Kostapanos, and MS Elisaf, "Association Between Omega-3 Fatty Acid Supplementation and Risk of Major Cardiovascular Disease Events: A Systematic Review and Meta-Analysis," *Journal of the American Medical Association,* September 12, 2012, 308(10):1024–33.

15. CE Ramsden, JR Hibbeln, SF Majchrzak, and JM Davis, "n-6 Fatty Acid-Specific and Mixed Polyunsaturated Dietary Interventions Have Different Effects on CHD Risk: A Meta-Analysis of Randomised Controlled Trials," *Br J Nutr,* December 2010, 104(11):1586–600.

16. M. Borkman, DJ Chisholm, SM Furler, LH Storlien, EW Kraegen, LA Simons, and CN Chesterman. "Effects of Fish Oil Supplementation on Glucose and Lipid Metabolism in NIDDM," *Diabetes,* October 1989, 38(10):1314–9.

17. B. Vessby, B. Karlstrom, M. Boberg, H. Lithell, and C. Berne, "Polyunsaturated Fatty Acids May Impair Blood Glucose Control in Type 2 Diabetic Patients," *Diabet Med,* March 1992, 9(2):126–33.

18. M. Anthony, "Linoleic Acid Has an Effect on Migraine Head Aches," *Clin Exp Neurol,* 1978, 15:190–6.

19. FJ Kok, G. van Poppel, J. Melse, E. Verheul, EG Schouten, DH Kruyssen, and A. Hofman, "Do Antioxidants and Polyunsaturated Fatty Acids Have a Combined Association with Coronary Atherosclerosis?" *Atherosclerosis,* January 1991, 86(1):85–90.

20. EC Rizos, EE Ntzani, E. Bika, MS Kostapanos, and MS Elisaf, "Association Between Omega-3 Fatty Acid Supplementation and Risk of Major Cardiovascular Disease Events: A Systematic Review and Meta-Analysis," *Journal of the American Medication Association,* September 12, 2012, 308(10):1024–33. doi: 10.1001/2012.jama.11374.

21. Thomas A. Trikalinos, MD; Jounghee Lee, PhD; Denish Moorthy, M.B.B.S., MS; Winifred W. Yu, MS, RD; Joseph Lau, MD; Alice H. Lichtenstein, D.Sc.; Mei Chung, PhD, M.P.H., "Volume 4: Effects of Eicosapentanoic Acid and Docosahexanoic Acid on Mortality Across Diverse Settings: Systematic Review and Meta-Analysis of Randomized Trials and Prospective Cohorts. Tufts Medical Center Evidence-based Practice Center," www.ahrq.gov/research/findings/evidence-based-reports/nutrtp4.pdf.

22. M. Meydani, F. Natiello, B. Goldin, N. Free, M. Woods, E. Schaefer, JB Blumberg, and SL Gorbach, "Effect of Long-Term Fish Oil Supplementation on Vitamin E Status and Lipid Peroxidation in Women," *J Nutr,* April 1991, 121(4):484–91.

23. MJ Gonzalez, JI Gray, RA Schemmel, L. Dugan Jr., and CW Welsch, "Lipid Peroxidation Products Are Elevated in Fish Oil Diets Even in thePresence of Added Antioxidants," *J Nutr,* November 1992, 122(11):2190–5.

24. KM Humphries, Y. Yoo, and LI Szweda, "Inhibition of NADH-Linked Mitochondrial Respiration by 4-hydroxy-2-nonenal," *Biochemistry*, January 13, 1998, 37(2):552–7.

25. JM Ramon, R. Bou, S. Romea, ME Alkiza, M. Jacas, J. Ribes, and J. Oromi, "Dietary Fat Intake and Prostate Cancer Risk: A Case-Control Study in Spain," *Cancer causes & control: CCC*, 2000, 11 (8):679–85.

26. IA Brouwer, MB Katan, and PL Zock, "Dietary Alpha-Linolenic Acid Is Associated with Reduced Risk of Fatal Coronary Heart Disease, but Increased Prostate Cancer Risk: A Meta-Analysis," *The Journal of Nutrition*, 2004, 134 (4):919–22.

27. M. Lucas, F. Mirzaei, E.J. O'Reilly, A. Pan, W.C. Willett, I. Kawachi, K. Koenen, and A. Ascherio, "Dietary Intake of n-3 and n-6 Fatty Acids and the Risk of Clinical Depression in Women: A 10-y Prospective Follow-Up Study," *American Journal of Clinical Nutrition, 2011,* 93 (6):1337–43.

28. Christopher Masterjohn, "Good Fats, Bad Fats: Separating Fact from Fiction," Weston A. Price Foundation, March 24, 2012.

29. Josh and Jeanne Rubin, www.EastWestHealing.com.

30. Dr. Ray Peat. "Unsaturated fatty acids: Nutritionally essential, or toxic?" www.raypeat.com

31. Dr. Ray Peat. "Unsaturated Vegetable Oils: Toxic", www.raypeat.com

32. Dr. Ray Peat, "Coconut Oil", www.raypeat.com

33. Dr. Ray Peat. "Cholesterol, longevity, intelligence, and health." www.raypeat.com

34. Dr. Ray Peat. "Glycemia, starch, and sugar in context." www.raypeat.com

35. Dr. Ray Peat. "Aspirin, Brain and cancer" www.raypeat.com

36. Dr. Ray Peat, "Mind and Tissues". Self Published. 1994.

37. Dr. Ray Peat, "Generative Energy". Self Published. 1994.

38. Dr. Ray Peat, "Nutrition for Women" Self Published. 1993.

Chapter 4

1. Johanna Burani, MS, RD, "Practical Use of the GI," American Diabetes Association, 2006.

2. MC Moore, SN Davis, SL Mann, and AD Cherrington, "Acute Fructose Administration Improves Oral Glucose Tolerance in Adults with Type 2 Diabetes," *Diabetes Care,* November 2001, 24(11):1882–7.h.

3. Dr. David Katz, "Sugar *Isn't* Evil: A Rebuttal," *Huffington Post,* October 12, 2012.

4. The University of Sidney GI listings, www.GlycemicIndex.com/index.p.

5. JA Welsh, AJ Sharma, L. Grellinger, and MB Vos, "Consumption of Added Sugars Is Decreasing in the United States," *American Journal of Clinical Nutrition*, September 2011, 94(3):726–34. Epub July 13, 2011.

6. MC Moore, AD Cherrington, SL Mann, and SN Davis, "Acute Fructose Administration Decreases the Glycemic Response to an Oral Glucose Tolerance Test in Normal Adults," *J Clin Endocrinol Metab,* December 2000, 85(12):4515–9.

7. RW Simpson, JI Mann, J. Eaton, RA Moore, R. Carter, and TD Hockaday, "Improved Glucose Control in Maturity-Onset Diabetes Treated with High-Carbohydrate-Modified Fat Diet," *Br Med J,* June 30, 1979, 1(6180):1753–6.

8. L. Tappy and E. Jequier, "Fructose and Dietary Thermogenesis," *American Journal of Clinical Nutrition,* November 1993, 58(5 Suppl):766S–770S.

9. I. Spasojević, A. Bajić, K. Jovanović, M. Spasić, and P. Andjus, "Protective Role of Fructose in the Metabolism of Astroglial C6 Cells Exposed to Hydrogen Peroxide," *Carbohydr Res,* September 8, 2009, 344(13):1676–81. Epub June 3, 2009.

10. T. Brundin and J. Wahren, "Whole Body and Splanchnic Oxygen Consumption and Blood Flow After Oral Ingestion of Fructose or Glucose," *AJP – Endo,* April 1993, vol. 264 no. 4, E504–E513.

11. E. Tsanzi, HR Light, and JC Tou, "The Effect of Feeding Different Sugar-Sweetened Beverages to Growing Female Sprague-Dawley Rats on Bone Mass and Strength," *Bone,* May 2008, 42(5):960–8. Epub February 15, 2008.

12. JT Holbrook, JC Smith Jr, and S. Reiser "Dietary Fructose or Starch: Effects on Copper, Zinc, Iron, Manganese, Calcium, and Magnesium Balances in Humans," *American Journal of Clinical Nutrition,* June 1989, 49(6):1290–4.

13. H. Ghanim, P. Mohanty, R. Pathak, A. Chaudhuri, CL Sia, and P. Dandona, "Orange Juice or Fructose Intake Does Not Induce Oxidative and Inflammatory Response," *Diabetes Care,* June 2007, 30(6):1406–11. Epub March 23, 2007.

14. J. Ruzzin, YC Lai, and J. Jensen, "Consumption of Carbohydrate Solutions Enhances Energy Intake Without Increased Body Weight and Impaired Insulin Action in Rat

Skeletal Muscles," *Diabetes Metab*, April 2005, 31(2):178–88.

15. I. Anundi, J. King, DA Owen, H. Schneider, JJ Lemasters, and RG Thurman, "Fructose Prevents Hypoxic Cell Death in Liver," *Am J Physiol*, September 1987, 253(3 Pt 1):G390–6.

16. Dr. Ray Peat, "Glycemia, Starch and Sugar in Context," www.RayPeat.com.

17. Dr. Ray Peat, "Sugar Issues," www.RayPeat.com.

18. T. Brundin and J. Wahren, "Whole Body and Splanchnic Oxygen Consumption and Blood Flow After Oral Ingestion of Fructose or Glucose," *Am J Physiol,* April 1993, 264(4 Pt 1):E504–13.

19. NS Al-Waili, "Natural Honey Lowers Plasma Glucose, C-Reactive Protein, Homocysteine, and Blood Lipids in Healthy, Diabetic, and Hyperlipidemic Subjects: Comparison with Dextrose and Sucrose," *J Med Food,* Spring 2004, 7(1):100–7.

20. D. Mascord, J. Smith, GA Starmer, and JB Whitfield, "The Effect of Fructose on Alcohol Metabolism and on the [Lactate]/[Pyruvate] Ratio in Man," *Alcohol Alcohol,* 1991, 26(1):53–9.

21. Husam Ghanim, Chang Ling Sia, Mannish Upadhyay, Kelly Korzeniewski, Prabhakar Viswanathan, Sanaa Abuaysheh, Priya Mohanty, and Paresh Dandona, "Orange Juice Neutralizes the Proinflammatory Effect of a High-Fat, High-Carbohydrate Meal and Prevents Endotoxin Increase and Toll-Like Receptor Expression," American Society for Nutrition, 2010.

22. PH Bisschop, HP Sauerwein, E. Endert, and JA Romijn, "Isocaloric Carbohydrate Deprivation Induces Protein

Catabolism Despite a Low T3-syndrome in Healthy Men," *Clin Endocrinol (Oxf),* January 2001, 54(1):75–80.

23. KA Lê and L. Tappy, "Metabolic Effects of Fructose," *Curr Opin Clin Nutr Metab Care,* July 2006, 9(4):469–75.

24. R. Crescenzo, F. Bianco, I. Falcone, P. Coppola, G. Liverini, and S. Iossa, "Increased Hepatic de Novo Lipogenesis and Mitochondrial Efficiency in a Model of Obesity Induced by Diets Rich in Fructose," *Eur J Nutr,* March 2013, 52(2):537–45.

25. L. Tappy and KA Lê, " "Does Fructose Consumption Contribute to Non-Alcoholic Fatty Liver Disease?" *Clin Res Hepatol Gastroenterol,* December 2012, 36(6):554–60.

26. T. Mizobe, Y. Nakajima, H. Ueno, and DI Sessler, "Fructose Administration Increases Intraoperative Core Temperature by Augmenting Both Metabolic Rate and the Vasoconstriction Threshold," *Anesthesiology,* June 2006, 104(6):1124–30.

27. RG Hendler, M. Walesky, and RS Sherwin, "Sucrose Substitution in Prevention and Reversal of the Fall in Metabolic Rate Accompanying Hypocaloric Diets," *Am J Med,* August 1986, 81(2):280–4.

28. L. Tappy, JP Randin, JP Felber, R. Chiolero, DC Simonson, E. Jequier, and DeFronzo, "Comparison of Thermogenic Effect of Fructose and Glucose in Normal Humans," *Am J Physiol,* June 1986, 250(6 Pt 1):E718–24.

29. G. Livesey and R. Taylor, "Fructose Consumption and Consequences for Glycation, Plasma Triacylglycerol, and Body Weight: Meta-Analyses and Meta-Regression Models of Intervention Studies," *American Journal of Clinical Nutrition,* November 2008, 88(5):1419–37.

30. LC Dolan, SM Potter, and GA Burdock, "Evidence-Based Review on the Effect of Normal Dietary Consumption of Fructose on Development of Hyperlipidemia and Obesity in Healthy, Normal Weight Individuals," *Crit Rev Food Sci Nutr,* January 2010, 50(1):53–84.

31. L. Tappy and KA Lê, "Metabolic Effects of Fructose and the Worldwide Increase in Obesity," *Physiol Rev,* January 2010, 90(1):23–46.

32. KA Lê, M. Ith, R. Kreis, D. Faeh, M. Bortolotti, C. Tran, c. Boesch, and L. Tappy, "Fructose Overconsumption Causes Dyslipidemia and Ectopic Lipid Deposition in Healthy Subjects with and Without a Family History of Type 2 Diabetes," *American Journal of Clinical Nutrition,* June 2009, 89(6):1760–5.

33. Salwa W. Rizkalla, "Health Implications of Fructose Consumption: A Review of Recent Data," *Nutr Metab* (London), 2010, 7:82. Published online November 4, 2010.

34. JL Sievenpiper, RJ de Souza, A. Mirrahimi, ME Yu, AJ Carleton, J. Beyene, L. Chiavaroli, M. Di Buono, AL Jenkins, LA Leiter, TM Wolever, CW Kendall, and DJ Jenkins, "Effect of Fructose on Body Weight in Controlled Feeding Trials: A Systematic Review and Meta-Analysis," *Ann Intern Med,* February 21, 2012, 156(4):291–304.

35. Dr. John Sievenpiper, interview, "Fate of Fructose," Mau 26, 2012, http://EvolvingHealthScience.blogspot.com/2012/05/fate-of-fructose-interview-with-dr-john.html.

36. Sabine Thuy, Ruth Ladurner, Valentina Volynets, Silvia Wagner, Stefan Strahl, Alfred Königsrainer, Klaus-Peter Maier, Stephan C. Bischoff, and Ina Bergheim, "Nonalcoholic Fatty Liver Disease in Humans Is Associated with Increased Plasma Endotoxin and Plasminogen

Activator Inhibitor 1 Concentrations and with Fructose Intake," Department of Nutritional Medicine, University of Hohenheim, *The Journal of Nutrition and Disease.*

Chapter 5

1. C. Catassi, JC Bai, B. Bonaz, G. Bouma, A. Calabrò, A. Carroccio, G. Castillejo, C. Ciacci, F. Cristofori, J. Dolinsek, R. Francavilla, L. Elli, P. Green, W. Holtmeier, P. Koehler, S. Koletzko, C. Meinhold, D. Sanders, M. Schumann, D. Schuppan, R. Ullrich, A. Vécsei, U. Volta, V. Zevallos, A. Sapone, and A. Fasano, "Non-Celiac Gluten Sensitivity: The New Frontier of Gluten Related Disorders," *Nutrients,* September 26, 2013, 5(10):3839–53. doi: 10.3390/nu5103839.

2. S. Currie, N. Hoggard, MJ Clark, DS Sanders, ID Wilkinson, PD Griffiths, and M. Hadjivassiliou, ""Alcohol Induces Sensitization to Gluten in Genetically Susceptible Individuals: A Case Control Study," *PLOS One,* October 15, 2013, 8(10):e77638.

3. VF Zevallos, HJ Ellis, T. Suligoj, LI Herencia, and PJ Ciclitira, " Variable Activation of Immune Response by Quinoa (Chenopodium Quinoa Willd.) Prolamins in Celiac Disease," *American Journal of Clinical Nutrition,* August 2012, 96(2):337–44.

4. JP Ortiz-Sánchez, F. Cabrera-Chávez, and AM de la Barca, "Maize Prolamins Could Induce a Gluten-Like Cellular Immune Response in Some Celiac Disease Patients," *Nutrients,* October 21, 2013, 5(10):4174–83.

5. F. Cabrera-Chávez, S. Iametti, M. Miriani, AM de la Barca, G. Mamone, and F. Bonomi, "Maize Prolamins Resistant to Peptic-Tryptic Digestion Maintain Immune-Recognition by

IgA from Some Celiac Disease Patients," *Plant Foods Hum Nutr*, March 2012, 67(1):24, 30.

6. Anna Sapone, Julio C. Bai, Carolina Ciacci, Jernej Dolinsek, Peter HR Green, Marios Hadjivassiliou, Katri Kaukinen, Kamran Rostami, David S. Sanders, Michael Schumann, Reiner Ullrich, Danilo Villalta, Umberto Volta, Carlo Catassi, and Alessio Fasano, "Spectrum of Gluten-Related Disorders: Consensus on New Nomenclature and Classification." *BMC Medicine* 2012, 10:13

7. Jeffrey M. Smith, "Can Genetically- Engineered Foods Explain the Exploding Gluten Sensitivity?" Institute for Responsible Technology Research support by Sayer Ji, GreenMedInfo.com; Dr. Tom O' Bryan, thedr.com; Tom Malterre, MS CN, nourishingmeals.com; and Stephanie Seneff, PhD, http://people.csail.mit.edu/seneff/.

8. SS Mehr, AM Kakakios, and AS Kemp, "Rice: A Common and Severe Cause of Food Protein-Induced Enterocolitis Syndrome," *Arch Dis Child*, March 2009, 94(3):220–3.

9. S. Mehr, A. Kakakios, K. Frith, and AS Kemp, "Food Protein-Induced Enterocolitis Syndrome: 16-Year Experience," *Pediatrics*, March 2009, 123(3):e459–64.

10. A. Nowak-Wegrzyn and A. Muraro, "Food Protein-Induced Enterocolitis Syndrome," *Curr Opin Allergy Clin Immunol*, August 2009, 9(4):371–7.

11. F. Mearin and M. Montoro, "Irritable Bowel Syndrome, Celiac Disease and Gluten," *Med Clin* (Barc), September 9, 2013. pii: S0025-7753(13)00459-4.

12. U. Volta, G. Caio, F. Tovoli, and R. De Giorgio., "Non-Celiac Gluten Sensitivity: Questions Still to Be Answered Despite Increasing Awareness," *Cell Mol Immunol*, September 2013, 10(5):383–92.

13. AJ Lucendo and A. García-Manzanares, "Bone Mineral Density in Adult Coeliac Disease: An Updated Review," *Rev Esp Enferm Dig*, May 2013, 105(3):154–162.

14. B. Bilgic, D. Aygun, AB Arslan, A. Bayram, F. Akyuz, S. Sencer, and HA Hanagasi, "Silent Neurological Involvement in Biopsy-Defined Coeliac Patients." *Neurol Sci*, December 2013, 34(12):2199–204.

15. NJ van Hees, W. Van der Does, and EJ Giltay, "Coeliac Disease, Diet Adherence and Depressive Symptoms," *J Psychosom Res*, February 2013, 74(2):155–60.

16. Fl Soares, R. de Oliveira Matoso, LG Teixeira, Z. Menezes, SS Pereira, AC Alves, NV Batista, AM de Faria, DC Cara, AV Ferreira, and JI Alvarez-Leite, "Gluten-Free Diet Reduces Adiposity, Inflammation and Insulin Resistance Associated with the Induction of PPAR-Alpha and PPAR-Gamma Expression," *J Nutr Biochem*, June 2013, 24(6):1105–11.

17. AM Johnson, RC Dale, L. Wienholt, M. Hadjivassiliou, D. Aeschlimann, and JA Lawson, "Coeliac Disease, Epilepsy, and Cerebral Calcifications: Association with TG6 Autoantibodies," *Dev Med Child Neurol*, January 2013, 55(1):90–3.

18. G. Ferretti, T. Bacchetti, L. Saturni, N. Manzella, C. Candelaresi, A. Benedetti, and A. Di Sario, "Lipid Peroxidation and Paraoxonase-1 Activity in Celiac Disease," *J Lipids*, 2012, 2012:587479.

19. A. Sapone, JC Bai, C. Ciacci, J. Dolinsek, PH Green, M. Hadjivassiliou, K. Kaukinen, K. Rostami, DS Sanders, M. Schumann, R. Ullrich, D. Villalta, U. Volta, C. Catassi, and A. Fasano, "Spectrum of Gluten-Related Disorders: Consensus on New Nomenclature and Classification," *BMC Med*, February 7, 2012, 10:13.

20. K. Sestak, L. Conroy, PP Aye, S. Mehra, GG Doxiadis, and D. Kaushal, "Improved Xenobiotic Metabolism and Reduced Susceptibility to Cancer in Gluten-Sensitive Macaques upon Introduction of a Gluten-Free Diet," *PLoS One,* April 12, 2011, 6(4):e18648.

21. R. Uibo, M. Panarina, K. Teesalu, I. Talja, E. Sepp, M. Utt, M. Mikelsaar, K. Heilman, O. Uibo, and T. Vorobjova, "Celiac Disease in Patients with Type 1 Diabetes: A Condition with Distinct Changes in Intestinal Immunity?" *Cell Mol Immunol,* March 2011, 8(2):150–6.

22. AV Stazi and B. Trinti, "Selenium Status and Over-Expression of Interleukin-15 in Celiac Disease and autoimmune Thyroid Diseases," *Ann Ist Super Sanita,* 2010, 46(4):389–99.

23. HJ Freeman, "Celiac Disease and Selected Long-Term Health Issues," *Maturitas,* November 2012, 73(3):206–11.

24. www.fda.gov/Food/GuidanceRegulation/GuidanceDocumentsRegulatoryInformation/Allergens/ucm362880.htm.

25. P R Shewry and N G. Halford "THE PROLAMIN STORAGE PROTEINS OF SORGHUM AND MILLETS." Long Ashton Research Station, Long Ashton, Bristol BS41 9AF, UK, 2003.

26. E.N. Clare Mills, "Plant Food Allergens." *Institute of Food Research Norwich, UK.* Peter R. Shewry, *Rothamsted Research Harpenden, UK.* Blackwell Science Ltd., a Blackwell Publishing Company. 2004.

27. Andrew Cassel, "Why U.S. Farm Subsidies Are Bad for the World: They Make it Possible for Us to Export Food So Cheaply that Farmers in Poorer Nations can't Possibley Compete," *Philadelphia Inquirer,* May 6, 2002.

28. National Foundation of Celiac Awareness, www.CeliacCentral.org/celiac-disease/facts-and-figures/.

29. José Xavier Filho, "Trypsin Inhibitors in Sorghum Grain," *Food Science Journal of Food Science,* March 1974, Volume 39, Issue 2, pp. 422–423.

30. "Protease Inhibitors in Plants: Genes for Improving Defenses Against Insects and Pathogens," *Annual Review of Phytopathology,* September 1990, 28:425–449.

31. DJ Jenkins, TM Wolever, RH Taylor, H. Barker, H. Fielden, JM Baldwin, AC Bowling, HC Newman, AL Jenkins, and DV Goff, "Glycemic Index of Foods: A Physiological Basis for Carbohydrate Exchange," The American Society for Clinical Nutrition, Inc, 1981.

32. Torsten Bohn, Lena Davidsson, Thomas Walczyk, and Richard F. Hurrell , "Phytic Acid Added to White-Wheat Bread Inhibits Fractional Apparent Magnesium Absorption in Humans," American Society for Clinical Nutrition, 2004.

33. TB Koerner, C. Cleroux, C. Poirier, I. Cantin, S. La Vieille, S. Hayward, and S. Dubois, "Gluten Contamination of Naturally Gluten-Free Flours and Starches Used by Canadians with Celiac Disease," *Food Addit Contam Part A Chem Anal Control Expo Risk Assess,* October 14, 2013.

34. W. Daniewski, A. Wojtasik, and H. Kunachowicz, "Gluten Content in Special Dietary Use Gluten-Free Products and Other Food Products," *Rocz Panstw Zakl Hig,* 2010, 61(1):51–5.

35. T. Thompson, AR Lee, and T. Grace, "Gluten Contamination of Grains, Seeds, and Flours in the United States: A Pilot Study," *J Am Diet Assoc,* June 2010, 110(6):937–40.

36. MS Calvo and YK Park, "Changing Phosphorus Content of the U.S. Diet: Potential for Adverse Effects on Bone, *J Nutr,* 1996, 126(4 Suppl):1168S–1180S.

37. MS Calvo, "The Effects of High Phosphorus Intake on Calcium Homeostasis," *Adv Nutr Res,* 1994, 9:183–207.

38. MS Calvo, "Dietary Phosphorus, Calcium Metabolism and Bone," *J Nutr,* September 1993, 123(9):1627–33.

39. "Phosphorus," Linus Pauling Institute, http://lpi.oregonstate.edu/infocenter/minerals/phosphorus/.

40. Dr. Ray Peat, "Glycemia, Starch, and Sugar in Context." www.raypeat.com.

41. Dr. Ray Peat, "Glucose and Sucrose for Diabetes." www.raypeat.com

42. http://AllButGluten.com/products/all-but-gluten-blueberry-muffins.

43. Weiwen Chai and Michael Liebman, "Oxalate Content of Legumes, Nuts, and Grain-Based Flours," *Journal of Food Composition and Analysis,* 2005, 18:723–729.

44. *Manual of Clinical Dietetics,* Chicago Dietetic Association, American Dietetic Association, Chicago, Illinois, 2000, p. 475.

Chapter 6

1. Loren Cordain, L. Toohey, M.J. Smith, and M.S. Hickey, "Modulation of Immune Function by Dietary Lectins in Rheumatoid Arthritis," Department of Health and Exercise Science, Colorado State University, Fort Collins, Colorado.

2. K. Miyake, T. Tanaka, and PL McNeil, "Lectin-Based Food Poisoning: A New Mechanism of Protein Toxicity," In Steinhardt, Richard, *PLoS ONE,* 2007, 2 (1): e687.

3. Fredric L. Coe, Andrew Evan, and Elaine Worcester, "Kidney Stone Disease," , *J Clin Invest,* October 1, 2005, 115(10):2598–2608.

4. U. Pabuccuoglu, "Aspects of Oxalosis Associated with Aspergillosis in Pathology Specimens," *Pathol Res Pract,* 2005, 201(5): 363–8.

5. "The Oxalate Content of Food," www.OHF.org/docs/Oxalate2008.pdf.

6. *Dietary Reference Intakes for Energy, Carbohydrate, Fiber, Fat, Fatty Acids, Cholesterol, Protein, and Amino Acids (Macronutrients),* Chapter 7: "Dietary, Functional and Total fiber," U,S, Department of Agriculture, National Agricultural Library and National Academy of Sciences, Institute of Medicine, Food and Nutrition Board, 2005.

7. A. Cassidy "Potential Risks and Benefits of Phytoestrogen-Rich Diets," Int J Vitam Nutr Res, March 2003, 73(2):120–6.

8. DA Sloan, DM Fleiszer, GK Richards, D Murray, and RA Brown, "The Effect of the Fiber Components Cellulose and Lignin on Experimental Colon Neoplasia," *J Surg Oncol,* February 1993, 52(2):77–82.

9. R. McPherson-Kay, "Fiber, Stool Bulk, and Bile Acid Output: Implications for Colon Cancer Risk," *Prev Med,* July 1987, 16(4):540–4.

10. WR Obermeyer, SM Musser, JM Betz, RE Casey, AE Pohland, and SW Page, "Chemical Studies of Phytoestrogens and Related Compounds in Dietary Supplements: Flax and

Chaparral," *Proc Soc Exp Biol Med,* January 1995, 208(1):6–12.

11. R.S. Markin, D. Blackwood, D.M.E. Harvell, J.D. Shull, and K.L. Pennington,"Dietary Lignin, an Insoluble Fiber, Enhanced Uterine Cancer but Did Not Influence Mammary Cancer Induced by N-methyl-N-nitrosourea in Rats," *Nutrition and cancer,* 1998, volume 31.

12. LR Jacobs, "Relationship Between Dietary Fiber and Cancer: Metabolic, Physiologic, and Cellular Mechanisms," Proc Soc Exp Biol Med, December 1986, 183(3):299–310.

13. JR Lupton and LJ Marchant, "Independent Effects of Fiber and Protein on Colonic Luminal Ammonia Concentration," *J Nutr,* February 1989, 119(2):235–41.

14. B. Reddy, A. Engle, S. Katsifis, B. Simi, HP Bartram, P. Perrino, and C. Mahan, "Biochemical Epidemiology of Colon Cancer: Effect of Types of Dietary Fiber on Fecal Mutagens, Acid, and Neutral sterols in healthy subjects," Cancer Res, August 15, 1989, 49(16):4629–35.

15. LR Jacobs, "Effect of Dietary Fiber on Colonic Cell Proliferation and its Relationship to Colon Carcinogenesis," *Prev Med,* July 1987, 16(4):5671.

16. LR Jacobs and JR Lupton, "Relationship Between Colonic Luminal pH, Cell Proliferation, and Colon Carcinogenesis in 1,2-dimethylhydrazine Treated Rats Fed High Fiber Diets," *Cancer Res,* April 1986, 46(4 Pt 1):1727–34.

17. RD Reynolds, "Bioavailability of Vitamin B-6 from Plant Foods," The American Society for Clinical Nutrition, Inc., 1988.

18. Pam Schoenfeld, "Vitamin B6: The Under-Appreciated Vitamin," Weston A. Price Foundation, April 1, 2011.

19. HC Lichtstein, IC Gunsalus, and WW Umbreit, "Function of the Vitamin B6 Group; Pyridoxal Phosphate (Codecarboxylase) in Transamination," *J Biol Chem,* 1945, 161 (1):311–20

19. JC Tou, J. Chen, and LU Thompson, "Flaxseed and its Lignan Precursor, Secoisolariciresinol Diglycoside, Affect Pregnancy Outcome and Reproductive Development in Rats," *J Nutr,* November 1998, 128(11):1861–8.

20. H. Sakagami, K. Asano, T. Yoshida, and Y. Kawazoe, "Organ Distribution and Toxicity of Lignin," *In Vivo,* January–February 1999, 13(1):41–4.

21. Konstantin Monastyrsky, *The Fiber Menace,* Ageless Press, 2008.

22. Dr. Ray Peat, "Vegetables etc. Who Defines Food?" www.RayPeat.com.

23. Dr. Ray Peat, "Unsaturated Vegetable Oil: Toxic," www.RayPeat.com.

24. Dr. Ray Peat, "Natural Estrogens," www.RayPeat.com.

25. Dr. Ray Peat, "Mind and Tissue", Self Published. 1994

26. Dr. Ray Peat. "Generative Energy." Self Published. 1994

27. Josh and Jeanne Rubin, "The Metabolic Blue Print," www.EastWestHealing.com.

28. Willy Blackmore, "Kale Bites Back: Turns Out the Popular Green Has a Potent Self-Defense System. Evolution Has Given This Popular Brassica, Like Most Every Other Vegetable, an Arsenal of Anti-Vegan Defenses," October 7, 2013, www.TakePart.com/article/2013/10/07/killer-kale?cmpid=foodinc-fb.

29. J. Robertson, WG Brydon, K. Tadesse, P. Wenham, A. Walls, and MA Eastwood, "The Effect of Raw Carrot on Serum Lipids and Colon Function," The American Society for Clinical Nutrition, Inc., 1979.

30. T. Betsche and B. Fretzdorff, "Biodegradation of Oxalic Acid from Spinach Using Cereal Radicles," *J Agric Food Chem,* December 14, 2005, 53(25):9751–8.

31. L. Brinkley, J. McGuire, J. Gregory, and CY Pak, "Bioavailability of Oxalate in Foods," *Urology,* June 1981, 17(6):534–8.

Chapter 7

1. E. Mezey, "Liver Disease and Protein Needs," *Annu Rev Nutr,* 1982;2:21–50.

2. LH Bernstein and Y. Ingenbleek, "Transthyretin: Its Response to Malnutrition and Stress Injury. Clinical Usefulness and Economic Implications," *Clin Chem Lab Med,* December 2002, 40(12):1344–8.

3. ShS Azimova, OS Petrova, and A. Abdukarimov, "The Role of Serum Thyroxine Binding Prealbumin in the Realization of the Hormonal Effect," *Biokhimiia,* January 1985, 50(1):114–121.

4. L. Bartalena and J. Robbins, "Thyroid Hormone Transport Proteins," *Clin Lab Med,* September 1993, 13(3):583–98.

5. GD Brinkworth, M. Noakes, JB Keogh, ND Luscombe, GA Wittert, and PM Clifton, "Long-Term Effects of a High-Protein, Low-Carbohydrate Diet on Weight Control and Cardiovascular Risk Markers in Obese Hyperinsulinemic Subjects," *Int J Obes Relat Metab Disord,* May 2004, 28(5):661–70.

6. Peter M. Clifton, Jennifer B. Keogh, and Manny Noakes. "Long-Term Effects of a High-Protein Weight-Loss Diet[1,2,3]," American Society for Clinical Nutrition, 2008.

7. Manny Noakes, Jennifer B. Keogh, Paul R. Foster, and Peter M. Clifton. "Effect of an Energy-Restricted, High-Protein, Low-Fat Diet Relative to a Conventional High-Carbohydrate, Low-Fat Diet on Weight Loss, Body Composition, Nutritional Status, and Markers of Cardiovascular Health in Obese Women[1,2,3]," American Society for Clinical Nutrition, 2005.

8. Sachiko T. St. Jeor, RD, PhD; Barbara V. Howard, PhD; T. Elaine Prewitt, RD, DrPH; Vicki Bovee, RD, MS; Terry Bazzarre, PhD; and Robert H. Eckel, MD, for the AHA Nutrition Committee, "Dietary Protein and Weight Reduction," A Statement for Healthcare Professionals from the Nutrition Committee of the Council on Nutrition, Physical Activity, and Metabolism of the American Heart Association.

9. M. Lepe, M. Bacardí Gascón, and A. Jiménez Cruz, "Long-Term Efficacy of High-Protein Diets: A Systematic Review." *Nutr Hosp,* November–December 2011, 26(6):1256–9.

10. Lukas Schwingshackl and Georg Hoffmann, "Long-Term Effects of Low-Fat Diets Either Low or High in Protein on Cardiovascular and Metabolic Risk Factors: A Systematic Review and Meta-Analysis," *Nutrition Journal,* 2013, 12:48.

11. TP Wycherley, LJ Moran, PM Clifton, M. Noakes, and GD Brinkworth, "Effects of Energy-Restricted High-Protein, Low-Fat Compared with Standard-Protein, Low-Fat Diets: A Meta-Analysis of Randomized Controlled Trials," *American Journal of Clinical Nutrition,* December 2012, 96(6):1281–98. doi: 10.3945/ajcn.112.044321. Epub October 24, 2012.

12. "Analysis of Health Problems Associated with High-Protein, High-Fat, Carbohydrate-Restricted Diets," reported via an Online Registry: A Report by the Physicians Committee for Responsible Medicine, May 2004.

13. D. Feskanich, WC Willett, MJ Stampfer, and GA Colditz, "Protein Consumption and Bone Fractures in Women, *Am J Epidemiol,* 1996, 143:472–479.

14. BJ Abelow, TR Holford, and KL Insogna, "Cross-Cultural Association Between Dietary Animal Protein and Hip Fracture: A Hypothesis," *Calcif Tissue Int,* January 1992, 50(1):14–8.

15. M. Koshihara, R. Masuyama, M. Uehara, and K. Suzuki, "Effect of Dietary Calcium:Phosphorus Ratio on Bone Mineralization and Intestinal Calcium Absorption in Ovariectomized Rats," *Biofactors,* 2004, 22(1-4):39–42.

16. ST Reddy, CY Wang, K. Sakhaee, L. Brinkley, and CY Pak, "Effect of Low-Carbohydrate High-Protein Diets on Acid-Base Balance, Stone-Forming Propensity, and Calcium Metabolism," *Am J Kidney Dis,* August 2002, 40(2):265–74.

17. MS Calvo, "The Effects of High Phosphorus Intake on Calcium Homeostasis," *Adv Nutr Res,* 1994, 9:183–207.

18. MS Calvo, "Dietary Phosphorus, Calcium Metabolism and Bone," *J Nutr,* September 1993, 123(9):1627–33.

19. C. Gaudichon, C. Bos, C. Morens, KJ Petzke, F. Mariotti, J. Everwand, R. Benamouzig, S. Daré, D. Tomé, and CC Metges, "Ileal Losses of Nitrogen and Amino Acids in Humans and Their Importance to the Assessment of Amino Acid Requirements," *Gastroenterology,* July 2002, 123(1):50–9.

20. SM Phillips and LJ Van Loon "Dietary Protein for Athletes: From Requirements to Optimum Adaptation," *J Sports Sci,* 2011, 29 Suppl 1:S29–38.

21. PW Lemon, "Effects of Exercise on Dietary Protein Requirements," *Int J Sport Nutr,* December 1998, 8(4):426–47.

22. RA Fielding and J. Parkington, "What Are the Dietary Protein Requirements of Physically Active Individuals? New Evidence on the Effects of Exercise on Protein Utilization During Post-Exercise Recovery," *Nutr Clin Care,* July–August 2002, 5(4):191–6.

23. LJ Van Loon and MJ Gibala, "Dietary Protein to Support Muscle Hypertrophy," *Nestle Nutr Inst Workshop Ser.,* 2011, 69:79–89, discussion 89–95. doi: 10.1159/000329287. Epub January 18, 2012.

24. WJ Evans, "Protein Nutrition, Exercise and Aging," *J Am Coll Nutr,* December 2004, 23(6 Suppl):601S–609S.

25. Kaayla T. Daniel, PhD, CCN, "Why Broth Is Beautiful: Essential Roles for Proline, Glycine and Gelatin," June 18, 2003, 16:43.

26. Thomas H. Creigthon, Chapter 1, *Proteins: Structures and Molecular Properties,* San Francisco, California: W.H. Freeman, 1993.

27. D. Joe Millward, "Human Amino Acid Requirements," *The Journal of Nutrition,* American Society for Nutritional Services, 1997.

28. Janice R. Hermann, "Protein and the Body," Oklahoma Cooperative Extension Service, Division of Agricultural Sciences and Natural Resources, Oklahoma State University.

29. S. Clejan and H. Schulz, "Does the GH-IGF Axis Play a Role in Cancer Pathogenesis?" *Growth Horm IGF Res,* December 2000, 10(6):297–305.

30. ML De Marte and HE Enesco, "Influence of Low Tryptophan Diet on Survival and Organ Growth in Mice," *Mech Ageing Dev,* October 1986, 36(2):161–71.

31. F. Meyer, JB Brown, AS Morrison, and B. MacMahon, "Endogenous Sex Hormones, Prolactin, and Breast Cancer in Premenopausal Women," *J Natl Cancer Inst,* September 1986, 77(3):613–6.

32. JP Raymond, R. Isaac, RE Merceron, and F. Wahbe, "Comparison Between the Plasma Concentrations of Prolactin and Parathyroid Hormone in Normal Subjects and in Patients with Hyperparathyroidism or Hyperprolactinemia," *J Clin Endocrinol Metab,* December 1982, 55(6):1222–5.

33. Charles Janeway, *Immunobiology,* 5th ed., Garland Publishing, 2001.

34. "The Biology of Malnutrition," Part 2. www.NutriSci.wisc.edu/ns350/PPTs/BioMalnutritionP2.pdf.

35. SW Olde Damink, NE Deutz, CH Dejong, PB Soeters, and R. Jalan, "Interorgan Ammonia Metabolism in Liver Failure," *Neurochem Int,* August–September 2002, 41(2–3):177–88.

36. Michelle Lane and David K. Gardner, "Ammonium Induces Aberrant Blastocyst Differentiation, Metabolism, pH Regulation, Gene Expression and Subsequently Alters Fetal Development in the Mouse. *Biology of Reproduction.*" 65(1):14-22. 2001

37. Stefan Walenta, Michael Wetterling, Michael Lehrke, Georg Schwickert, Kolbein Sundfør, Einar K. Rofstad, and Wolfgang Mueller-Klieser. "High Lactate Levels Predict Likelihood of Metastases, Tumor Recurrence, and Restricted Patient Survival in Human Cervical Cancers," *Cancer Research,* March 1999.

38. P.J. Watkins, J.S. Smith, M.G. Fitzgerald, and J.M. Malins, "Lactic Acidosis in Diabetes," *Br Med J,* March 22, 1969, 1(5646):744–747.

39. "Foods High in Tryptophan," http://NutritionData.self.com/foods-000079000000000000000-20.html?

40. Strakie Sowers, "A Primer on Branched Chain Amino Acids," Huntington College of Health Sciences, Retrieved March 22, 2011.

41. DL Brandon, AH Bates, and M. Friedman, "ELISA Analysis of Soybean Trypsin Inhibitors in Processed Foods," *Adv Exp Med Biol,* 1991;289:321–37.

42. *Dietary Reference Intakes for Energy, Carbohydrate, Fiber, Fat, Fatty Acids, Cholesterol, Protein, and Amino Acids (Macronutrients),* National Academies Press, 2005, www.nap.edu/books/0309085373/html/.

43. K. Shibata and S. Toda, "Effects of Sex Hormones on the Metabolism of Tryptophan to Niacin and to Serotonin in Male Rats," *Biosci Biotechnol Biochem,* July 1997, 61(7):1200–2.

44. L.B. Carew, Jr., F.A. Alster, D.C. Foss, and C.G. Scanes, "Effect of a Tryptophan Deficiency on Thyroid Gland, Growth Hormone and Testicular Functions in Chickens," *J. Nutr,* 1983, 113:1756–1765.

45. I. Gonzalez-Burgos, MI Perez-Vega, AR Del Angel-Meza, and A. Feria-Velasco, Centro de Investigacion Biomedica de Michoacan, Instituto Mexicano del Seguro Social, Morelia, "Effect of tryptophan restriction on short-term memory." *Physiol Behav,* January 1998, 63(2):165–9.

46. BJa Medovar, KJ Petzke, TG Semesko, V. Albrecht, and JuG Grigorov, Institut fur Gerontologie, AMW, UdSSR, Kiev, "The Effect of Different Protein Diets on Longevity and Various Biochemical Parameters of Aged Rats," *Nahrung,* 1991, 35(9):961–7.

47. "Alert: Protein drinks You don't need the extra protein or the heavy metals our tests found", *Consumer Reports,* July 2010.

48. E. Blomstrand, "Amino Acids and Central Fatigue," *Amino Acids,* 2001, 20(1):25–34.

49. EA Newsholme and E. Blomstrand, "Tryptophan, 5-hydroxytryptamine and a Possible Explanation for Central Fatigue," *Adv Exp Med Biol,* 1995, 384:315–20.

50. LM Castell, T. Yamamoto, J. Phoenix, and EA Newsholme, "The Role of Tryptophan in Fatigue in Different Conditions of Stress," *Adv Exp Med Biol,* 1999, 467:697–704.

51. J D Schaechter and RJ Wurtman, "Serotonin Release Varies with Brain Tryptophan Levels," *Brain Res,* November 5, 1990, 532(1–2):203–10.

52. M. Biasiolo, A. Bertazzo, CV Costa, and G. Allegri, "Correlation Between Tryptophan and Hair Pigmentation in Human Hair," *Adv Exp Med Biol,* 1999, 467:653–7.

53. A. Bertazzo, M. Biasiolo, CV Costa, E. Cardin de Stefani, and G. Allegri, "Tryptophan in Human Hair: Correlation with Pigmentation," *Farmaco,* August 2000, 55(8):521–5.

54. DP Carvalho, AC Ferreira, SM Coelho, JM Moraes, MA Camacho, and D. Rosenthal, "The Low-Methionine Content of Vegan Diets May Make Methionine Restriction Feasible as a Life Extension Strategy," *Braz J Med Biol Res,* March 2000, 33(3):355–61

55. L. Maintz and N. Novak, "Histamine and Histamine Intolerance," *American Journal of Clinical Nutrition,* 2007, 85:1185–96.

56. S. Wöhrl et al., "Histamine Intolerance-Like Symptoms in Healthy Volunteers After Oral Provocation with Liquid Histamine," *Allergy Asthma Proc,* 2004, 25(5):305–311.

57. Katherine L. Tucker, Kyoko Morita, Ning Qiao, Marian T. Hannan, L. Adrienne Cupples, and Douglas P. Kiel, "Colas, but Not Other Carbonated Beverages, Are Associated with Low Bone Mineral Density in Older Women," The Framingham Osteoporosis Study[1,2,3].

Chapter 8

1. Niva Shapira and Joseph Pinchasov. "Modified Egg Composition to Reduce Low-Density Lipoprotein Oxidizability: High Monounsaturated Fatty Acids and Antioxidants Versus Regular Highn–6 Polyunsaturated Fatty Acids," *Journal of Agricultural and Food Chemistry,* 2008, 56 (10): 3688. DOI: 10.1021/jf073549r

2. I. Staprans, JH Rapp, XM Pan, KY Kim, and KR Feingold, "Oxidized Lipids in the Diet Are a Source of Oxidized Lipid in Chylomicrons of Human Serum," *Arterioscler Thromb,* December 1994, 14(12):1900–5.

3. FA Kummerow, Y. Kim, J. Hull, J. Pollard, P. Ilinov, DL Drossiev, and J. Valek, "The Influence of Egg Consumption

on the Serum Cholesterol Level in Human Subjects," *American Journal of Clinical Nutrition,* 1977, 30:664–73.

4. TR Dawber, RJ Nickerson, FN Brand, and J. Pool, "Eggs, Serum Cholesterol, and Coronary Heart Disease," *American Journal of Clinical Nutrition,* 1982, 36:617–25.

5. AI Qureshi, FK Suri, S. Ahmed, A. Nasar, AA Divani, and JF Kirmani, "Regular Egg Consumption Does Not Increase the Risk of Stroke and Cardiovascular Diseases," *Med Sci Monit,* 2007, 13:CR1–8.

6. PJ Jones, AS Pappu, L. Hatcher, ZC Li, DR Illingworth, and WE Connor, "Dietary Cholesterol Feeding Suppresses Human Cholesterol Synthesis Measured by Deuterium Incorporation and Urinary Mevalonic Acid Levels," *Arterioscler Thromb Vasc Biol,* 1996, 16:1222.

7. Dr. Joseph Raffaele, "The Candaian Yolk Study's Scrambled Science, "Raffaele Reports, August 25, 2012.

8. Frank B. Hu, MD; Meir J. Stampfer, MD; Eric B. Rimm, ScD; JoAnn E. Manson, MD; Alberto Ascherio, MD; Graham A. Colditz, MD; Bernard A. Rosner, PhD; Donna Spiegelman, ScD; Frank E. Speizer, MD; Frank M. Sacks, MD; Charles H. Hennekens, MD; and Walter C. Willett, MD, "A Prospective Study of Egg Consumption and Risk of Cardiovascular Disease in Men and Women," *Journal of the American Medical Association,* April 21, 1999;281(15):1387-1394

9. DJ McNamara, "The Impact of Egg Limitations on Coronary Heart Disease Risk: Do the Numbers Add Up?" *J Am Coll Nutr,* October 2000, 19(5 Suppl):540S–548S.

10. Eggs and Heart Disease," Harvard School of Public Health: The Nutrition Source, www.hsph.harvard.edu/nutritionsource/what-should-you-eat/eggs/#1.

11. Cheryl Long and Tabitha Alterman, "Meet Real Free Range Eggs," Mother Earth News, October/November 2007, www.motherearthnews.com/Real-Food/2007-10-01/Tests-Reveal-Healthier-Eggs.aspx#ixzz27yFbfsJn.

12. I. Zazpe, JJ Beunza, M. Bes-Rastrollo, J. Warnberg, C. de la Fuente-Arrillaga, S. Benito, Z. Vázquez, and MA Martínez-González, SUN Project Investigators, "Egg Consumption and Risk of Cardiovascular Disease in the SUN Project," *Eur J Clin Nutr*, June 2011, 65(6):676–82. Epub March 23, 2011.

13. E. Eguchi, H. Iso, N. Tanabe, Y. Wada, H. Yatsuya, S. Kikuchi, Y. Inaba, and A. Tamakoshi, Japan Collaborative Cohort Study Group, "Healthy Lifestyle Behaviours and Cardiovascular Mortality Among Japanese Men and Women: The Japan Collaborative Cohort Study," *Eur Heart J*, February 2012, 33(4):467–77.

14. ML Fernandez, "Dietary Cholesterol Provided by Eggs and Plasma Lipoproteins in Healthy Populations," *Curr Opin Clin Nutr Metab Care*, January 2006, 9(1):8–12.

15. DK Houston, J. Ding, JS Lee, M. Garcia, AM Kanaya, FA Tylavsky, AB Newman, M. Visser, and SB Kritchevsky, "Dietary Fat and Cholesterol and Risk of Cardiovascular Disease in Older Adults: The Health ABC Study," *Nutr Metab Cardiovasc Dis*, June 2011, 21(6):430–7.

16. JM Rueda and P. Khosla, "Impact of Breakfasts (With or Without Eggs) on Body Weight Regulation and Blood Lipids in University Students over a 14-Week Semester," *Nutrients*, December 16, 2013, 5(12):5097–113.

17. E. Rodríguez-Rodríguez, LG González-Rodríguez, RM Ortega Anta, and AM López-Sobaler, "Consumption of Eggs

May Prevent Vitamin D Deficiency in Schoolchildren," *Nutr Hosp,* May–June 2013, 28(3):794–801.

18. CJ Andersen, CN Blesso, J. Lee, J. Barona, D. Shah, MJ Thomas, and ML Fernandez, "Egg Consumption Modulates HDL Lipid Composition and Increases the Cholesterol-Accepting Capacity of Serum in Metabolic Syndrome," *Lipids,* June 2013, 48(6):557–67.

19. Y. Rong, L. Chen, T. Zhu, Y. Song, M. Yu, Z. Shan, A. Sands, FB Hu, and L. Liu, "Egg Consumption and Risk of Coronary Heart Disease and Stroke: Dose-Response Meta-Analysis of Prospective Cohort Studies," *BMJ,* January 7, 2013, 346:e8539.

20. CN Blesso, CJ Andersen, J. Barona, JS Volek, and ML Fernandez, "Whole Egg Consumption Improves Lipoprotein Profiles and Insulin Sensitivity to a Greater Extent Than Yolk-Free Egg Substitute in Individuals with Metabolic Syndrome," *Metabolism,* March 2013, 62(3):400–10.

21. LL Smith, "Another Cholesterol Hypothesis: Cholesterol as Antioxidant," *Free Radic. Biol. Med,* 1991, 11(1):47–61.

22. Dr. Ray Peat, "Cholesterol, Longevity, Intelligence, and Health," www.RayPeat.com.

23. Dr. Ray Peat, "Tryptophan, Serotonin, and Aging," www.RayPeat.com.

24. "The Incredible Egg," Egg Nutrition, www.aeb.org/food-manufacturers/egg-nutrition-and-trends/nutrient-composition#5.

25. Leslie M. Fischer, Kerry-Ann da Costa, Lester Kwock, Joseph Galanko, and Steven H, Zeisel, "Dietary Choline Requirements of Women: Effects of Estrogen and Genetic Variation," *American Journal of Clinical Nutrition,* 2010.

26. SH Zeisel and KA da Costa, "Choline: An Essential Nutrient for Public Health," *Nutr Rev*, November 2009, 67(11):615–23.

27. Paraskevi Detopoulou, Demosthenes B. Panagiotakos, Smaragdi Antonopoulou, Christos Pitsavos, and Christodoulos Stefanadis, "Dietary Choline and Betaine Intakes in Relation to Concentrations of Inflammatory Markers in Healthy Adults: The ATTICA Study," American Society for Clinical Nutrition, 2008.

28. "Selenium," National Institute of Health, http://ods.od.nih.gov/factsheets/Selenium-HealthProfessional/.

29. MB Zimmermann and J. Köhrle, "The Impact of Iron and Selenium Deficiencies on Iodine and Thyroid Metabolism: Biochemistry and Relevance to Public Health," *Thyroid*, October 2002, 12(10):867–78.

30. "Beef, Variety Meats and By-Products, Liver, Cooked, Braised," SELF Nutritional Data, http://nutritiondata.self.com/facts/beef-products/3469/2.

31. Anna J. Duffield, Christine D. Thomson, Kristina E. Hill, and Sheila Williams, "An Estimation of Selenium Requirements for New Zealander," American Society for Clinical Nutrition, 1999.

32. "What You Need to Know About Mercury in Fish and Shellfish" (brochure), Food and Drug Administration, March 2004, www.fda.gov/food/resourcesforyou/consumers/ucm110591.htm.

33. L. Penumarthy, Dr. F. W. Oehme, and R.H. Hayes, "Lead, Cadmium, and Mercury Tissue Residues in Healthy Swine, Cattle, Dogs, and Horses from the Midwestern United States," Archives of Environmental Contamination and Toxicology, 1980, Volume 9, Issue 2, pp. 193–206.

34. M. López Alonso, J.L. Benedito, M. Miranda, C. Castillo, J. Hernández, and R.F. Shore, "Mercury Concentrations in Cattle from NW Spain," *Science of The Total Environment,* January 20, 2003, Volume 302, Issues 1–3, pp. 93–100.

35. L.B. Carew, Jr., F.A. Alster, D.C. Foss, and C.G. Scanes, "Effect of a Tryptophan Deficiency on Thyroid Gland, Growth Hormone and Testicular Functions in Chickens," *J. Nutr,* 1983, 113: 1756–1765.

36. Dr. Ray Peat, "Cholesterol, Longevity, Intelligence and Health," www.RayPeat.com.

37. M. Guéguen, JC Amiard, N. Arnich, PM Badot, D. Claisse, T. Guérin, and JP Vernoux, "Shellfish and Residual Chemical Contaminants: Hazards, Monitoring, and Health Risk Assessment Along French Coasts," *Rev Environ Contam Toxicol,* 2011, 213:55–111.

38. Faye M. Dong, "The Nutritional Value of Shellfish," Department of Food Science and Human Nutrition, College of Agricultural, Consumer and Environmental Sciences, University of Illinois, Urbana, Illinois. A Washington Sea Grant publication. 2001

39. Lorraine DiBella, "Is Our Seafood Safe to Eat?" NC State University Seafood Laboratory, http://ncsu.edu/foodscience/extension_program/documents/seafood_is_it_safe_to_eat.pdf.

40. M. Borkman, DJ Chisholm, SM Furler, LH Storlien, EW Kraegen, LA Simons, and CN Chesterman. "Effects of Fish Oil Supplementation on Glucose and Lipid Metabolism in NIDDM," *Diabetes,* October 1989, 38(10):1314–9.

41. NW Istfan and RB Khauli, "Evaluation of the Effect of Fish Oil on Cell Kinetics: Implications for Clinical Immunosuppression," Boston University School of

Medicine, Massachusetts, USA, *Cancer Res,* April 15, 1989, 49(8):1931–6.

42. L. Klieveri, O. Fehres, P. Griffini, CJ Van Noorden, and WM Frederiks, "Promotion of Colon Cancer Metastases in Rat Liver by Fish Oil Diet Is Not Due to Reduced Stroma Formation," *Clin Exp Metastasis,* 2000, 18(5):371–7.

43. Homer Adkins and W.H. Hartung, "Acrolein"," *Org. Synth.; Coll.,* 1941, Vol. 1:15.

44. Dr. Ray Peat, "The Great Fish Oil Experiment," www.RayPeat.com.

45. FDA Letter about EPA and DHA need. Agency Response Letter GRAS Notice No. GRN 000102, CFSAN/Office of Food Additive Safety, September 3, 2002, www.fda.gov/Food/IngredientsPackagingLabeling/GRAS/NoticeInventory/ucm153701.htm.

46. "Serotonin and Endotoxin," East West Healing Interview with Ray Peat. www.eastwesthealing.com

47. Byb. P. Hughes, "The Amino-Acid Composition of Potato Protein and of Cooked Potato," Medical Research Council Department of Experimental Medicine, Universityof Cambridge, September 7, 1957, http://journals.cambridge.org/download.php?file=%2FBJN%2FBJN12_02%2FS0007114558000271a.pdf&code=719bbdcea9569804ae713db408d36660.

48. D. Breese Jones and E.M. Nelson, "Nutritive Value of Potato Protein and of Gelatin," *J Biol. Chem,* 1931, 91:705–713.

49. Stephen Daniells, "Potato Proteins Offer Blood Pressure Benefits. Proteins Isolated from the Humble Potato May Be Biologically Active and Capable of Reducing Blood Pressure,

as well as Having Antioxidant Activity", Finnish Researchers Report. March 12, 2008, www.nutraingredients.com/Research/Potato-proteins-offer-blood-pressure-benefits

50. GA Di Lullo, SM Sweeney, J. Korkko, L. Ala-Kokko, and JD San Antonio, "Mapping the Ligand-Binding Sites and Disease-Associated Mutations on the Most Abundant Protein in the Human, Type I Collagen," *J Biol Chem,* February 8, 2002, 277(6):4223–31.

51. FM Pottenger, "Hydrophilic Colloid Diet, Health and Healing Wisdom," *Price Pottenger Nutrition Foundation Health Journal,* Spring 1997, 21, 1, 17.

52. NR Gotthoffer, *Gelatin in Nutrition and Medicine,* Grayslake, Illinois: Grayslake Gelatin Company, 1945.

53. Kaalya Daniel, "Why Broth Is Beautiful: Essential Roles for Proline, Glycine and Gelatin," *Wise Traditions,* Spring 2003, 25–36.

54. Kaayla T. Daniel, PhD, C.C.N., "Taking Stock: Soup for Healing Body, Mind, Mood, and Soul Soup: The Surprising Secret to Staying Juicy for Life," Naughty Nutrition, February 20, 2012.

55. Frank Petrat, Kerstin Boengler, Rainer Schulz, and Herbert de Groot, "Glycine, a Simple Physiological Compound Protecting by Yet Puzzling Mechanism(s) Against Ischaemia–Reperfusion Injury: Current Knowledge," *Br J Pharmacol,* April 2012, 165(7):2059–2072.

56. "Gelatin Treats Ulcers," [online] Medical News Today. August 22, 2006.

57. Z. Zhong, MD Wheeler, X. Li, M. Froh, P. Schemmer, M. Yin, H. Bunzendaul, B. Bradford, and JJ Lemasters,

"L-Glycine: A Novel Antiinflammatory, Immunomodulatory, and Cytoprotective Agent," *Curr Opin Clin Nutr Metab Care,* March 2003, 6(2):229–40.

58. B. Matilla, JL Mauriz, JM Culebras, J. González-Gallego, and P. González, "Glycine: A Cell-Protecting Anti-Oxidant Nutrient," *Nutr Hosp,* January–February 2002, 17(1):2–9.

59. M. Yin, K. Ikejima, GE Arteel, V. Seabra, BU Bradford, H. Kono, I. Rusyn, and RG Thurman, "Glycine Accelerates Recovery from Alcohol-Induced Liver Injury," *J Pharmacol Exp Ther,* August 1998, 286(2):1014–9.

60. M.L. , J. Madren, H. Bunzendahl, and R.G. Thurman, "Dietary Glycine Inhibits the Growth of B16 Melanoma Tumors in Mice," *Carcinogenesis,* May 1999, Vol. 20, No. 5, pp. 793–798.

61. M. Minuskin, et al., "Nitrogen Retention, Muscle Creatine and Orotic Acid Excretion in Traumatized Rats Fed Argenine and Glycine Enriched Diets," *Journal of Nutrition*, 1981, III, 1265–1274.

62. Jaksic, et al., "Plasma Proline Kinetics and Concentrations in Young Men in Response to Dietary Proline Deprivation," *American Journal of Clinical Nutrition*, 1990, 52, 307–312.

63. A. Cherkin, et al., "L-Proline and Related Compounds: Correlation of Structure, Amnesiac Potency, and Anti-Spreading Depression Potency," *Brain Research*, 1978, 156, 2, 265–273.

64. O. Bruyereand JY Reginster, "Glucosamine and Chondroitin Sulfate as Therapeutic Agents for Knee and Hip Osteoarthritis," *Drugs Aging,* 2007, 24(7):573–80.

65. AD Sawitzke, Helen Shi,Martha F. Finco, Dorothy D. Dunlop. Clifton O. Bingham, Crystal L. Harris, Nora G.

Singer, John D. Bradley, et al., "The Effect of Glucosamine and/or Chondroitin Sulfate on the Progression of Knee Osteoarthritis: A Report from the Glucosamine/Chondroitin Arthritis Intervention Trial," *Arthritis Rheum,* October 2008, 58 (10):3183–91.

67. Ray Peat, PhD, "Gelatin, Stress, Longevity," www.RayPeat.com.

68. "Questions and Answers: NIH Glucosamine/Chondroitin Arthritis Intervention Trial Primary Study," National Center for Complementary and Alternative Medicine, http://nccam.nih.gov/research/results/gait/qa.htm.

Chapter 9

1. A. Aro, et al., Kuopio University, Finland; P. Bougnoux; R. Lavillonniere; and E. Riboli, "Inverse Relation between CLA in Adipose Breast Tissue and Risk of Breast Cancer. A Case-Control Study in France," *Inform,* 1999, 10;5:S43.

2. S.K. Jensen, "Quantitative Secretion and Maximal Secretion Capacity of Retinol, Beta-Carotene and Alpha-Tocopherol into Cows' Milk," *J Dairy Res,* 1999, 66, no. 4: 511–22.

3. T.R. Dhiman, G. R. Anand, et al., "Conjugated Linoleic Acid Content of Milk from Cows Fed Different Diets," *J Dairy Sci,* 1999, 82(10): 2146–56.

4. U. Riserus, P. Arner, et al., "Treatment with Dietary Trans10cis12 Conjugated Linoleic Acid Causes Isomer-Specific Insulin Resistance in Obese Men with the Metabolic Syndrome," *Diabetes Care,* 2002, 25(9): 1516–21.

5. WJ Crinnion, "Organic Foods Contain Higher Levels of Certain Nutrients, Lower Levels of Pesticides, and May

Provide Health Benefits for the Consumer," *Altern Med Rev*, Aprl 2010, 15(1):4–12.

6. E. Palupi, A. Jayanegara, A. Ploeger, and J. Kahl, "Comparison of Nutritional Quality Between Conventional and Organic Dairy Products: A Meta-Analysis," *J Sci Food Agric*, November 2012, 92(14):2774–81.

7. Charles M. Benbrook, Gillian Butler, Maged A. Latif, Carlo Leifert, and Donald R. Davis, "Organic Production Enhances Milk Nutritional Quality by Shifting Fatty Acid Composition: A United States–Wide, 18-Month Study," published online December 9, 2013.

8. JK Lorenzen, SK Jensen, and A. Astrup, "Milk Minerals Modify the Effect of Fat Intake on Serum Lipid Profile: Results from an Animal and a Human Short-Term Study" *Br J Nutr*, November 25, 2013, 1–9.

9. FI Arnaldezand LJ Helman, "Targeting the Insulin Growth Factor Receptor 1, " *Hematol. Oncol. Clin. North Am.*, June 2012, 26 (3): 527–42, vii–viii.

10. SS Epstein, "Unlabeled Milk from Cows Treated with Biosynthetic Growth Hormones: A Case of Regulatory Abdication," *Int J Health Serv.*, 1996, 26(1):173–85.

11. J. Guevara-Aguirre, P. Balasubramanian, M. Guevara-Aguirre, M. Wei, F. Madia, CW Cheng, D. Hwang, A. Martin-Montalvo, J. Saavedra, S. Ingles, R. de Cabo, P. Cohen, and VD Longo, "Growth Hormone Receptor Deficiency Is Associated with a Major Reduction in Pro-Aging Signaling, Cancer, and Diabetes in Humans, " *Sci Transl Med*, February 2011, 3 (70):70ra13.

12. Helena Lindmark Månsson,"Fatty Acids in Bovine Milk Fat," *Food Nutr Res*, 2008; 52: 10.3402/fnr.v52i0.1821.

13. RJ van Neerven, EF Knol, JM Heck, and HF Savelkoul, "Which Factors in Raw Cow's Milk Contribute to Protection Against Allergies?" *J Allergy Clin Immunol,* October 2012, 130(4):853–8.

14. ME Mangino and JR Brunner, "Homogenized Milk: Is it Really the Culprit in Dietary-Induced Atherosclerosis?" *J Dairy Sci,* August 1976, 59(8):1511–2.

15. A. Zamora, AJ Trujillo, E. Armaforte, DS Waldron, and AL Kelly, "Effect of Fat Content and Homogenization Under Conventional or Ultra-High-Pressure Conditions on Interactions Between Proteins in Rennet Curds," *J Dairy Sci,* September 2012, 95(9):4796–803.

16. AA Tribst, PE Augusto, and M. Cristianini, "The Effect of High Pressure Homogenization on the Activity of a Commercial β-galactosidase," *J Ind Microbiol Biotechnol,* November 2012, 39(11):1587–96.

17. MA Augustin and P. Udabage, "Influence of Processing on Functionality of Milk and Dairy Proteins," *Adv Food Nutr Res.,* 2007, 53:1–38.

18. MB Let, C. Jacobsen, AD Sørensen, and AS Meyer, "Homogenization Conditions Affect the Oxidative Stability of Fish Oil Enriched Milk Emulsions: Lipid Oxidation," *J Agric Food Chem.,* March 7, 2007, 55(5):1773–80.

19. TR Neyestani, M. Hajifaraji, N. Omidvar, B. Nikooyeh, MR Eshraghian, N. Shariatzadeh, A. Kalayi, N. Khalaji, M. Zahedirad, M. Abtahi, and S. Asadzadeh, "Calcium-Vitamin D-Fortified Milk Is as Effective on Circulating Bone Biomarkers as Fortified Juice and Supplement but Has Less Acceptance: A Randomised Controlled School-Based Trial," *J Hum Nutr Diet,* November 25, 2013. doi: 10.1111/jhn.12191.

20. KJ Murphy, GE Crichton, KA Dyer, AM Coates, TL Pettman, C. Milte, AA Thorp, NM Berry, JD Buckley, M. Noakes, and PR Howe, "Dairy Foods and Dairy Protein Consumption Is Inversely Related to Markers of Adiposity in Obese Men and Women," *Nutrients,* November 20, 2013, 5(11):4665–84.

21. LC Muniz, SW Madruga, and CL Araújo, "Consumption of Dairy Products by Adults and the Elderly in the South of Brazil: A Population-Based Study," *Cien Saude Colet,* December 2013, 18(12):3515–22.

22. PJ Huth and KM Park, "Influence of Dairy Product and Milk Fat Consumption on Cardiovascular Disease Risk: A Review of the Evidence," *Adv Nutr,* May 1, 2012, 3(3):266–85.

23. DI Givens, "Milk in the Diet: Good or Bad for Vascular Disease?" *Proc Nutr Soc.,* February 2012, 71(1):98–104.

24. KM Livingstone, JA Lovegrove, JR Cockcroft, PC Elwood, JE Pickering, and DI Givens, "Does Dairy Food Intake Predict Arterial Stiffness and Blood Pressure in Men?: Evidence from the Caerphilly Prospective Study," *Hypertension,* January 2013, 61(1):42–7.

25. SA de Albuquerque Fernandes, AP Magnavita, SP Ferrao, SA Gualberto, AS Faleiro, AJ Figueiredo, and SV Matarazzo, "Daily Ingestion of Tetracycline Residue Present in Pasteurized Milk: A Public Health Problem," *Environ Sci Pollut Res Int.,* November 17, 2013.

26. F. Fumeron, A. Lamri, N. Emery, N. Bellili, R. Jaziri, I. Porchay-Baldérelli, O. Lantieri, B. Balkau, and M. Marre; DESIR Study Group, "Dairy Products and the Metabolic Syndrome in a Prospective Study, DESIR." *J Am Coll Nutr,* October 2011, 30.

27. F. Fumeron, A. Lamri, C. Abi Khalil, R. Jaziri, I. Porchay-Baldérelli, O. Lantieri, S. Vol, . Balkau, and M. Marre, "Dairy Consumption and the Incidence of Hyperglycemia and the Metabolic Syndrome: Results from a French Prospective Study, Data from the Epidemiological Study on the Insulin Resistance Syndrome (DESIR), *Diabetes Care,* April 2011, 34(4):813–7.

28. P. Drouillet, B. Balkau, MA Charles, S. Vol, M. Bedouet, P. Ducimetière; DESIR Study Group, "Calcium Consumption and Insulin Resistance Syndrome Parameters. Data from the Epidemiological Study on the Insulin Resistance Syndrome (DESIR)," *Nutr Metab Cardiovasc Dis,* September 2007, 17(7):486–92.

29. CM Benbrook, G. Butler, MA Latif, C. Leifert, and DR Davis, "Organic Production Enhances Milk Nutritional Quality by Shifting Fatty Acid Composition: A United States-Wide, 18-Month Study." *PLoS One.* 2013 Dec 9;8(12)

30. Y. Kim, OJ Kelly, and JZ Ilich, "Synergism of α-linolenic Acid, Conjugated Linoleic Acid and Calcium in Decreasing Adipocyte and Increasing Osteoblast Cell Growth," *Lipids,* August 2013, 48(8):787–802.

31. G. Zurera-Cosano, R. Moreno-Rejas, and M. Amaro-Lopez, "Effects of Processing on Contents and Relationship of Mineral Elements of Milk," *Food Chemistry,* 1994, V51, Issue 1, pp. 75–78.

32. HM Said, DE Ong, and JL Shingleton, "Intestinal Uptake of Retinol: Enhancement by Bovine Milk Beta-Lactoglobulin," The American Society for Clinical Nutrition, Inc., 1989.

33. CDC, www.CDC.gov/foodsafety/rawmilk/raw-milk-questions-and-answers.html#benefits.

34. Ted Beals, MS, MD, "Pilot Survey of Cow Share Consumer/Owners Lactose Intolerance Section," February 2014. http://www.realmilk.com/health/lactose-intolerance-survey/

35. K. Rahmani, A. Djazayery, MI Habibi, H. Heidari, AR Dorosti-Motlagh, M. Pourshahriari, and L. Azadbakht, "Effects of Daily Milk Supplementation on Improving the Physical and Mental Function as well as School Performance Among Children: Results from a School Feeding Program," *J Res Med Sci,* April 2011 , 16(4):469–76.

36. L. Paajanen, T. Tuure, T. Poussa, and R. Korpela, "No Difference in Symptoms During Challenges with Homogenized and Unhomogenized Cow's Milk in Subjects with Subjective Hypersensitivity to Homogenized Milk," *J Dairy Res,* May 2003, 70(2):175–9.

37. RW Hubbard, Y. Ono, and A. Sanchez, "Atherogenic Effect of Oxidized Products of Cholesterol," *Prog Food Nutr Sci,* 1989, 13(1):17–44.

38. RM Bostick, JD Potter, TA Sellers, DR McKenzie, LH Kushi, and AR Folsom, "Relation of Calcium, Vitamin D, and Dairy Food Intake to Incidence of Colon Cancer Among Older Women. The Iowa Women's Health Study," *Am J Epidemiol,* June 15, 1993, 137(12):1302–17.

39. CE Dugan, J. Barona, and ML Fernandez, "Increased Dairy Consumption Differentially Improves Metabolic Syndrome Markers in Male and Female Adults," *Metab Syndr Relat Disord,* November 15 2013.

40. SJ Park, SE Joo, H. Min, JK Park, Y. Kim, SS Kim, and Y. Ahn, "Dietary Patterns and Osteoporosis Risk in Postmenopausal Korean Women," *Osong Public Health Res Perspect,* December 2012, 3(4):199–205.

41. H. Shin, YS Yoon, Y. Lee, CI Kim, and SW Oh., "Dairy Product Intake Is Inversely Associated with Metabolic Syndrome in Korean Adults: Anseong and Ansan Cohort of the Korean Genome and Epidemiology Study," *J Korean Med Sci,* October 2013, 28(10):1482–8.

42. S. Naik, V. Bhide, A. Babhulkar, N. Mahalle, S. Parab, R. Thakre, and M. Kulkarni, "Daily Milk Intake Improves Vitamin B-12 Status in Young Vegetarian Indians: An Intervention Trial." Nutr J, October 9, 2013, 12(1):136.

43. RK Bailey, CP Fileti, J. Keith, S. Tropez-Sims, W. Price, and SD Allison-Ottey, "Lactose Intolerance and Health Disparities Among African Americans and Hispanic Americans: An Updated Consensus Statement," *J Natl Med Assoc,* Summer 2013, 105(2):112–27.

44. BA Pribila, SR Hertzler, BR Martin, CM Weaver, and DA Savaiano, "Improved Lactose Digestion and Intolerance Among African-American Adolescent Girls Fed a Dairy-Rich Diet," *J Am Diet Assoc,* May 2000, 100(5):524–8.

45. Andrew Curry, "Archaeology: The Milk Revolution: When a Single Genetic Mutation First Let Ancient Europeans Drink Milk, it Set the Stage for a Continental Upheaval," July 31, 2013.

46. N. Murphy, T. Norat, P. Ferrari, M. Jenab, B. Bueno-de-Mesquita, G. Skeie, A. Olsen, A. Tjønneland, CC Dahm, K. Overvad, MC Boutron-Ruault, F. Clavel-Chapelon, L. Nailler, R. Kaaks, B. Teucher, H. Boeing, MM Bergmann, A. Trichopoulou, P. Lagiou, D. Trichopoulos, D. Palli, V. Pala, R. Tumino, P. Vineis, S. Panico, PH Peeters, VK Dik, E. Weiderpass, E. Lund, JR Garcia, R. Zamora-Ros, MJ Pérez, M. Dorronsoro, C. Navarro, E. Ardanaz, J. Manjer, M. Almquist, I. Johansson, R. Palmqvist, KT Khaw, N. Wareham, TJ Key, FL Crowe, V. Fedirko, MJ Gunter, and

E. Riboli, "Consumption of Dairy Products and Colorectal Cancer in the European Prospective Investigation into Cancer and Nutrition (EPIC)," PLoS One, September 2, 2013, 8(9):e72715.

47. KD Ballard, E. Mah, Y. Guo, R. Pei, JS Volek, and RS Bruno, "Low-Fat Milk Ingestion Prevents Postprandial Hyperglycemia-Mediated Impairments in Vascular Endothelial Function in Obese Individuals with Metabolic Syndrome," *J Nutr,* October 2013, 143(10):1602–10.

48. SH Kim, WK Kim, and MH Kang, "Effect of Milk and Milk Products Consumption on Physical Growth and Bone Mineral Density in Korean Adolescents," *Nutr Res Pract,* August 2013,7(4):309–14.

49. T. Eysteinsdottir, TI Halldorsson, I. Thorsdottir, G. Sigurdsson, S. Sigurðsson, T. Harris, LJ Launer, V. Gudnason, I. Gunnarsdottir, and L. Steingrimsdottir, "Milk Consumption Throughout Life and Bone Mineral Content and Density in Elderly Men and Women," *Osteoporos Int.,* August 16, 2013.

50. MS Calvo and YK Park, "Changing Phosphorus Content of the U.S. Diet: Potential for Adverse Effects on Bone," *J Nutr,* 1996, 126(4 Suppl):1168S–1180S.

51. MS Calvo, "The Effects of High Phosphorus Intake on Calcium Homeostasis," *Adv Nutr Res,* 1994, 9:183–207.

52. MS Calvo, "Dietary Phosphorus, Calcium Metabolism and Bone," *J Nutr,* September 1993, 123(9):1627–33.

53. M. Koshihara, R. Masuyama, M. Uehara, and K. Suzuki, "Effect of Dietary Calcium:Phosphorus Ratio on Bone Mineralization and Intestinal Calcium Absorption in Ovariectomized Rats," *Biofactors,* 2004, 22(1–4):39–42.

54. S. Radavelli-Bagatini, K. Zhu, JR Lewis, SS Dhaliwal, and RL Prince, "Association of Dairy Intake with Body Composition and Physical Function in Older Community-Dwelling Women," *J Acad Nutr Diet,* December 2013, 113(12):1669–74.

55. BH Rice, EE Quann, and GD Miller, "Meeting and Exceeding Dairy Recommendations: Effects of Dairy Consumption on Nutrient Intakes and Risk of Chronic Disease," *Nutr Rev,* April 2013, 71(4):209–23. doi: 10.1111/nure.12007. Epub January 30, 2013.

56. T. Fujita, "Calcium, Parathyroids and Aging," *Contrib Nephrol,* 1991, 90:206–11.

57. DA McCarron, CD Morris, and R. Bukoski, "The Calcium Paradox of Essential Hypertension,"*Am J Med,* January 26, 1987, 82(1B):27–33.

58. KF Hilpert, SG West, DM Bagshaw, V. Fishell, L. Barnhart, M. Lefevre, MM Most, MB Zemel, M. Chow, AL Hinderliter, and PM Kris-Etherton, "Effects of Dairy Products on Intracellular Calcium and Blood Pressure in Adults with Essential Hypertension," *J Am Coll Nutr,* April 2009, 28(2):142–9.

59. S. Bel-Serrat, T. Mouratidou, D. Jiménez-Pavón, I. Huybrechts, M. Cuenca-García, L. Mistura, F. Gottrand, M. González-Gross, J. Dallongeville, A. Kafatos, Y. Manios, P. Stehle, M. Kersting, S. De Henauw, M. Castillo, L. Hallstrom, D. Molnár, K. Widhalm, A. Marcos, and L. Moreno; HELENA study group, "Is Dairy Consumption Associated with Low Cardiovascular Disease Risk in European Adolescents? Results from the HELENA Study," *Pediatr Obes,* July 15, 2013.

60. MP Villeneuve, Y. Lebeuf, R. Gervais, GF Tremblay, JC Vuillemard, J. Fortin, and PY Chouinard, "Milk Volatile Organic Compounds and Fatty Acid Profile in Cows Fed Timothy as Hay, Pasture, or Silage," *J Dairy Sci,* November 2013, 96(11):7181–94.

61. Lisa Ferguson-Stegall, Erin McCleave, Phillip G. Doerner, Zhenping Ding, Benjamin Dessard, Lynne Kammer, Bei Wang, Yang Liu, and John L. Ivy, FACSM, "Effects of Chocolate Milk Supplementation on Recovery from Cycling Exercise and Subsequent Time Trial Performance." Exercise Physiology and Metabolism Laboratory, Department of Kinesiology, University of Texas at Austin.

62. Jason R. Karp, Jeanne D. Johnston, Sandra Tecklenburg, Timothy D. Mickleborough, Alyce D. Fly, and Joel M. Stager, "Chocolate Milk as a Post-Exercise Recovery Aid," *International Journal of Sport Nutrition and Exercise Metabolism*, 2006, 16, 78–91.

63. S. Mahé, P. Marteau, JF Huneau, F. Thuillier, and D. Tomé, "Intestinal Nitrogen and Electrolyte Movements Following Fermented Milk Ingestion in Man," *Br J Nutr,* February 1994, 71(2):169–80.

64. L. Ebringer, M. Ferencík, and J. Krajcovic, "Beneficial Health Effects of Milk and Fermented Dairy Products—Review," *Folia Microbiol* (Praha), 2008, 53(5):378–94.

65. A. Haug, OA Christophersen, AT Høstmark, and OM Harstad, "Milk and Health," *Tidsskr Nor Laegeforen,* October 4, 2007, 127(19):2542–5.

66. MH Shin, MD Holmes, SE Hankinson, K. Wu, GA Colditz, and WC Willett, "Intake of Dairy Products, Calcium, and Vitamin D and Risk of Breast Cancer," *J Natl Cancer Inst,* September 4, 2002, 94(17):1301–11.

67. MA Rakib, WS Lee, GS Kim, JH Han, JO Kim, and YL Ha, "Antiproliferative Action of Conjugated Linoleic Acid on Human MCF-7 Breast Cancer Cells Mediated by Enhancement of Gap Junctional Intercellular Communication Through Inactivation of NF- κ B," *Evid Based Complement Alternat Med*, November 25, 2013.

68. Dr. Ray Peat, "Milk in Context: Allergies, Ecology, and Some Myths." www.raypeat.com

69. Dr. Ray Peat, "Calcium and Disease: Hypertension, Organ Calcification, & Shock, vs. Respiratory Energy." www.raypeat.com

70. Josh Rubin, "The Metabolic Blueprint," www.EastWestHealing.com.

71. Weston A. Price, "Nutrition and Physical Degeneration." Published by The Price-Pottinenger Nutrition Foundation Inc. 2009.

72. www.WorldLifeExpectancy.com/cause-of-death/coronary-heart-disease/by-country/.

73. "Current Worldwide Total Milk Consumption per Capita," http://chartsbin.com/view/1491.

74. Danny Roddy, "The Peat Whisperer," www.DannyRoddy.com.

75. Sara Holmberg, Anders Thelin, and Eva-Lena Stiernström, "Food Choices and Coronary Heart Disease: A Population Based Cohort Study of Rural Swedish Men with 12 Years of Follow-up," *Int. J. Environ. Res. Public Health*, 2009, 6, pp. 2626–2638.

Chapter 10

1. W. W. Campbell and M. Tang. "Protein Intake, Weight Loss, and Bone Mineral Density in Postmenopausal Women," *The Journals of Gerontology Series A: Biological Sciences and Medical Sciences,* 2010.

2. Dr. Colin Campbell and Thomas M. Campbell, *The China Study,* Benbella Books, 2006.

3. Dr. Loren Cordain, *The Paleo Diet,* John Wiley and Sons, 2002.

4. Cordain, Loren, and T. Colin Campbell, "The Protein Debate," *Performance Menu: Journal of Nutrition & Athletic Excellence,* 2008, accessed August 28, 2011.

5. Sally Fallon Morell and Mary Enig, *Australian Aborigines: Living Off the Fat of the Land,* Weston A Price Foundation, 2000.

6. Cynthia A. Daley, Amber Abbott, Patrick S. Doyle, Glenn A. Nader, and Stephanie Larson, "A Review of Fatty Acid Profiles and Antioxidant Content in Grass-Fed and Grain-Fed Beef," *Nutrition Journal,* 2010.

7. H.K. Biesalski, "Meat as a Component of a Healthy Diet: Are There Any Risks or Benefits if Meat Is Avoided in the Diet?" *Meat Science,* July 2005, Volume 7, Issue 3, pp. 509–524.

8. P.T. Garcia, N.A. Pensel, A.M. Sancho, N.J. Latimori, A.M. Kloster, M.A. Amigone, and J.J. Castol "Beef Lipids in Relation to Animal Breed and Nutrition in Argentina," *Meat Science,* Volume 79, Issue 3, Pages 500–508.

9. JM Leheska, LD Thompson, JC Howe, e. Hentges, J. Boyce, JC Brooks, B. Shriver, L. Hoover, and MF Miller, "Effects of Conventional and Grass-Feeding Systems on the Nutrient

Composition of Beef," *Journal Animal Science,* 2008, 86:3575–85.

10. "Foods High in Tryptophan," http://NutritionData.self.com/foods-000079000000000000000-20.html?

11. MS Calvo and YK Park, "Changing Phosphorus Content of the U.S. Diet: Potential for Adverse Effects on Bone," *J Nutr,* 1996;126(4 Suppl):1168S–-1180S.

12. MS Calvo, "The Effects of High Phosphorus Intake on Calcium Homeostasis," *Adv Nutr Res,* 1994;9:183–207.

13. MS Calvo, "Dietary Phosphorus, Calcium Metabolism and Bone," *J Nutr,* September 1993, 123(9):1627–33.

14. M. Koshihara, R. Masuyama, M. Uehara, and K. Suzuki, "Effect of Dietary Calcium:Phosphorus Ratio on Bone Mineralization and Intestinal Calcium Absorption in Ovariectomized Rats," *Biofactors,* 2004, 22(1-4):39–42.

15. Danny Roddy, "Ray Peat's Brain: Building a Foundation for Better Understanding," www.DannyRoddy.com/main/2011/12/29/ray-peats-brain-building-a-foundation-for-better-understandi.html.

16. Ray Peat, PhD, "Gelatin, Stress, Longevity," www.RayPeat.com.

17. Ray Peat, PhD, "Tryptophan, Serotonin, and Aging," www.RayPeat.com.

Chapter 11

1. Rita Yaacoub, Rachad Saliba, Bilal Nsouli, Gaby Khalaf, and Inès Birlouez-Aragon, "Formation of Lipid Oxidation and Isomerization Products During Processing of Nuts and

Sesame Seeds," *J. Agric. Food Chem.,* 2008, 56 (16):7082–7090.

2. Thomas Richardson and John W. Finley, "Chemical Changes in Food During Processing", pp. 206–209.

3. E. Pelvan, C. Alasalvar, and SJ Uzman, "Agric. Effects of Roasting on the Antioxidant Status and Phenolic Profiles of Commercial Turkish Hazelnut Varieties," *Food Chem,* February 8, 2012, 60(5):1218–23. Epub January 27, 2012.

4. "The Why, How and Consequences of Cooking Our Food" EUFIC review, November 2010. [online] http://www.eufic.org/article/en/expid/cooking-review-eufic/

5. T. Bohn, L. Davidsson, T. Walczyk, and RF Hurrell, "Phytic Acid Added to White-Wheat Bread Inhibits Fractional Apparent Magnesium Absorption in Humans," *The American Journal of Clinical Nutrition,* 2004, 79(3):418–423.

6. SEO Mahgoub and SA Elhag, "Effect of Milling, Soaking, Malting, Heat-Treatment and Fermentation on Phytate Level of Four Sudanese Sorghum Cultivars" *Food Chemistry,* 1998, 61(1–2):77–80.

7. BJ Macfarlane, WR Bezwoda, TH Bothwell, RD Baynes, JE Bothwell, AP MacPhail, RD Lamparelli, and F. Mayet, "Inhibitory Effect of Nuts on Iron Absorption," *The American Journal of Clinical Nutrition,* 1988, 47:270–274.

8. Fanbin Kong and R. Paul Singh, "Digestion of Raw and Roasted Almonds in Simulated Gastric Environment," *Food Biophys,* December 2009, 4(4): 365–377.

9. P. Pandey, RB Raizada, and LP Srivastava, "Level of Organochlorine Pesticide Residues in Dry Fruit Nuts," *J Environ Biol,* September 2010, 31(5):705–7.

10. Ricardo Bessin, Gerald R. Brown, John R. Hartman, and James R. Martin, "Food Safety: Pesticide Residues in Grains, Vegetables, Fruits, and Nuts," Issued 7-90, www.ca.uky.edu/agc/pubs/ip/ip9/ip9.htm.

11. JP Allard, R. Kurian, E. Aghdassi, R. Muggli, and D. Royall, "Lipid Peroxidation During n-3 Fatty Acid and Vitamin E Supplementation in Humans," *Lipids,* May 1997, 32(5):535–41.

12. M. Meydani, F. Natiello, B. Goldin, N. Free, M. Woods, E. Schaefer, JB Blumberg, and SL Gorbach, "Effect of Long-Term Fish Oil Supplementation on Vitamin E Status and Lipid Peroxidation in Women," *J Nutr,* April 1991, 121(4):484–91.

13. MJ Gonzalez, JI Gray, RA Schemmel, L. Dugan Jr., and CW Welsch, "Lipid Peroxidation Products Are Elevated in Fish Oil Diets Even in the Presence of Added Antioxidants," *J Nutr,* November 1992, 122(11):2190–5.

14. KM Humphries, Y. Yoo, and LI Szweda, "Inhibition of NADH-lLinked Mitochondrial Respiration by 4-hydroxy-2-nonenal," *Biochemistry,* January 13, 1998, 37(2):552–7.

15. "Nuts, Grains & Seeds Chart," Dr. Decuypere's Nutrient Charts™. www.health-alternatives.com/nut-seed-nutrition-chart.html.

16. Dr. Ray Peat, "Unsaturated Vegetable Oils: Toxic," www.RayPeat.com.

17. Fritz Geiser, "Metabolic Rate and Body Temperature Reduction During Hibernation and Daily Torpor," *Annu. Rev. Physiol,* 2004, (66): 239–274.

18. Ray Peat, PhD, "Thyroid, Insomnia, and the Insanities: Commonalities in Disease." www.RayPeat.com.

19. Emilio Ros, "Health Benefits of Nut Consumption," *Nutrients,* July 2010, 2(7):652–682.

20. Loren Cordain, L. Toohey, M.J. Smith, and M.S. Hickey, "Modulation of Immune Function by Dietary Lectins in Rheumatoid Arthritis," Department of Health and Exercise Science, Colorado State University, Fort Collins, Colorado.

21. K. Miyake, T. Tanaka, PL McNeil, "Lectin-Based Food Poisoning: A New Mechanism of Protein Toxicity," In Steinhardt, Richard, PLoS ONE, 2007, 2(1): e687.

22. Pragya Pandey, R.B. Raizada, and L.P. Srivastava, "Level of Organochlorine Pesticide Residues in Dry Fruit Nuts," Pesticide Toxicology Laboratory, Indian Institute of Toxicology Research, India.

23. "Nuts", *Websters Dictionary.*

24. "Seeds", *Websters Dictionary.*

25. A. Wakatsuki, N. Ikenoue, and Y. Sagara, "Estrogen-Induced Small Low-Density Lipoprotein Particles in Postmenopausal Women," *Obstet Gynecol,* February 1998, 91(2):234–40.

26. FJ Kok, G. van Poppel, J. Melse, E. Verheul, EG Schouten, DH Kruyssen, and A. Hofman, "Do Antioxidants and Polyunsaturated Fatty Acids Have a Combined Association with Coronary Atherosclerosis?" *Atherosclerosis,* January 1991, 86(1):85–90.

27. Weiwen Chai and Michael Liebman, "Oxalate Content of Legumes, Nuts, and Grain-Based Flours," *Journal of Food Composition and Analysis,* 2005, 18:723–729.

28. *Manual of Clinical Dietetics,* Chicago Dietetic Association, Chicago, Illinois: American Dietetic Association, 2000, p. 475.

29. LJ Brinkley, J. Gregory, and CY Pak, "A Further Study of Oxalate Bioavailability in Foods," *J Urol.,* July 1990, 144(1):94–6.

Chapter 12

1. Dr. Kaayla Daniel, PhD, "The Whole Soy Story." NewTrends Publishing, Inc. 2005.

2. Alicia A. Thorp, Peter RC Howe, Trevor A. Mori, Alison M. Coates, Jonathan D. Buckley, Jonathan Hodgson, Jackie Mansour, and Barbara J. Meyer, "Soy Food Consumption Does Not Lower LDL Cholesterol in Either Equol or Nonequol Producers," American Society for Clinical Nutrition, 2008.

3. Aaron J. Michelfelder, MD, "Soy: A Complete Source of Protein," Loyola University Chicago Stritch School of Medicine, Maywood, Illinois, *Am Fam Physician,* January 1, 2009, 79(1):43–47.

4. FM Sacks, A. Lichtenstein, L. Van Horn, W. Harris, P. Kris-Etherton, and M. Winston, "Soy Protein, Isoflavones, and Cardiovascular Health: An American Heart Association Science Advisory for Professionals from the Nutrition Committee," American Heart Association Nutrition Committee, February 21, 2006, 113(7):1034–44. Epub January 17, 2006.

5. J. Vanderpas, "Nutritional Epidemiology and Thyroid Hormone Metabolism," *Annu. Rev. Nutr,* 2006, 26:293–322. doi:10.1146/annurev.nutr.26.010506.103810. PMID 16704348.

6. RL Divi, HC Chang, and DR Doerge, "Anti-Thyroid Isoflavones from Soybean: Isolation, Characterization, and

Mechanisms of Action," *Biochem Pharmacol.,* November 15, 1997, 54(10):1087–96.

7. Dr. Ray Peat, "Natural Estrogen," www.RayPeat.com.

8. D. Ingram, "Phytoestrogens and Their Role in Breast Cancer," *Lancet,* 1997, 350:990–994; *Breast NEWS: Newsletter of the NHMRC National Breast Cancer Centre,* Winter 1997, Vol. 3, No. 2.

9. Van Rensburg, et al., "Nutritional Status of African Populations Predisposed to Esophageal Cancer," *Nutrition and Cancer,* 1983, vol. 4, pp. 206–216.

10. P.B. Moser, et al., "Copper, Iron, Zinc and Selenium Dietary Intake and Status of Nepalese Lactating Women and Their Breastfed infants," *American Journal of Clinical Nutrition,* April 1988, 47:729–734.

11. B.F. Harland et al., "Nutritional Status and Phytate: Zinc and Phytate X Calcium: Zinc Dietary Molar Ratios of Lacto-Ovovegetarian Trappist Monks: 10 Years Later," *Journal of the American Dietetic Association,* December 1988, 88:1562–1566.

12. A.H. Tiney, "Proximate Composition and Mineral and Phytate Contents of Legumes Grown in Sudan," *Journal of Food Composition and Analysis,* 1989, 2:6778.

13. RF Hurrell, "Influence of Vegetable Protein Sources on Trace Element and Mineral Bioavailability," *The Journal of Nutrition,* September 2003, 133(9):2973S–7S.

14. B. Lönnerdal, "Dietary Factors Influencing Zinc Absorption," Department of Nutrition, University of California at Davis, *J Nutr,* May 2000, 130(5S Suppl):1378S–83S.

15. http://www.soyconnection.com/sites/default/files/Consumer%20Attitudes_Med_062714.pdf

16. AL Tan-Wilson and KA Wilson, "Relevance of Multiple Soybean Trypsin Inhibitor Forms to Nutritional Quality," *Adv Exp Med Biol.,* 1986, 199:391–411.

17. www.westonaprice.org/soy-alert/ploy-of-soy.

18. "Risks and Benefits of Estrogen Plus Progestin in Healthy Postmenopausal Women. Principal Results From the Women's Health Initiative Randomized Controlled Trial," *FJAMA,* July 2002, 288(3):321–333.

19. "Questions and Answer Regarding the Women's Health Initiative on Hormonal Therapy Trials," www.nhlbi.nih.gov/whi/whi_faq.htm.

20. "Soybean and Oil Crops," USDA Economic Research Service, www.ers.usda.gov/topics/crops/soybeans-oil-crops/related-data-statistics.aspx#.UoQFhxbvzEY.

21. G. Ma, Y. Li, Y. Jin, F. Zhai, FJ Kok, and X. Yang, "Phytate Intake and Molar Ratios of Phytate to Zinc, Iron and Calcium in the Diets of People in China," *Eur J Clin Nutr.,* March 2007, 61(3):368–74. Epub August 23, 2006.

22. Institute of Responsible Technology, www.responsibletechnology.org/health-risks#32.

23. Chris Masterjohn, "Thyroid Toxins: The Double-Edged Swords of the Kingdom *Plantae,"* Cholesterol-And-Health. Com Special Reports, Volume 1, Issue 1.

24. Julia R. Barrett, "The Science of Soy: What Do We Really Know?" *Environ Health Perspect,* June 2006, 114(6):A352–A358.

25. "Food Labeling: Health Claims; Soy Protein and Coronary Heart Disease. Food and Drug Administration, HHS. Final Rule," *Fed Regist,* 1999, 64:57700–33.

26. JM Hodgson, IB Puddey, LJ Beilin, TA Mori, and KD Croft, "Supplementation with Isoflavonoid Phytoestrogens Does Not Alter Serum Lipid Concentrations: A Randomized Controlled Trial in Humans," *J Nutr,* 1998, 128:728–32.

27. WL Hall, K. Vafeiadou, J. Hallund, et al., "Soy-Isoflavone-Enriched Foods and Markers of Lipid and Glucose Metabolism in Postmenopausal Women: Interactions with Genotype and Equol Production," *American Journal of Clinical Nutrition,* 2006, 83:592–600.

28. BJ Meyer, TA Larkin, AJ Owen, LB Astheimer, LC Tapsell, and PR Howe, "Limited Lipid-Lowering Effects of Regular Consumption of Whole Soybean Foods," *Ann Nutr Metab,* 2004, 48:67–78.

29. NR Matthan, SM Jalbert, LM Ausman, JT Kuvin, RH Karas, and AH Lichtenstein, "Effect of Soy Protein from Differently Processed Products on Cardiovascular Disease Risk Factors and Vascular Endothelial Function in Hypercholesterolemic Subjects," *American Journal of Clinical Nutrition,* 2007, 85:960–6.

30. Stephan Sinatra and Jonny Bowden, "The Great Cholesterol Myth." Fair Winds Press. 2012.

31. Uffe Ravnskov, "Ignore the Awkward! How the Cholesterol Myths Are Kept Alive." Self Published. 2010.

32. Dr. Ray Peat, "Cholesterol, Longevity, Intelligence and Health," www.RayPeat.com.

33. Dr. Dwight Lundell, "The Great Cholesterol Lie."

34. Y. Birk, "Protein Proteinase Inhibitors in Legume Seeds—Overview," *Arch Latinoam Nutr.,* December 1996, 44(4 Suppl 1):26S–30S.

35. FM Lajolo and MI Genovese, "Nutritional Significance of Lectins and Enzyme Inhibitors from Legumes," *J Agric Food Chem,* October 23, 2002, 50(22):6592–8.

36. GS Gilani, KA Cockell, and E. Sepehr, "Effects of Antinutritional Factors on Protein Digestibility and Amino Acid Availability in Foods," *J AOAC Int.,* May–June 2005, 88(3):967–87.

37. hulam Sarwar, "The Protein Digestibility Corrected Amino Acid Score Method Overestimates Quality of Proteins Containing Anti-nutritional Factors and of Poorly Digestible Proteins Supplemented with Limiting Amino Acids in Rats," American Society for Nutritional Sciences, *The Journal of Nutrition,* 1997.

38. Gertjan Schaafsma. "The Protein Digestibility–Corrected Amino Acid Score[1]," The American Society for Nutritional Sciences, *The Journal of Nutrition,* 2000.

39. "Protein Digestibility Corrected Amino Acid Score (PDCAAS)", Wikipedia

40. Journal of Food Composition and Analysis 18 (2005) 723–729. www.elsevier.com/locate/jfca

41. Weiwen Chai and Michael Liebman, "Short Communication: Oxalate Content of Legumes, Nuts, and Grain-Based Flours," Department of Family and Consumer Sciences (Human Nutrition), University of Wyoming, University Station, Wyoming.

42. "Phytic Acid: Tips for the Consumers From Food Science," www.phyticacid.org/soaking-beans/.

Chapter 13

1. Ghulam Sarwar, "The Protein Digestibility–Corrected Amino Acid Score Method Overestimates Quality of Proteins Containing Antinutritional Factors and of Poorly Digestible Proteins Supplemented with Limiting Amino Acids in Rats," *The Journal of Nutrition.* May 1, 1997 vol. 127 no. 5 758-764

2. Yvette C. Luiking, Nicolaas E.P. Deutz[3], Martin Jäkel, and Peter B. Soeters, "Casein and Soy Protein Meals Differentially Affect Whole-Body and Splanchnic Protein Metabolism in Healthy Humans," The American Society for Nutritional Sciences, 2005.

3. JM Bell and PK Lundberg, "Effects of a Commercial Soy Lecithin Preparation on Development of Sensorimotor Behavior and Brain Biochemistry in the Rat," *Dev Psychobiol,* January 1985, 18(1):59–66.

4. "Soybeans and Soy Lecithin," University of Nebraska-Lincoln (UNL), accessed March 14, 2013, http://farrp.unl.edu/resources/gi-fas/opinion-and-summaries/soy-lecithin.

5. E. Reverchon, M. Poletto, L. Sesti Osséo, and M. Somma, "Hexane Elimination from Soybean Oil by Continuous Packed Tower Processing with Supercritical CO2," *Journal of the American Oil Chemists' Society,* 2000, Volume 77, Issue 1, pp. 9–14.

6. Stephen R. Clough and Leyna Mulholland, ""Hexane," *Encyclopedia of Toxicology 2* (2nd ed.), Elsevier, 2005, pp. 522–525.

7. BA Magnuson, GA Burdock, J. Doull, RM Kroes, GM Marsh, MW Pariza, PS Spencer, WJ Waddell, R. Walker, and GM Williams, "Aspartame: A Safety Evaluation Based

on Current Use Levels, Regulations, and Toxicological and Epidemiological Studies," *Crit Rev Toxicol,* 2007, 37(8):629–727.

8. P. Humphries, E. Pretorius, and H, Naudé, "Direct and Indirect Cellular effects of Aspartame on the Brain," *Eur J Clin Nutr,* April 2008, 62(4):451–62. Epub August 8, 2007.

9. Mohamed B. Abou-Donia*, Eman M. El-Masry, Ali A. Abdel-Rahman, Roger E. McLendon, and Susan S. Schiffman, "Splenda Alters Gut Microflora and Increases Intestinal P-Glycoprotein and Cytochrome P-450 in Male Rats," *Journal of Toxicology and Environmental Health,* Part A: Current Issues. Volume 71, Issue 21, 2008.

10. Qing Yang, "Gain Weight by 'Going Diet?' Artificial Sweeteners and the Neurobiology of Sugar Cravings," *Yale J Biol Med,* June 2010, 83(2): 101–108.

11. SD Stellman and L. Garfinkel, "Artificial Sweetener Use and One-Year Weight Change Among Women," *Prev Med.,* 1986, 15:195–202.

12. SP Fowler, K. Williams, RG Resendez, KJ Hunt, HP Hazuda, and MP Stern, "Fueling the Obesity Epidemic? Artificially Sweetened Beverage Use and Long-Term Weight Gain," *Obesity* (Silver Spring, Md.) 2008, 16:1894–1900.

13. RG Hendler, M. Walesky, and RS Sherwin, "Sucrose Substitution in Prevention and Reversal of the Fall in Metabolic Rate Accompanying Hypocaloric Diets," *Am J Med.,* August 1986, 81(2):280–4.

14. M. Yanina Pepino, PhD; Courtney D. Tiemann, MPH, MS, RD; Bruce W. Patterson, PhD; Burton M. Wice, PhD; and Samuel Klein, MD, "Sucralose Affects Glycemic and Hormonal Responses to an Oral Glucose Load," *Diabetic Care.*

15. PB Jeppesen, S. Gregersen, CR Poulsen, and K. Hermansen, "Stevioside Acts Directly on Pancreatic Beta Cells to Secrete Insulin: Actions Independent of Cyclic Adenosine Monophosphate and Adenosine Triphosphate-Sensitive K+-Channel Activity," *Metabolism,* February 2000, 49(2):208–14.

16. B. Geeraert, F. Crombé, M. Hulsmans, N. Benhabilès, JM Geuns, and P. Holvoet, "Stevioside Inhibits Atherosclerosis by Improving Insulin Signaling and Antioxidant Defense in Obese Insulin-Resistant Mice," *Int J Obes* (Lond), March 2010, 34(3):569–77. doi: 10.1038/ijo.2009.261. Epub December 15, 2009.

17. "Alert: Protein Drinks. You Don't Need the Extra Protein or the Heavy Metals Our Tests Found," *Consumer Report,* 2010, www.consumerreports.org/cro/magazine-archive/2010/july/food/protein-drinks/overview/index.htm.

18. Carolanne Wright. "Dying to Be Healthy: Many Protein Powders Laced with Heavy Metals, MSG," *Natural News,* August 8, 2013.

19. WH Yang, MA Drouin, M. Herbert, Y. Mao, and J. Karsh, "The Monosodium Glutamate Symptom Complex: Assessment in a Double-Blind, Placebo-Controlled, Randomized Study," *J Allergy Clin Immunol,* June 1997, 99(6 Pt 1):757–62.

20. National Center for Complimentary Care and Alternative Care, http://nccam.nih.gov/news/2009/073009.htm.

21. "The CHEK Institute Position Statement on Whey Protein," www.ppssuccess.com/foodforthought/articlesbypaul/articlesbypaulchekdetailpage/tabid/496/smid/2144/articleid/90/reftab/104/t/whey%20products%20%20supplement%20or%20detriment/default.aspx.

22. Great Lakes Gelatin, www.greatlakesgelatin.com.

Chapter 14

Eliseo Guallar, MD, DrPH; Saverio Stranges, MD, PhD; Cynthia Mulrow, MD, MSc, Senior Deputy Editor; Lawrence J. Appel, MD, MPH; and Edgar R. Miller III, MD, PhD, "Enough Is Enough: Stop Wasting Money on Vitamin and Mineral Supplements," *Annals of Internal Medicine*, December 17, 2013.

Stephen P. Fortmann, MD; Brittany U. Burda, MPH; Caitlyn A. Senger, MPH; Jennifer S. Lin, MD, MCR; and Evelyn P. Whitlock, MD, MPH, "Vitamin and Mineral Supplements in the Primary Prevention of Cardiovascular Disease and Cancer: An Updated Systematic Evidence Review for the U.S. Preventive Services Task Force," *Annals of Internal Medicine,* December 2013.

G. Bjelakovic, D. Nikolova, and C. Gluud, "Antioxidant Supplements to Prevent Mortality," *Journal of the American Medical Association,* 2013, 310:1178–9.

Salt

1. AM Sharma, U. Schorr, HM Thiede, and A. Distler, "Effect of Dietary Salt Restriction on Urinary Serotonin and 5-hydroxyindoleacetic Acid Excretion in Man," *J Hypertens*, December 1993, 11(12):1381–6.

2. Matt Stone, "Eat for Heat," E-Book. November 2012.

3. Dr. Ray Peat, "Water Swelling, Pain, Tension, Fatigue, Aging," www.RayPeat.com.

4. Dr. Ray Peat, "Salt, Energy, Metabolic Rate, and Longevity," www.RayPeat.com.

5. Dr. Pablo Pelegrin, "A Solution to Reducing Inflammation," University of Manchester, September 20, 2012, www.manchester.ac.uk/aboutus/news/display/?id=8723.

6. Richard E. Klabunde, PhD, "Cardiovascular Physiological Concepts," Blood Volume, revised April 1, 2007, www.cvphysiology.com/Blood%20Pressure/BP025.htm.

7. R.S. Taylor, K.E. Ashton, T. Moxham, L. Hooper, and S. Ebrahim, "Reduced Dietary Salt for the Prevention of Cardiovascular Disease," Cochrane Database of Systematic Reviews (online), 2011, vol. (7), no. 7, pp. CD009217.

8. M.G. Nicholls, W. Kiowski, A.J. Zweifler, S. Julius, M.A. Schork, and J. Greenhouse, "Plasma Norepinephrine Variations with Dietary Sodium Intake," *Hypertension*, 1980, vol. 2, no. 1, pp. 29–32.

9. J. Park, "Cardiovascular Risk in Chronic Kidney Disease: Role of the Sympathetic Nervous System," *Cardiology Research and Practice*, 2012, vol. 2012, pp. 319432.

10. R.M. Carey, G.R. Van Loon, A.D. Baines, and D.L. Kaiser, "Suppression of Basal and Stimulated Noradrenergic Activities by the Dopamine Agonist Bromocriptine in Man," *The Journal of Clinical Endocrinology and Metabolism*, 1983, vol. 56, no. 3, pp. 595–602.

11. R.M. Carey, G.R. Van Loon, A.D. Baines, and E.M. Ortt, "Decreased Plasma and Urinary Dopamine During Dietary Sodium Depletion in Man," *The Journal of Clinical Endocrinology and Metabolism*, 1981, vol. 52, no. 5, pp. 903–909.

12. Gary Taubes, "Salt We Misjudged You," *The New York Times*, www.nytimes.com/2012/06/03/opinion/sunday/we-only-think-we-know-the-truth-about-salt.html?pagewanted=all&_r=1&.

13. MH Alderman, S. Madhavan, H. Cohen, JE Sealey, and JH Laragh, "Low Urinary Sodium Is Associated with Greater Risk of Myocardial Infarction Among Treated Hypertensive Men," *Hypertension,* 1995, 25: 1144–1152.

14. MH Alderman, H. Cohen, and S. Madhavan, "Dietary Sodium Intake and Mortality," The National Health and Nutrition Examination Survey (NHANES I), *Lancet,* 1998, 351:781–785.

15. Katarzyna Stolarz-Skrzypek, MD, PhD; Tatiana Kuznetsova, MD, PhD; Lutgarde Thijs, MSc; Valérie Tikhonoff, MD, PhD; Jitka Seidlerová, MD, PhD; Tom Richart, MD; Yu Jin, MD; Agnieszka Olszanecka, MD, PhD; Sofia Malyutina, MD, PhD; Edoardo Casiglia, MD, PhD; Jan Filipovský, MD, PhD; Kalina Kawecka-Jaszcz, MD, PhD; Yuri Nikitin, MD, PhD; and Jan A. Staessen, MD, PhD, "Fatal and Nonfatal Outcomes, Incidence of Hypertension, and Blood Pressure Changes in Relation to Urinary Sodium Excretion," *Journal of the American Medical Association*, 2011, 305(17):1777–1785. doi:10.1001/jama.2011.574.

17. Jairo de Jesus Mancilha-Carvalho and Nelson Albuquerque de Souza e Silva, "The Yanomami Indians in the INTERSALT Study," Rio de Janeiro, Brazil, www.scielo.br/pdf/abc/v80n3/a05v80n3.pdf.

18. Frank M. Sacks, MD; Laura P. Svetkey, MD; William M. Vollmer, PhD; Lawrence J. Appel, MD; George A. Bray, MD; David Harsha, PhD; Eva Obarzanek, PhD; Paul R. Conlin, MD; Edgar R. Miller, MD, PhD; Denise G. Simons-Morton, MD, PhD; Njeri Karanja, PhD; Pao-Hwa Lin, PhD; Mikel Aickin, PhD; Marlene M. Most-Windhauser, PhD; Thomas J. Moore, MD; Michael A. Proschan, PhD; and Jeffrey A. Cutler, MD, for the DASH–Sodium Collaborative Research Group, "Effects on Blood

Pressure of Reduced Dietary Sodium and the Dietary Approaches to Stop Hypertension (DASH) Diet," *N Engl J Med,* 2001, 344:3–10, January 4, 2001. DOI: 10.1056/NEJM2001010434401.

19. B.R. Walker, "Cortisol–Cause and Cure for Metabolic Syndrome?" *Diabetic Medicine: A Journal of the British Diabetic Association,* 2006, vol. 23, no. 12, pp. 1281–1288.

20. FG Orr, PN Johnstone, and RL Haden, "Hypertonic Saline and Peristalsis," *Surg. Gynec. Obst.,* May 1931, 52, 941.

21. DA McCarron and CD Morris, "Calcium, Parathyroid Hormone, and Hypertension," *Adv Nephrol Necker Hosp,* 1985; 14:479–501.

22. Martin O'Donnell, M.B., PhD' Andrew Mente, PhD; Sumathy Rangarajan, M.Sc., Matthew J. McQueen, M.B., PhD; Xingyu Wang, PhD; Lisheng Liu, MD; Hou Yan, PhD; Shun Fu Lee, PhD; Prem Mony, MD; Anitha Devanath, MD; Annika Rosengren, MD; Patricio Lopez-Jaramillo, MD, PhD; Rafael Diaz, MD; Alvaro Avezum, MD, PhD; Fernando Lanas, MD; Khalid Yusoff, M.B., BS; Romaina Iqbal, PhD; Rafal Ilow, PhD; Noushin Mohammadifard, M.Sc.; Sadi Gulec, MD; Afzal Hussein Yusufali, MD; Lanthe Kruger, PhD; Rita Yusuf, PhD; Jephat Chifamba, M.Phil.; Conrad Kabali, PhD; Gilles Dagenais, MD; Scott A. Lear, PhD; Koon Teo, M.B., PhD; and Salim Yusuf, D.Phil., for the PURE Investigators, "Urinary Sodium and Potassium Excretion, Mortality, and Cardiovascular Events," *N Engl J Med,* August 14, 2014; 371:612–623.

Coffee

1. A. Linos, DA Linos, N. Vgotza, A. Souvatzoglou, and DA Koutras, "Does Coffee Consumption Protect Against

Thyroid Disease?" *Acta Chir Scand,* June–July 1989, 155(6-7):317–20.

2. CE Ruhland JE Everhart, "Coffee and Caffeine Consumption Reduce the Risk of Elevated Serum Alanine Aminotransferase Activity in the United States," *Gastroenterology,* January 2005, 128(1):24–32.

3. E. Casiglia, P. Spolaore, G. Ginocchio, and GB Ambrosio, Istituto di Medicina Clinica, Universita di Padova, Italy, "Unexpected Effects of Coffee Consumption on Liver Enzymes," *Eur J Epidemiol,* May 1993, 9(3):293–7.

4. GW Ross, RD Abbott, H. Petrovitch, DM Morens, A. Grandinetti, KH Tung, CM Tanner, KH Masaki, PL Blanchette, JD Curb, JS Popper, and LR White, "Association of Coffee and Caffeine Intake with the Risk of Parkinson Disease," *JAMA* May 24–31, 2000, 283(20):2674–9.

5. TM Chouand NL Benowitz, "Caffeine and Coffee: Effects on Health and Cardiovascular Disease," *Comp Biochem Physiol C Pharmacol Toxicol Endocrinol,* October 1994, 109(2):173–89.

6. Francesca Bravi, Cristina Bosetti, Alessandra Tavani, Silvano Gallus, and Carlo La Vecchia, "Coffee Reduces Risk for Hepatocellular Carcinoma: An Updated Meta-Analysis," *Clinical Gastroenterology and Hepatology,* 2013; 11 (11).

7. Rohit Anthony Sinha, Benjamin L. Farah, Brijesh K. Singh, Monowarul Mobin Siddique, Ying Li, Yajun Wu, Olga R. Ilkayeva, Jessica Gooding, Jianhong Ching, Jin Zhou, Laura Martinez, Sherwin Xie, Boon-Huat Bay, Scott A. Summers, Christopher B. Newgard, and Paul M. Yen, "Caffeine Stimulates Hepatic Lipid Metabolism via Autophagy-Lysosomal Pathway," *Hepatology,* 2013.

8. "Coffee and Tea May Contribute to a Healthy Liver," *Science Daily*, Duke-NUS Graduate Medical School Singapore, August 16, 2013.

9. GW Arendash and C. Cao, "Caffeine and coffee as therapeutics against Alzheimer's Disease," *J Alzheimers Dis.*, 2010, 20 Suppl 1:S117–26. doi: 10.3233/JAD-2010-091249.

10. Shilpa N. Bhupathiraju, An Pan, JoAnn E. Manson, Walter C. Willett, Rob M. van Dam, and Frank B. Hu, "Changes in Coffee Intake and Subsequent Risk of Type 2 Diabetes: Three Large Cohorts of US Men and Women," *Diabetologia*. October 22, 2013.

11. TA Morck, SR Lynch, and JD Cook, "Inhibition of Food Iron Absorption by Coffee," The American Society for Clinical Nutrition, Inc., 1983.

12. L. Hallberg and L. Rossander, "Effect of Different Drinks on the Absorption of Non-Heme Iron from Composite Meals," *Hum Nutr Appl Nutr*, April 1982, 36(2):116–23.

13. Margaret Giles and John Birkbeck, "Tea and Coffee as Sources of Some Minerals in the New Zealand Diet," *American Journal of Clinical Nutrition*, 1983, 936–942.

Eggshell Calcium

1. A. Schaafsma, I. Pakan, G.J.H. Hofstede, F.A. Muskiet, E. Van Der Veer, and P.J.F. De Vries, "Mineral, Amino Acid, and Hormonal Composition of Chicken Eggshell Powder and the Evaluation of its Use in Human Nutrition," *Poulty Science,* 01/2001; 79(12):1833-8.

2. N. Gongruttananun, "Effects of Eggshell Calcium on Productive Performance, Plasma Calcium, Bone

Mineralization, and Gonadal Characteristics in Laying Hens," *Poultry Science,* 02/2011; 90(2):524-9.

3. "Eggshell Calcium Found to Have Extreme Low Levels of Heavy Metals: Eggshell Calcium (ESC®): The Ideal Natural Calcium Source," www.esmingredients.com/wp-content/uploads/ESC%20Heavy%20Metals%20White%20Paper%20New%20Chart.pdf.

4. J. Rovenský, M. Stancíková, P. Masaryk, K. Svík, and R. Istok, "Eggshell Calcium in the Prevention and Treatment of Osteoporosis," *Int J Clin Pharmacol Res.,* 2003, 23(2–3):83–92.

5. Y. Masuda, "Hen's Eggshell Calcium," *Clin Calcium,* January 2005, 15(1):95–100.

6. A. Schaafsma, JJ van Doormaal, FA Muskiet, GJ Hofstede, I. Pakan, and E. van der Veer, "Positive Effects of a Chicken Eggshell Powder-Enriched Vitamin-Mineral Supplement on Femoral Neck Bone Mineral Density in Healthy Late Post-Menopausal Dutch Women," *Br J Nutr,* March 2002, 87(3):267–75.

7. Dr. Ray Peat, "Osteoporosis, Aging, Tissue Renewal, and Product Science." www.raypeat.com

8. R. Heaney MD, M.S. Dowel, Phd, J Bierman, C. Hale, and A. Bendich, "Absorbability and Cost Effectiveness in Calcium Supplementation," Creighton University, December 11, 2000.

9. George W. Bo-Linn, Glenn R. Davis, David J. Buddrus, Stephen G. Morawski, Carol Santa Ana, and John S. Fordtran, "An Evaluation of the Importance of Gastric Acid Secretion in the Absorption of Dietary Calcium," Department of Internal Medicine, Baylor University Medical Center, Dallas, Texas.

10. MB Zemel, W. Thompson, A. Milstead, K. Morris, and P. Campbell, "Calcium and Dairy Acceleration of Weight and Fat Loss During Energy Restriction in Obese Adults," *Obes Res,* April 2004, 12(4):582–90.

Vitamins and minerals

1. RD Semba, "On the 'Discovery' of Vitamin A," *Annals of Nutrition & Metabolism,* 2012, 61 (3):192–198.

2. NM Niren, "Pharmacologic Doses of Niacinamide in the Treatment of Inflammatory Skin Conditions: A Review." *Cutis,* 2006, 77 (1 Suppl):11–16.

3. http://www.vitamins-supplements.org/vitamin-B6-pyridoxine.php.

4. R. Brigelius-Flohé and MG Traber MG, "Vitamin E: Function and Metabolism," *FASEB J.,* 1999, 13(10):1145–1155.

5. MG Traber, "The Biological Activity of Vitamin E," The Linus Pauling Institute, 1998, Retrieved March 6, 2011.

6. SJ Padayatty, A. Katz, Y. Wang, P. Eck, O. Kwon, JH Lee, S. Chen, C. Corpe, A. Dutta, SK Dutta, and M. Levine, "Vitamin C as an Antioxidant: Evaluation of its Role in Disease Prevention". *J Am Coll Nutr,* February 2003, 22(1):18–35.

7. A. Cranney, T. Horsley, S. O'Donnell, H. Weiler, L. Puil, D. Ooi, S. Atkinson, L. Ward, D. Moher, D. Hanley, M. Fang, F. Yazdi, C. Garritty, M. Sampson, N. Barrowman, A. Tsertsvadze, and V. Mamaladze, "Effectiveness and Safety of Vitamin D in Relation to Bone Health," *Evidence Report/Technology Assessment,* August 2007, (158):1–235.

8. D. Feskanich, P. Weber, WC Willett, H. Rockett, SL Booth, and GA Colditz, "Vitamin K Intake and Hip Fractures in Women: A Prospective Study," *American Journal of Clinical Nutrition,* 1999, 69:74–79.

9. C. Vermeerand E. Theuwissen, "Vitamin K, Osteoporosis and Degenerative Diseases of Aging," *Menopause Int.,* March 2011, 17(1):19–23.

10. KS Jie, ML Bots, C. Vermeer, JC Witteman, and DE Grobbee, "Vitamin K Intake and Osteocalcin Levels in Women with and Without Aortic Atherosclerosis: A Population-Based Study," *Atherosclerosis.,* July 1995, 116(1):117–23.

11. Dr. Kate Rheaume-Bleue, ND, *Vitamin K2 and the Calcium Paradox: How a Little-Known Vitamin Could Save Your Life,* Wiley, 2012.

12. Lothar Rink, "Zinc and the Immune System," Institute of Immunology and Transfusion Medicine, University of Lübeck School of Medicine, Lübeck, Germany.

13. Copper information, www.copper.org/consumers/health/papers/cu_health_uk/cu_health_uk.html.

14. Dr. Ray Peat, "Iron Dangers," www.RayPeat.com.

15. "Selenium," Linus Pauling Institute at Oregon State University, retrieved January 5, 2009.

16. FJ Heand GA MacGregor, "Beneficial Effects of Potassium on Human Health," *Physiol Plant,* August 2008, 133(4):725–35.

17. Chou-Long Huang and Elizabeth Kuo, "Mechanism of Hypokalemia in Magnesium Deficiency," *JASN,* 2007.

Chapter 15

1. Stephen Kreitzman, Ann Coxon, and Kalmon Szaz, "Glycogen Stores: Illusions of Easy Weight Loss, Excessive Weight Regain, and Distortions in Estimates of Body Composition," *The American Journal of Clinical Nutrition.*

2. Constance Martin, *Endocrine Physiology,* Oxford University Press, 1985, pp. 118, 120–122, 124, 132, 216, 273.

3. William D. McArdle, Frank Katch, and Victor Katch, *Exercise Physiology: Energy, Nutrition, and Human Performance,* 3rd edition, Lea and Febiger, 1991, pp. 9–10, 208–209, 517.

4. "Study Shows Eating Alone Is Bad for Your Health," Huffington Post, www.HuffingtonPost.com/2013/10/29/loneliness-affects-diet_n_4173944.html.

5. Konstantin Monastyrsky, *The Fiber Menace,* Ageless Press, 2005.

6. Broda Barnes, MD, and Laurence Galton, *Hypothyroidism: The Unsuspected Illness,* Harper and Row Publishing, 1976.

7. Cron-o-meter Food logging, www.Cronometer.com.

8. Dr. Ray Peat, "TSH, Temperature, Pulse Rate, and Other Indicators in Hypothyroidism," www.raypeat.com.

Chapter 16

1. Jeffrey M. Joneshttp, "In U.S., 40% Get Less Than Recommended Amount of Sleep. Hours of Sleep Similar to Recent Decades, but Much Lower Than in 1942," December 19, 2013, www.gallup.com/poll/166553/less-recommended-amount-sleep.aspx.

2. JJ Reilly, J. Armstrong, AR Dorosty, PM Emmett, A. Ness, I. Rogers, C. Steer, and A. Sherriff, "Early Life Risk Factors for Obesity in Childhood: Cohort Study. Avon Longitudinal Study of Parents and Children Study Team," *BMJ,* June 11, 2005, 330(7504):1357. Epub May 20, 2005.

3. SR Patel, A. Malhotra, DP White, DJ Gottlieb, and FB Hu, "Association Between Reduced Sleep and Weight Gain in Women," *Am J Epidemiol,* November 15, 2006, 164(10):947–54. Epub August 16, 2006.

4. JP Chaput, JP Després, C. Bouchard, and A. Tremblay, "The Association Between Sleep Duration and Weight Gain in Adults: A 6-Year Prospective Study from the Quebec Family Study," *Sleep,* April 2008, 31(4):517–23.

5. Eve Van Cauter, PhD; Kristen Knutson, PhD; Rachel Leproult, PhD; and Karine Spiegel, PhD, Faculty and Disclosures, "The Impact of Sleep Deprivation on Hormones and Metabolism," www.Medscape.org/viewarticle/502825.

6. Karine Spiegel, PhD ,, Rachel Leproult, BS, and Eve Van Cauter, PhD, "Impact of Sleep Debt on Metabolic and Endocrine Function," *The Lancet,* October 23, 1999, Volume 354, Issue 9188, pp. 1435–1439.

7. Karine Spiegel, Rachel Leproult, Mireille L'Hermite-Balé Raiux, Georges Copinschi, Plamen D. Penev, and Eve van Cauter, "Leptin Levels Are Dependent on Sleep Duration: Relationships with Sympathovagal Balance, Carbohydrate Regulation, Cortisol, and Thyrotropin," Department of Medicine (K.S., R.L., P.D.P., E.V.C.), University of Chicago, Illinois; and Laboratory of Physiology (K.S., M.L.-B., G.C)

8. David Nutt, DM, FRCP, FRCPsych, FMedSci; Sue Wilson, PhD; and Louise Paterson, PhD, "Sleep Disorders as Core Symptoms of Depression," *Dialogues Clin Neurosci,* September 2008, 10(3): 329–336.

9. Dr. Ray Peat, "Thyroid, Insomnia, and the Insanities: Commonalities in Disease," www.RayPeat.com.

10. Dr. Ray Peat, "Protective CO2 and Aging," www.RayPeat.com.

11. Dr. Ray Peat, "Glycemia, Starch, and Sugar in Context," www.RayPeat.com.

12. A.B. Loucks and E.M. Heath, "Induction of low-T3 syndrome in exercising women occurs at a threshold of energy availability," *American Journal of Physiology - Regulatory, Integrative and Comparative Physiology,* March 1, 1994, Vol.

13. PK Opstad, D. Falch, O. Oktedalen, F. Fonnum, and R. Wergeland, "The Thyroid Function in Young Men During Prolonged Exercise and the Effect of energy and Sleep Deprivation," *Clin Endocrinol (Oxf),* June 1984, 20(6):657–69.

14. A. Wirth, G. Holm, G. Lindstedt, PA Lundberg, and P. Björntorp, "Thyroid Hormones and Lipolysis in Physically Trained Rats." *Metabolism,* March 1981, 30(3):237–41.

15. D. Rosołowska-Huszcz, "The Effect of Exercise Training Intensity on Thyroid Activity at Rest," *J Physiol Pharmacol,* September 1998, 49(3):457–66.

16. "Endurance Training with Constant Energy Intake in Identical Twins: Changes over Time in Energy Expenditure and Related Hormones," Metabolism, May 1997, 46(5):499–503.

17. A. Pakarinen, K. Häkkinen, and M. Alen, "Serum Thyroid Hormones, Thyrotropin and Thyroxine Binding Globulin in Elite Athletes During Very Intense Strength Training of One Week," *J Sports Med Phys Fitness,* June 1991, 31(2):142–6.

18. A. Pakarinen, M. Alén, K. Häkkinen, and P. Komi, "Serum Thyroid Hormones, Thyrotropin and Thyroxine Binding Globulin During Prolonged Strength Training," *Eur J Appl Physiol Occup Physiol.,* 1988, 57(4):394–8.

19. A. Pakarinen, M. Alén, K. Häkkinen, and P. Komi, "Serum Thyroid Hormones, Thyrotropin and Thyroxine Binding Globulin During Prolonged Strength Training," *Eur J Appl Physiol Occup Physiol.,* 1988, 57(4):394–8.

20. Figen Ciloglu, Ismail Peker, Aysel Pehlivan, Kursat Karacabey, Nevin İlhan, Ozcan Saygin, and Recep Ozmerdivenli, "Exercise Intensity and its Effects on Thyroid Hormones," *Neuroendocrinology* Letters No. 6, December 2005, Vol. 26.

21. EE Hill, E. Zack, C. Battaglini, M. Viru, A. Viru, and AC Hackney, "Exercise and Circulating Cortisol Levels: The Intensity Threshold Effect," *J Endocrinol Invest,* July 2008, 31(7):587–91.

22. AC Hackney, KP Hosick, A. Myer, DA Rubin, and CL Battaglini, "Testosterone Responses to Intensive Interval Versus Steady-State Endurance Exercise," *J Endocrinol Invest,* December 2012, 35(11):947–50.

23. Tsutomu Kamei, Yoshitaka Toriumi, Hiroshi Kimura, Satoshi Ohno, Hiroaki Kumano, and Keishin Kimura, "Decrease in Serum Cortisol During Yoga Exercise is Correlated with Alpha Wave Activation." *Perceptual and Motor Skills,* 2000, Volume 90, Issue 3, pp. 1027–1032.

24. Dr. Ray Peat, "Bleeding, Clotting, Cancer," www.RayPeat.com.

25. LB Borghouts and HA Keizer, "Exercise and Insulin Sensitivity: A Review," *Int J Sports Med,* January 2000, 21(1):1–12.

26. TA Elliot, MG Cree, AP Sanford, RR Wolfe, and KD Tipton, "Milk Ingestion Stimulates Net Muscle Protein Synthesis Following Resistance Exercise," *Med Sci Sports Exerc,* April 2006, 38(4):667–74.

27. NJ Cook, A. Ng, GF Read, B. Harris, and D. Riad-Fahmy, "Salivary Cortisol for Monitoring Adrenal Activity During Marathon Runs," *Horm Res.,* 1987, 25(1):18–23.

28. Hans Selye, "Stress and the General Adaptation Syndrome," *Br Med J.,* June 17, 1950, 1(4667):1383–1392.

29. Floyd R. Skelton and Paul M. Hyde, "Functional Response of Regenerating Adrenal Glands to Stress," *Exp Biol Med* (Maywood) 1961, 106:142.

30. "This 122 Year Old Woman Has The Most Important Secret To A Life of Longevity," www.collective-evolution.com/2014/05/02/this-122-year-old-woman-has-the-most-important-secret-to-a-life-of-longevity/.

31. Dan Buettner, *The Blue Zones,* Published by the National Geography Society. 2008.

32. Dr Ray Peat, "Water: Swelling, Tension, Pain, Fatigue, Aging," www.RayPeat.com.

33. Christopher S.D. Almond, MD, M.P.H.; Andrew Y. Shin, MD; Elizabeth B. Fortescue, MD; Rebekah C. Mannix, MD; David Wypij, PhD; Bryce A. Binstadt, MD, PhD; Christine N. Duncan, MD; David P. Olson, MD, PhD; Ann E. Salerno, MD; Jane W. Newburger, MD, M.P.H.; and David S. Greenes, MD; "Hyponatremia Among Runners in the Boston Marathon," *N Engl J Med,* 2005, 352:1550–1556.

34. Harminder S. Sandhu, Emmanuelle Gilles, Maria V. DeVita, Georgia Panagopoulos, and Michael F. Michelis, "Hyponatremia Associated with Large-Bone Fracture in Elderly Patients," *International Urology and Nephrology,* September 2009, Volume 41, Issue 3, pp. 733–737.

35. Matt Stone, "Eat for Heat". Published by Archangel. 2012.

Remember to get your FREE monthly newsletter

Continued knowledge and education are musts in the health and fitness industry. Join Kate's list of thousands of current readers and receive a FREE monthly newsletter with the most updated scientific based nutritional information.

You will find information on:
- Why "green juicing" may be doing you more harm than good.
- Why a low-carb diet is killing your metabolism.
- Why avoiding sugar is the worst thing you can do for a high metabolic rate.
- How to increase your sleep time and quality.
- Why too much exercise can encourage a low metabolic rate.

To join the community of the "out of the box" nutritionally minded people, go to **www.KateDeering.com/Blog** *and enter your name and e-mail.*

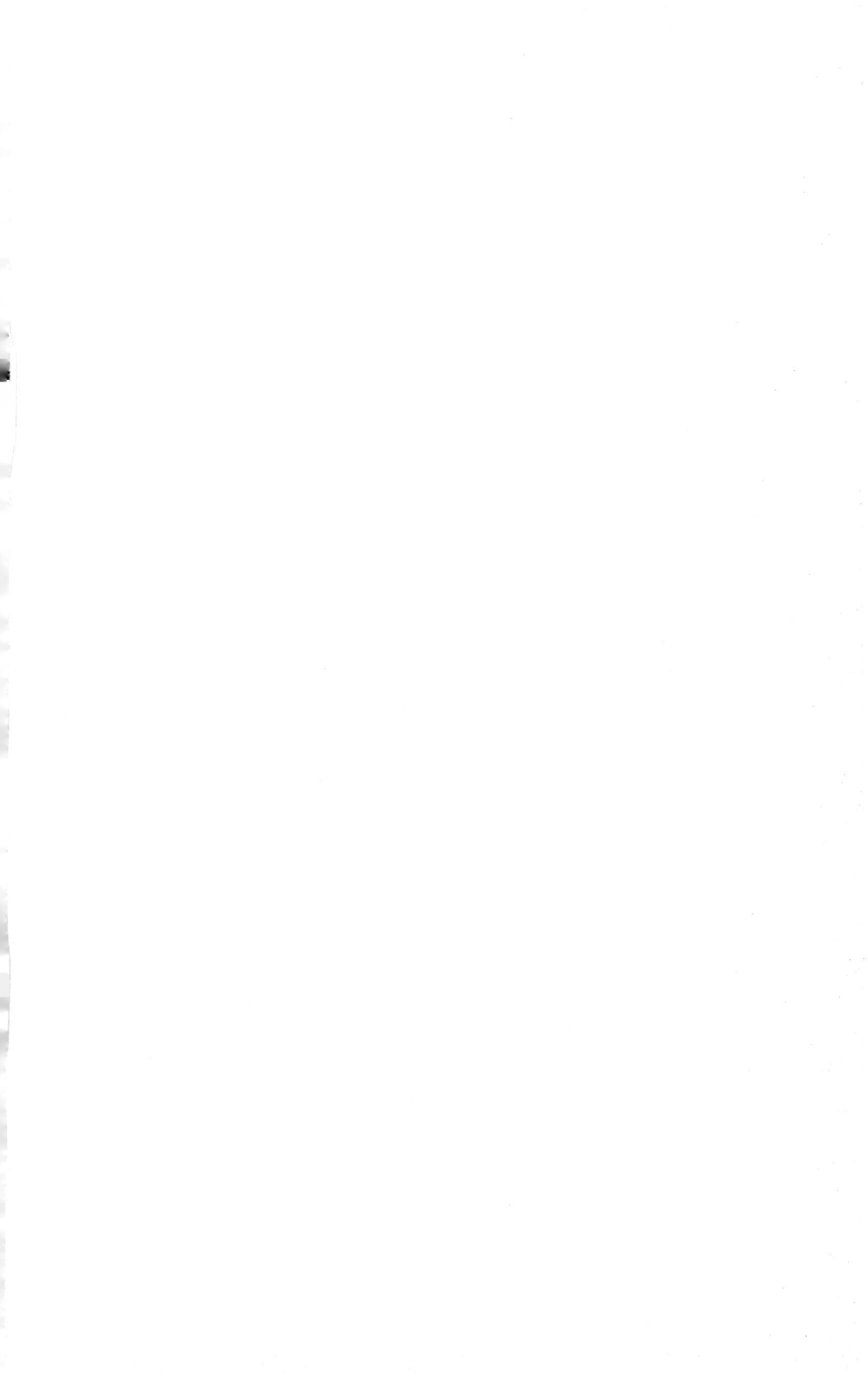

Printed in Great Britain
by Amazon